AML in the Molecular Age:
From Biology to Clinical Management

AML in the Molecular Age:
From Biology to Clinical Management

Special Issue Editors

Celalettin Ustun
Lucy A. Godley

MDPI • Basel • Beijing • Wuhan • Barcelona • Belgrade

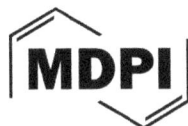

MDPI

Special Issue Editors

Celalettin Ustun
University of Minnesota
USA

Lucy A. Godley
The University of Chicago
USA

Editorial Office
MDPI
St. Alban-Anlage 66
Basel, Switzerland

This is a reprint of articles from the Special Issue published online in the open access journal *Journal of Clinical Medicine* (ISSN 2077-0383) from 2014 to 2015 (available at: http://www.mdpi.com/journal/jcm/special_issues/aml)

For citation purposes, cite each article independently as indicated on the article page online and as indicated below:

LastName, A.A.; LastName, B.B.; LastName, C.C. Article Title. *Journal Name* **Year**, *Article Number, Page Range.*

ISBN 978-3-03897-280-8 (Pbk)
ISBN 978-3-03897-281-5 (PDF)

Contents

About the Special Issue Editors

Celalettin Ustun is a hematologist, trained in Turkey and then in the US. His focus of interest is on acute myeloid leukemia treatment, including allogeneic hematopoietic cell transplantation. He has worked in Ankara University Medical School, Medical College of Georgia, University of Minnesota, and Rush University.

Lucy A. Godley developed her deep respect for science through her work in the Marchesi laboratories at Yale University, with Dr. Don Wiley (Harvard), and Dr. Harold Varmus (University of California, San Francisco; National Institutes of Health). She completed her medical training at Northwestern University followed by an Internal Medicine/Hematology-Oncology residency/fellowship at The University of Chicago. After postdoctoral research with Dr. Michelle Le Beau, Dr. Godley joined the faculty at The University of Chicago in 2003. Her laboratory has focused on understanding the molecular drivers of abnormal patterns of modified cytosines that characterize cancer cells as well as the molecular drivers of inherited hematopoietic malignancies. As a physician-scientist with both research and clinical responsibilities, Dr. Godley seeks to understand disease on a molecular basis and is able to bring that perspective to the care of her patients.

Preface to "AML in the Molecular Age: From Biology to Clinical Management"

In this issue, we have covered the new era in acute myeloid leukemia (AML). Molecular abnormalities have become increasingly important, not only in prognostication but also management of AML. The rationale of targeted therapies, hypomethylating agents were reviewed. While we are emphasizing management of AML regarding molecular abnormalities, we also tackled treatment differences regarding age, and disease status. Allogeneic hematopoietic cell transplantation has been the most important means to cure AML; however, in this issue we focused on alternative donor sources that has becoming highly important. In the same regard, T-cell depletion and its pros and cons were reviewed. Lastly, what is the place of radiology for diagnosis of central nervous system leukemia was discussed.

Celalettin Ustun, Lucy A. Godley

Special Issue Editors

Journal of
Clinical Medicine

MDPI

Review

Molecular Genetic Markers in Acute Myeloid Leukemia

Sophia Yohe

Department of Laboratory Medicine and Pathology, Divisions of Hematopathology and Molecular Genetic Pathology, University of Minnesota, MMC Box 609 Mayo, 420 Delaware St. SE. Minneapolis, MN 55455, USA; yohe0001@umn.edu; Tel.: +1-612-273-3098; Fax: +1-612-624-6662

Academic Editors: Celalettin Ustun and Lucy A. Godley
Received: 5 January 2015; Accepted: 3 February 2015; Published: 12 March 2015

Abstract: Genetics play an increasingly important role in the risk stratification and management of acute myeloid leukemia (AML) patients. Traditionally, AML classification and risk stratification relied on cytogenetic studies; however, molecular detection of gene mutations is playing an increasingly important role in classification, risk stratification, and management of AML. Molecular testing does not take the place of cytogenetic testing results, but plays a complementary role to help refine prognosis, especially within specific AML subgroups. With the exception of acute promyelocytic leukemia, AML therapy is not targeted but the intensity of therapy is driven by the prognostic subgroup. Many prognostic scoring systems classify patients into favorable, poor, or intermediate prognostic subgroups based on clinical and genetic features. Current standard of care combines cytogenetic results with targeted testing for mutations in *FLT3*, *NPM1*, *CEBPA*, and *KIT* to determine the prognostic subgroup. Other gene mutations have also been demonstrated to predict prognosis and may play a role in future risk stratification, although some of these have not been confirmed in multiple studies or established as standard of care. This paper will review the contribution of cytogenetic results to prognosis in AML and then will focus on molecular mutations that have a prognostic or possible therapeutic impact.

Keywords: acute myeloid leukemia (AML); gene mutation; *FLT3*-ITD; *NPM1*; *CEBPA*

1. Introduction

There is a well-established role for genetic classification of acute myeloid leukemia (AML) into different prognostic groups. Traditionally, this classification has relied on detection of large chromosomal abnormalities by cytogenetics; however, detection of smaller scale mutations is playing an increasingly important role in classification and prognostication of AML. These mutations do not take the place of cytogenetic testing results but play a complementary role to help refine prognosis, especially within specific AML subgroups.

With the exception of acute promyelocytic leukemia, therapy for AML is not targeted and the intensity of therapy is driven by the prognostic subgroup. Many prognostic scoring systems classify patients into favorable, poor, or intermediate prognosis based on clinical and cytogenetic features. Research on molecular testing has generally tried to refine the prognosis of intermediate cases or to find mutations that explain why some patients in a favorable prognosis category have resistant disease. If identified, these patient could potential receive more aggressive therapy upfront. This paper will briefly review the contribution of cytogenetic results to prognosis in AML and then will focus on molecular mutations that change prognostic subgrouping. Gene mutations that appear to have prognostic effect but have not been confirmed in multiple studies or established as standard of care will also be explored.

2. Genetics and AML Classification

The current World Health Organization (WHO) 2008 classifies AML based on patient history, morphologic findings, and the presence or absence of specific genetic abnormalities. Genetic abnormalities play the biggest role in two categories: AML with recurrent genetic abnormalities and AML with myelodysplasia related changes (AML-MRC) [1]. (Table 1) AML-MRC can also be diagnosed in patients with a history of a myelodysplastic syndrome (MDS) or based on the presence of significant morphologic dysplasia in two cell lineages at the time of AML diagnosis. However, current treatment guidelines for AML use only a subset of the AML-MRC genetic abnormalities to guide therapy in the absence of a history of MDS (Table 2) [2]. The presence of morphologic dysplasia alone does not affect therapy.

3. Cytogenetic Abnormalities and Prognosis

Most of the prognostic cytogenetic abnormalities in AML are either chromosomal rearrangements or large genomic deletions. (Table 2) Acute promyelocytic leukemia with t(15;17) and the core binding factor leukemias with inv(16)/t(16;16) or t(8;21) have a better prognosis. In contrast, complex or monosomal karyotypes, deletions of chromosomes 5 or 7, and some other specific chromosomal rearrangements have a poorer prognosis. Other changes including normal cytogenetics, t(9;11) and isolated +8 have an intermediate prognosis. However, the presence of certain molecular mutations may modify these prognostic groups. Isolated *NPM1* or biallelic *CEBPA* mutations improve the prognosis of AML with normal cytogenetics from intermediate to favorable; whereas a *FLT3* ITD changes it to poor. The presence of a *KIT* mutation in core binding factor leukemia worsens the prognostic category to intermediate.

Table 1. Genetic abnormalities that affect acute myeloid leukemia (AML) classification.

AML with Recurrent Genetic Abnormalities	AML with Myelodysplasia Related Changes
*RUNX1-RUNX1*T1 t(8;21)(q22;q22)	Complex karyotype ($\geq$3 unrelated abnormalities)
CBFB-MYH11 inv(16)(p12.1q22) or t(16;16)(p13.1;q22)	-7/del(7q), -5/del(5q)
PML-RARA t(15;17)(q22;q12)	-13/del(13q), del(11q), del(12p)/t(12p), del(9q)
MLLT3-MLL/KMT2A t(9;11)(q22;q23)	i(17q)/t(17p), idic(X)(q13)
DEK-NUP214 t(6;9)(p23;q34)	t(5;12)(q33;p12), t(5;7)(q33;q11.2) t(5;17)(q33;p13), t(5;10)(q33;q21)
RPN-EVI1 inv(3)(q21q26.2) or t(3;3)(q21;q26.2)	t(1;3)(p36.3;q21.2), t(3;5)(q25;q34)
RBM15-MKL1 t(1;22)(p13;q13)	t(11;16)(q23;p13.3) *, t(3;21)(q26.2;q22.1) *
NPM1 gene mutation (provisional entity)	t(2;11)(p21;q23) *
Mutated *CEBPA* (provisional entity)	

* Rule out therapy related AML before using any of these three translocations to make a diagnosis of AML with myelodysplasia related changes.

Table 2. Cytogenetic and molecular findings used in risk stratification for AML.

Risk	Cytogenetics	Molecular
Favorable	inv(16) or t(16;16) t(8;21) t(15;17)	Normal cytogenetics with: Isolated biallelic *CEBPA* mutation *NPM1* mutation without *FLT3* ITD
Intermediate	Normal cytogenetics Isolated +8 t(9;11) Other non-good and non-poor changes	*KIT* mutation in core binding factor leukemia: inv(16) or t(16;16) t(8;21)
Poor	Complex (≥3 clonal abnormalities) Monosomal karyotype * −5/−5q or −7/−7q 11q23 rearrangements other than t(9;11) inv(3) or t(3;3) t(6;9) t(9;22)	Normal cytogenetics with: *FLT3* ITD

* Monosomal: ≥2 monosomies or 1 monosomy and additional 1 or more structural abnormalities (Breems JCO 2008; 26:4791); ITD: internal tandem duplication. (Adapted with permission from the NCCN Clinical Practice Guidelines in Oncology (NCCN Guidelines®) for Acute Myeloid Leukemia V.1.2015 © National Comprehensive Cancer Network, Inc 2014. All rights reserved. Accessed January 13, 2015. To view the most recent and complete version of the guideline, go online to NCCN.org. NATIONAL COMPREHENSIVE CANCER NETWORK®, NCCN®, NCCN GUIDELINES®, and all other NCCN Content are trademarks owned by the National Comprehensive Cancer Network, Inc.)

4. Established Gene Mutations Associated with Prognosis

Refining the prognosis for AML in the cytogenetic intermediate risk category has received the most attention. As this group is heterogeneous, the best treatment for an individual patient in the intermediate risk category is uncertain. Favorable risk patients are treated with standard chemotherapy while patients in the poor risk category should undergo allogeneic hematopoietic stem cell transplant. However, 40%–50% of adult AML falls into the intermediate category and most of these have a normal karyotype. *FLT3*, *NPM1* and *CEBPA* mutations were the first to be found useful in helping stratify cytogenetically intermediate risk patients with a normal karyotype. Mutations in *KIT* help to refine prognosis in core binding factor leukemia.

4.1. FLT3 (Fms-like Tyrosine Kinase 3)

FLT3 is a receptor tyrosine kinase involved in hematopoiesis and commonly mutated in AML. There are two common mutations that occur in *FLT3*: an internal tandem duplication (ITD) in the juxtamembrane domain and a point mutation of the tyrosine kinase domain (TKD). Both mutations lead to constitutive activation; however only the *FLT3* ITD is definitively associated with a poorer prognosis. About 20% of all AMLs harbor a *FLT3* ITD mutation, but the mutation is more common in AML with t(15;17) and AML with a normal karyotype (cytogenetically normal AML or CN-AML), accounting for approximately 30% of these cases [3,4]. AML with a normal karyotype and *FLT3* ITD mutation has a poorer prognosis [3–5].

Testing of patients by PCR followed by size analysis, reveals variability in the size of the *FLT3* ITD, the number of *FLT3* ITD mutations, and the amount of *FLT3* ITD mutation compared to wild type. Some of these have prognostic implications. Studies have shown that patients with a higher *FLT3* ITD mutant:wild type allelic ratio have a worse prognosis than patients with a lower ratio [6,7]. Although the ratio may reflect disease burden to a certain extent, a high allelic ratio of >0.5 (or ratio ≥1 using area under the curve) is presumed to be due to biallelic *FLT3* ITD mutations in at least a subset of the blasts [7,8]. Despite the prognostic impact, current risk stratification does not include the allelic ratio. Approximately 14%–25% of *FLT3* ITD positive patients will have more than one *FLT3* ITD mutation, in these cases the mutant:wild type ratio of the most prevalent mutation should be used for the allelic ratio [6,7,9]. Most studies have not shown a prognostic effect of having multiple *FLT3* ITD mutations [6–8,10]. The *FLT3* ITD size can vary from a few base pairs to over 1000 base pairs [7]. A correlation between size and prognosis has been demonstrated in some studies but not others [6,7,11–13].

Sequencing of *FLT3* ITD reveals that there is also variability in the site and sequence of the mutations, in fact some mutations are not true tandem duplications and not all *FLT3* ITD are in the juxtamembrane domain. The term *FLT3* length mutation (*FLT3* LM) has been proposed as a more accurate term [7]. Only about two-thirds of *FLT3* mutations are actual duplications while the remaining third are insertions or complex duplications and insertions [7]. Despite the sequence differences, mutations appear to remain in-frame [7,10]. The insertion site of the *FLT3* mutation is highly variable, one study found 91 unique insertion sites in 689 patients [7]. Approximately 30% of *FLT3* ITD occur outside the juxtamembrane domain and instead occur in the first tyrosine kinase domain (TKD1), usually in the β1 sheet [7,10,14]. At least some of these *FLT3* ITD in the TKD1 domain have been shown to lead to constitutive activation [14]. Kayser *et al.* in 2009 and Schlenk have shown worse prognosis with insertion in the TKD1 domain, but the 2012 study by Schnittger did not [7–9]. The Schnittger study did show a trend to worse prognosis with a more 3′ location of the insertion and the TKD1 domain is more 3′ than the juxtamembrane domain [7]. Further studies are needed to evaluate the different *FLT3* mutations and insertion sites to determine whether specific mutations have different prognostic impacts.

Allogeneic transplant is usually recommended for *FLT3* ITD positive AML with a normal karyotype; however, even with transplant there is a high risk of relapse. There is also interest in targeting *FLT3* ITD mutations with *FLT3* inhibitors; unfortunately, to date success in this area has been limited [15]. Possible reasons include coexistence or development of *FLT3* TKD mutations, activation of downstream signaling molecules, up-regulation of *FLT3*, or activation of other pathways [15].

The less common *FLT3* TKD mutation is found in about 10% of AML and also leads to constitutive activation of *FLT3* [3,4]. However, despite a seemingly similar mechanism of action the *FLT3* TKD has not clearly been shown to have an effect on prognosis. Some studies suggested an adverse prognostic risk; however, other studies have not confirmed this [3,4]. It is unclear at this time whether this mutation is targetable with *FLT3* inhibitors, although some studies suggest that it is not [15].

4.2. NPM1 (Nucleophosmin 1)

NPM1 encodes a phosphoprotein that normally shuttles between the nucleus and cytoplasm and plays a role in ribosome biogenesis, centrosome duplication during mitosis, and cell proliferation and apoptosis through p53 and p19Arf [16]. Mutations in *NPM1* occur in the C-terminus of the gene leading to loss of the nucleolar localization signal and gain of a nuclear export signal ultimately leading to cytoplasmic localization of this protein. The most common mutation is a 4 base pair insertion. *NPM1* mutations are found in about 30% of all AML and 50%–60% of AML with a normal karyotype making it the most common genetic mutation in AML [3]. *NPM1* rarely occurs with the any of the recurrent genetic abnormalities, *BCOR*, or *CEBPA* but frequently co-exist with *FLT3*, *DNMT3A*, and IDH [17–19].

The presence of an *NPM1* mutation in AML with normal karyotype in the absence of a *FLT3* ITD mutation portends a favorable prognosis similar to the core-binding factor leukemias [5,17]. Some studies have suggested that an *NPM1* mutation with a *FLT3* ITD mutation has a prognosis intermediate compared to either mutation in isolation; while some studies suggest this may only be the case when the *FLT3* ITD mutation load is low [6,20]. There is limited data suggesting that the presence of multi-lineage dysplasia or an adverse karyotype do not affect the favorable prognosis of *NPM1* mutations as long as *FLT3* ITD is absent [21,22].

4.3. CEBPA (CCAAT Enhancer Binding Protein)

CEBPA is a transcription factor involved in neutrophil differentiation. *CEBPA* mutations are found in approximately 10% of AML and are more common in AML with a normal karyotype or with 9q deletions [4]. *CEBPA* mutations in AML may be biallelic, which accounts for approximately two-thirds of cases, or monoallelic, accounting for the remaining cases. In AML with a normal karyotype, isolated biallelic *CEBPA* mutations clearly confer a better prognosis, whereas a monoallelic mutation likely does not confer the same favorable prognosis [23–25]. A recent meta-analysis does not show a better prognosis with monoallelic *CEBPA* and in long term follow-up, biallelic *CEBPA* mutations show a longer overall survival (9.6 years) *versus* monoallelic *CEBPA* mutations (1.7 years) [23,24]. Biallelic mutations usually include one C-terminus and one N-terminus mutation and lead to absent expression of normal *CEBPA* [26,27]. The truncating N-terminal mutations result in a shortened *CEBPA* protein with a dominant negative effect [28]. The C-terminal mutations decrease dimerization or DNA binding [25].

4.4. KIT (v-KIT Hardy-Zuckerman 4 Feline Sa12rcoma Viral Oncogene Homolog)

KIT is a receptor tyrosine kinase involved in proliferation, differentiation, and survival. *KIT* mutations affect predominantly exons 8 or 17, lead to a gain of function, and occur in 2%–14% of all cases of AML [18,29–31]. The incidence of *KIT* mutations is higher in core-binding factor leukemia, being found in about 7%–46% of cases [32–34]. The presence of *KIT* mutations in core binding factor leukemia is generally accepted to be associated with a worse prognosis [35,36]. However, some studies have shown this to be the case only in t(8;21) AML [37,38] and other studies have failed to show a prognostic effect at all [18,39,40].

5. Other Gene Mutations in AML

With the advent of next generation sequencing, the number of genes found to be mutated in AML has drastically increased. However, the significance of many of these gene mutations is unclear as the genes that are independent predictors of poor outcome differ between studies. (Table 3) Some of these differences may be due to the methods used for mutation detection, but often the statistically significant findings are based on a relatively small subset of patients and therefore may not be reproducible. Additionally, a gene found to be significant in one study may not have been tested in earlier or concurrent studies. Many of these significant genes are also mutated in other myeloid neoplasms; therefore, the presence of one of these mutations is not specific or diagnostic of leukemia.

All of these genes affect transcription either directly or through epigenetic regulation. (See Figure 1) *DNMT3A, TET2,* and *IDH1/2* are involved in DNA methylation. The DNA methyl transferases (DNMT) add a methyl group to CpG islands leading to DNA methylation, the TET proteins convert the methyl group to a hydroxymethyl group. 5-Hydroxymethylation appears to have different effects than methylation and is also an intermediate step to de-methylation. Isocitrate dehydrogenase inhibits TET proteins through 2-hydroxyglutarate. *NRAS, KRAS, BCOR, RUNX1,* and *WT1* all affect transcription. *NRAS* and *KRAS* affect transcription through the MEK/ERK pathway; while *BCOR* affects transcription by repression of BCL6. *RUNX1* and *WT1* are transcription factors; in addition, some *WT1* isoforms appear to regulate mRNA. *ASXL1, KMT2A (MLL),* and *PHF6* all affect chromatin remodeling. *TP53* is a gatekeeper that monitors DNA repair and regulates apoptosis and the cell cycle.

The role of testing for these other genes is not well established. Although routine testing of all AML cases is not recommended at this time, testing may be useful to better stratify individual patients. Several studies have proposed alternative stratification of AML patients using some of these genes [19,29,41]. These alternative algorithms risk stratify at least as well as the standard risk stratification given in Table 2 and the scheme proposed by Patel *et al.* appears to perform better than the standard risk stratification [29]. However, these are single studies that need to be confirmed before any of these algorithms are implemented as standard care.

Table 3. Other gene mutations in AML.

Gene	Frequency	Effect
ASXL1	3%–5%	Associated with MDS, AML-MRC. Worse prognosis [19,29,42–44].
BCOR	4% CN-AML	Possible worse prognosis [45].
DNMT3A	20%	Possible worse prognosis. May respond to high dose anthracyclines [18,29].
IDH1	6%–9% adult 1% pediatric	Possible worse prognosis [29,46,48,48,49].
IDH2	8%–12% adult 1%–2% pediatric	Controversial. *IDH2* R140 mutation with *NPM1* associated with a favorable prognosis in one study [29,46,48,48,49].
MLL/KMT2A	4%–14%	*MLL* PTD shows worse prognosis in CN-AML [18,19,29–31].
NRAS	8%–13% adult and pediatric	No clear impact on prognosis [50,51].
KRAS	2% adult 9% pediatric	No clear impact on prognosis [52].
PHF6	2%–3%	Associated with adverse outcome [29].
RUNX1	5%–18%	Possibly poorer prognosis. May do better with allogeneic transplant [19,29,53].
TET2	7%–10% adult 1.5%–4% pediatric	Unclear, some studies show adverse outcome especially in intermediate risk AML with isolated *CEBPA* or *NPM1* [18,29,54,55].
TP53	2%–9% adult 1% pediatric	Unfavorable prognosis [18,19]. Mutations may be germline (Li-Fraumeni syndrome) and this possibility should be considered when testing especially in younger individuals.
WT1	4%–11%	Poorer outcome, especially in CN-AML [56,57].

MDS: myelodysplastic syndrome, AML-MRC: acute myeloid leukemia with myelodysplasia related changes, PTD: partial tandem duplication, CN-AML: cytogenetically normal acute myeloid leukemia.

5.1. ASXL1 (Additional Sex Combs like Transcriptional Regulator 1)

ASXL1 encodes a chromatin binding protein, which may enhance or repress gene transcription in localized areas by modification of chromatin structure. *ASXL1* mutations are frequently found in myelodysplastic syndromes (MDS) and in AML but appear to be enriched in secondary AML, AML-MRC, and intermediate risk AML [42,43]. The overall frequency in AML is 3%–5% [18,29,30] but is 11%–17% in intermediate risk AML (including AML with a normal karyotype) [31,58]. *ASXL1* mutations also increase with age, being more prevalent in patients over 60 and quite rare in children (approximately 1%) [58–60]. Most studies have shown that *ASXL1* mutations are associated with a worse prognosis; however, studies have not always controlled for a history of MDS or presence of AML-MRC [19,29,44]. *ASXL1* mutation status may change with relapse with both gains and losses of mutations being reported [61].

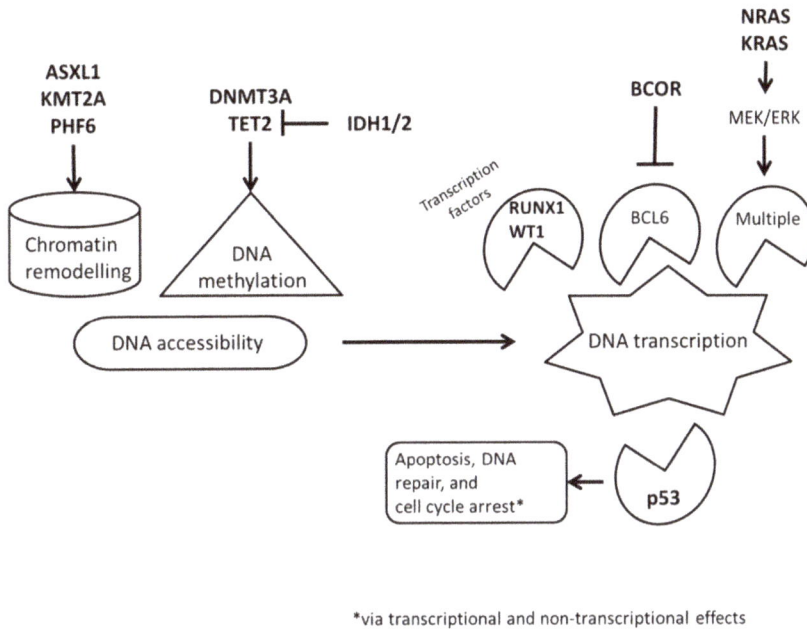

*via transcriptional and non-transcriptional effects

Figure 1. Direct and indirect effects of *ASXL1, BCOR, DNMT3A, IDH1, IDH2, KMT2A (MLL), KRAS, NRAS, PHF6, RUNX1, TET2, TP53,* and *WT1* on DNA transcription.

5.2. BCOR (BCL6 Corepressor)

The *BCOR* gene is located on the X chromosome and, as its name suggests, plays a role in repression of BCL6 [62]. The BCOR protein interacts with histone deacetylases (HDAC) which may explain its role in AML. *BCOR* mutations in AML have been described in a limited number of studies [45,63,64]. *BCOR* mutations occur in about 4% of CN-AML and frequently coexist with *DNMT3A* mutations [45]. *BCOR* mutations have also been described in 25% of AML cases with trisomy 13 [63]. The effect of *BCOR* mutations in prognosis is unclear at this time. One study showed decreased event free survival but no difference in overall survival in multivariate analysis [45].

5.3. DNMT3A (DNA Methyltransferase 3A)

DNMT3A is a DNA methyltransferase involved in the epigenetic regulation of the genome through methylation. Mutations in *DNMT3A* are quite common in AML, occurring in approximately 20% of patients. The most common mutation is a substitution of the amino acid arginine at position 882 (R882) [65]. *DNMT3A* mutations often co-occur with *FLT3* ITD, *NPM1, IDH1,* and *IDH2* mutations but are rare with t(15;17) and core binding factor rearrangements [65]. *DNMT3A* mutations in some studies have been associated with worse prognosis; however, this may be overcome by high dose anthracycline chemotherapy [18,29].

5.4. IDH1 and IDH2 (Isocitrate Dehydrogenase 1 and 2)

IDH1 and *IDH2* are genes involved in metabolism that appear to play an epigenetic role in histone and possibly DNA methylation [66]. Mutations in *IDH1* and *IDH2* occur at the active isocitrate binding site and lead to increased level of 2-hydroxyglutarate [67]. IDH mutations often occur with *NPM1* mutations and some studies have shown an impact only with *NPM1* but others have not [29,46,68]. When evaluated together, *IDH1* and *IDH2* mutations have been reported to have a favorable, neutral, and adverse effect on prognosis in AML with a normal karyotype [29,46–48]. However, despite an apparently similar biological effect, different mutations may have disparate prognostic impact. This fact makes it difficult to evaluate studies that grouped *IDH1* and *IDH2* mutations and the different *IDH2* mutations together.

IDH1 mutations affect either the arginine residue at position 132 or 170 (R132 or R170) and occur in 6%–9% of adult AML cases but only 1% of pediatric AML [29–31,46,49,59]. These mutations are exclusive of each other and exclusive of the *IDH2* mutation. When evaluated as a separate group, mutations in *IDH1* appear to have an unfavorable prognosis [49].

IDH2 mutations may affect either the arginine residue at position 140 or 172 (R140 or R172) and occur in 8%–12% of adult AML cases but only 1%–2% of pediatric cases [29–31,46,49,59,69]. However, only the R140 mutation appears to have prognostic significance [29,70]. The R140 mutation in *IDH2* has been shown to be associated with a favorable outcome in intermediate risk AML with *NPM1* mutation [29].

5.5. MLL/KMT2A (Mixed Lineage Leukemia/Lysine (K)-Specific Methyltransferase 2A)

The *MLL* gene (recently renamed to *KMT2A*) is a histone methyltransferase that regulates gene transcription through histone modification. Rearrangements involving *MLL* are well-known to cause acute lymphoblastic leukemia (ALL), AML, or mixed phenotype acute leukemia. However, partial tandem duplications of *MLL* (*MLL* PTD) occur predominantly in AML and are rare in ALL [71]. Approximately 4%–14% of AML cases will have an *MLL* PTD, which has been associated with a poor prognosis especially in AML with a normal karyotype [18,19,29–31].

5.6. NRAS and KRAS (Neuroblastoma RAS Viral (v-ras) Oncogene Homolog and Kirsten Rat Sarcoma Viral Oncogene Homolog)

KRAS and *NRAS* belong to the RAS GTPase family of genes. *NRAS* mutations in AML are fairly common being found in 8%–13% of cases in adults and children [17,29–31,59]. *KRAS* mutations are less common in adults being found in only 2% of cases but are more common in children where they account for about 9% of cases [29,59]. RAS mutations are more common in core binding factor leukemia, especially inv(16) [38,72]. Although some smaller studies have suggested a worse outcome; in large adult and pediatric studies, *NRAS* mutations have had no clear impact on outcome [50,51]. *KRAS* mutations also do not appear to have an impact on outcome [52].

5.7. PHF6 (Plant Homeodomain Finger 6)

PHF6 is an X-linked gene that appears to play a role in chromatin remodeling although its precise functions have not yet been elucidated [73]. Germline loss of function mutations are associated with X-linked intellectual disability disorders [74]. *PHF6* mutations occur in 2%–3% of adult AML and occur more frequently in males than females [29,75,76]. *PHF6* mutations are associated with adverse outcome in intermediate risk AML patients who are negative for *FLT3* ITD and it has been suggested that mutations in *PHF6* as well as other genes may be useful in stratifying this subgroup of AML patients [29]. Although this study result appears promising, further studies are needed as these conclusions were drawn on a limited number of patients. Only 14 patients had *PHF6* mutations in the test cohort of 398 patients and only 10 patients had *PHF6* mutations and were *FLT3* ITD negative (Patel, *et al.*, 2012 supplemental material) [29].

5.8. RUNX1 (Runt Related Transcription Factor 1)

RUNX1 (previously known as AML1) encodes the alpha subunit of core binding factor. Core binding factor is a heterodimer composed of an alpha and beta subunit that is in involved in transcription. Translocations involving *RUNX1* are found in AML with recurrent cytogenetic abnormalities (AML with t(8;21), *RUNX1-RUNX1T1*) and also in ALL. Mutations of *RUNX1* also occur in 5%–18% of AML, but are more common in intermediate risk AML and poor risk AML without a complex karyotype [19,29,31,53]. Germline *RUNX1* mutations are found in familial platelet disorder which predisposes to AML and less frequently T-lymphoblastic leukemia (TALL) [77]. Although several studies have shown a poorer prognosis with *RUNX1*, some studies have failed to show an effect [19,29,53]. A study by Gaidzik, *et al.* suggested that patients with *RUNX1* mutations did better with allogeneic transplant compared to autologous transplant or chemotherapy alone [53].

5.9. TET2 (Tet Methylcytosine Dioxygenase 2)

TET2 is an epigenetic modifier that converts methylcytosine to 5-hydroxymethylcytosine and plays a role in myelopoiesis. Mutations in *TET2* are found in 7%–10% of adult AML patients and 1.5%–4% of pediatric AML [59,78,79]. Mutations in *TET2* are highly variable and include nonsense mutations, deletions (frameshift and non-frameshift), missense mutations, and splice site mutations. All mutations, however, appear to cause loss of function and decreased hydroxymethylation of DNA [78]. *NPM1* and *TET2* defects are significantly correlated and *FLT3*-ITD and *FLT3*-TKD aberrations are often present together with *TET2* mutations [54,78]. *TET2* and IDH mutations seldom co-existed in the same patient as may be expected since IDH mutations abrogate the activity of *TET2* [31,54]. The frequency of *TET2* mutations in AML increases with age [31]. Of note, *TET2* mutations have been found in elderly females with no clear evidence of hematologic disease [80]. The prognostic effect of *TET2* is unclear with some studies showing an inferior survival in AML with a normal karyotype, especially those with favorable genetic mutations (isolated *CEBPA* and *NPM1*), and other studies showing no effect [18,29,54,55].

5.10. TP53 (Tumor Protein p53)

TP53 is a well-known tumor suppressor gene that regulates the cell cycle in response to cellular stress. Mutations in *TP53* occur in 2%–9% of adult AML and approximately 1% of pediatric AML [18,19,29,59]. *TP53* mutations are highly associated with a complex karyotype and rarely occur with *CEBPA*, *NPM1*, *FLT3* ITD, *ASXL1*, or *RUNX1* mutations [19]. As in other cancers, mutations of *TP53* in AML are associated with an unfavorable prognosis [18,19]. The presence of *TP53* mutation in a young person with AML brings up the possibility of a germline mutation and underlying Li-Fraumeni syndrome. If testing for *TP53* will be performed, the patient should be counselled regarding this possibility.

5.11. WT1 (Wilms Tumor 1)

WT1 encodes a transcription factor that plays an important role in urogenital development and appears to have a tumor suppressor role in renal tissues but an oncogenic role in leukemia [81]. Overexpression of *WT1* in AML is linked with poor outcome and relapse in several studies especially in AML with a normal karyotype [82,83]. Monitoring levels of *WT1* also has shown usefulness in monitoring for minimal residual disease [84,85]. Mutations in *WT1* also occur, being found 4%–11% of AML cases [29–31,43,59]. *WT1* mutations also appear to have an association with poor outcome in AML with a normal karyotype [56,57].

6. Conclusions

Genetics play an increasingly important role in the risk stratification and management of AML patients. Current standard of care combines cytogenetic results with testing for mutations in *FLT3*, *NPM1*, *CEBPA*, and *KIT*. The presence of *FLT3* ITD, *NPM1*, or *CEBPA* mutations refines the prognosis of patient with AML with normal karyotype which is normally intermediate risk. *FLT3* ITD modifies the risk to poor, while *NPM1* and biallelic *CEBPA* mutations improve the prognosis to favorable. *KIT* mutations in one of the core binding factor leukemias worsen the prognosis from good to intermediate.

As molecular testing methods advance, routinely testing multiple genes for mutations becomes more feasible and, indeed, gene panels that look for mutations in multiple genes are already available. Mutations in several genes appear to have prognostic impact. However, studies in the literature do not always agree on which mutations have independent prognostic effect and our understanding of the

J. Clin. Med. **2015**, *4*, 460–478

impact of co-existing mutations and the interplay with cytogenetic abnormalities is limited. Mutations in *ASXL1, MLL, TP53,* and *WT1* have been shown in multiple studies to be independently associated with a poorer prognosis. Mutations in *BCOR, DNMT3A, IDH1, PHF6, RUNX1* and *TET2* are possibly associated with a poorer prognosis but have either not been confirmed in multiple studies or have some conflicting results. *KRAS* and *NRAS* mutations do not appear to have an effect on prognosis. As prognosis guides therapy, these gene mutations could play a role in guiding therapy in the future. Two genes appear promising for more specifically guiding therapy in the future. AML with *DNMT3A* mutations may respond better to high dose anthracyclines and AML with *RUNX1* mutations may have better outcomes with allogeneic transplant. These findings are promising that testing for mutations in these additional genes can improve the current risk stratification and patient care; however, they need to be confirmed in additional studies before routine clinical implementation.

Author Contributions: Sophia Yohe is the sole author of this work.

Conflicts of Interest: The author declares no conflict of interest.

References

1. Swerdlow, S.H.; Campo, E.; Harris, N.L.; Jaffe, E.S.; Pileri, S.A.; Stein, H.; Thiele, J.; Vardiman, J.W. *Who Classification of Tumours of Hematopoietic and Lymphoid Tissues*, 4th ed.; International Agency for Research on Cancer: Lyon, France, 2008.
2. O'Donnel, M.R.; Tallman, M.S.; Abboud, C.N.; Altman, J.K.; Appelbaum, F.R.; Arber, D.A.; Attar, E.; Borate, U.; Damon, L.E.; Gregory, K.; *et al.* National comprehensive cancer network: NCCN categories of evidence and consensus. Available online: http://www.nccn.org/professionals/physician_gls/categories_of_consensus.asp (accessed on 13 January 2015).
3. Ofran, Y.; Rowe, J.M. Genetic profiling in acute myeloid leukaemia—Where are we and what is its role in patient management. *Br. J. Haematol.* **2013**, *160*, 303–320.
4. Martelli, M.P.; Sportoletti, P.; Tiacci, E.; Martelli, M.F.; Falini, B. Mutational landscape of AML with normal cytogenetics: Biological and clinical implications. *Blood Rev.* **2013**, *27*, 13–22. [PubMed]
5. Whitman, S.P.; Archer, K.J.; Feng, L.; Baldus, C.; Becknell, B.; Carlson, B.D.; Carroll, A.J.; Mrózek, K.; Vardiman, J.W.; George, S.L.; *et al.* Absence of the wild-type allele predicts poor prognosis in adult *de novo* acute myeloid leukemia with normal cytogenetics and the internal tandem duplication of *FLT3*: A cancer and leukemia group B study. *Cancer Res.* **2001**, *61*, 7233–7239. [PubMed]
6. Gale, R.E.; Green, C.; Allen, C.; Mead, A.J.; Burnett, A.K.; Hills, R.K.; Linch, D.C.; Party, M.R.C.A.L.W. The impact of *FLT3* internal tandem duplication mutant level, number, size, and interaction with *NPM1* mutations in a large cohort of young adult patients with acute myeloid leukemia. *Blood* **2008**, *111*, 2776–2784. [CrossRef] [PubMed]
7. Schnittger, S.; Bacher, U.; Haferlach, C.; Alpermann, T.; Kern, W.; Haferlach, T. Diversity of the juxtamembrane and TKD1 mutations (exons 13–15) in the *FLT3* gene with regards to mutant load, sequence, length, localization, and correlation with biological data. *Genes Chromosomes Cancer* **2012**, *51*, 910–924. [CrossRef] [PubMed]
8. Schlenk, R.F.; Kayser, S.; Bullinger, L.; Kobbe, G.; Casper, J.; Ringhoffer, M.; Held, G.; Brossart, P.; Lübbert, M.; Salih, H.R.; *et al.* Differential impact of allelic ratio and insertion site in *FLT3*-ITD positive AML with respect to allogeneic transplantation. *Blood* **2014**, *124*, 3441–3449. [CrossRef] [PubMed]
9. Kayser, S.; Schlenk, R.F.; Londono, M.C.; Breitenbuecher, F.; Wittke, K.; Du, J.; Groner, S.; Späth, D.; Krauter, J.; Ganser, A.; *et al.* Insertion of *FLT3* internal tandem duplication in the tyrosine kinase domain-1 is associated with resistance to chemotherapy and inferior outcome. *Blood* **2009**, *114*, 2386–2392. [CrossRef] [PubMed]
10. Blau, O.; Berenstein, R.; Sindram, A.; Blau, I.W. Molecular analysis of different *FLT3*-ITD mutations in acute myeloid leukemia. *Leuk. Lymphoma* **2013**, *54*, 145–152. [CrossRef] [PubMed]
11. Meshinchi, S.; Stirewalt, D.L.; Alonzo, T.A.; Boggon, T.J.; Gerbing, R.B.; Rocnik, J.L.; Lange, B.J.; Gilliland, D.G.; Radich, J.P. Structural and numerical variation of *FLT3*-ITD in pediatric AML. *Blood* **2008**, *111*, 4930–4933. [CrossRef] [PubMed]

12. Stirewalt, D.L.; Kopecky, K.J.; Meshinchi, S.; Engel, J.H.; Pogosova-Agadjanyan, E.L.; Linsley, J.; Slovak, M.L.; Willman, C.L.; Radich, J.P. Size of *FLT3* internal tandem duplication has prognostic significance in patients with acute myeloid leukemia. *Blood* **2006**, *107*, 3724–3726. [CrossRef] [PubMed]

13. Ponziani, V.; Gianfaldoni, G.; Mannelli, F.; Leoni, F.; Ciolli, S.; Guglielmelli, P.; Antonioli, E.; Longo, G.; Bosi, A.; Vannucchi, A.M. The size of duplication does not add to the prognostic significance of *FLT3* internal tandem duplication in acute myeloid leukemia patients. *Leukemia* **2006**, *20*, 2074–2076. [CrossRef] [PubMed]

14. Breitenbuecher, F.; Schnittger, S.; Grundler, R.; Markova, B.; Carius, B.; Brecht, A.; Duyster, J.; Haferlach, T.; Huber, C.; Fischer, T. Identification of a novel type of itd mutations located in nonjuxtamembrane domains of the *FLT3* tyrosine kinase receptor. *Blood* **2009**, *113*, 4074–4077. [CrossRef] [PubMed]

15. Alvarado, Y.; Kantarjian, H.M.; Luthra, R.; Ravandi, F.; Borthakur, G.; Garcia-Manero, G.; Konopleva, M.; Estrov, Z.; Andreeff, M.; Cortes, J.E. Treatment with *FLT3* inhibitor in patients with *FLT3*-mutated acute myeloid leukemia is associated with development of secondary *FLT3*-tyrosine kinase domain mutations. *Cancer* **2014**, *120*, 2142–2149. [CrossRef] [PubMed]

16. Falini, B.; Albiero, E.; Bolli, N.; De Marco, M.F.; Madeo, D.; Martelli, M.; Nicoletti, I.; Rodeghiero, F. Aberrant cytoplasmic expression of C-terminal-truncated NPM leukaemic mutant is dictated by tryptophans loss and a new NES motif. *Leukemia* **2007**, *21*, 2052–2054. [CrossRef] [PubMed]

17. Schlenk, R.F.; Döhner, K.; Krauter, J.; Fröhling, S.; Corbacioglu, A.; Bullinger, L.; Habdank, M.; Späth, D.; Morgan, M.; Benner, A.; *et al.* Mutations and treatment outcome in cytogenetically normal acute myeloid leukemia. *N. Engl. J. Med.* **2008**, *358*, 1909–1918. [CrossRef] [PubMed]

18. Kihara, R.; Nagata, Y.; Kiyoi, H.; Kato, T.; Yamamoto, E.; Suzuki, K.; Chen, F.; Asou, N.; Ohtake, S.; Miyawaki, S.; *et al.* Comprehensive analysis of genetic alterations and their prognostic impacts in adult acute myeloid leukemia patients. *Leukemia* **2014**, *28*, 1586–1595. [CrossRef] [PubMed]

19. Grossmann, V.; Schnittger, S.; Kohlmann, A.; Eder, C.; Roller, A.; Dicker, F.; Schmid, C.; Wendtner, C.M.; Staib, P.; Serve, H.; *et al.* A novel hierarchical prognostic model of AML solely based on molecular mutations. *Blood* **2012**, *120*, 2963–2972. [CrossRef] [PubMed]

20. Schnittger, S.; Bacher, U.; Kern, W.; Alpermann, T.; Haferlach, C.; Haferlach, T. Prognostic impact of *FLT3*-ITD load in *NPM1* mutated acute myeloid leukemia. *Leukemia* **2011**, *25*, 1297–1304. [CrossRef] [PubMed]

21. Falini, B.; Macijewski, K.; Weiss, T.; Bacher, U.; Schnittger, S.; Kern, W.; Kohlmann, A.; Klein, H.U.; Vignetti, M.; Piciocchi, A.; *et al.* Multilineage dysplasia has no impact on biologic, clinicopathologic, and prognostic features of aml with mutated nucleophosmin (*NPM1*). *Blood* **2010**, *115*, 3776–3786. [CrossRef] [PubMed]

22. Haferlach, C.; Mecucci, C.; Schnittger, S.; Kohlmann, A.; Mancini, M.; Cuneo, A.; Testoni, N.; Rege-Cambrin, G.; Santucci, A.; Vignetti, M.; *et al.* AML with mutated *NPM1* carrying a normal or aberrant karyotype show overlapping biologic, pathologic, immunophenotypic, and prognostic features. *Blood* **2009**, *114*, 3024–3032. [CrossRef] [PubMed]

23. Li, H.Y.; Deng, D.H.; Huang, Y.; Ye, F.H.; Huang, L.L.; Xiao, Q.; Zhang, B.; Ye, B.B.; Lai, Y.R.; Mo, Z.N.; *et al.* Favorable prognosis of biallelic *CEBPA* gene mutations in acute myeloid leukemia patients: A meta-analysis. *Eur. J. Haematol.* **2014**, in press.

24. Pastore, F.; Kling, D.; Hoster, E.; Dufour, A.; Konstandin, N.P.; Schneider, S.; Sauerland, M.C.; Berdel, W.E.; Buechner, T.; Woermann, B.; *et al.* Long-term follow-up of cytogenetically normal *CEBPA*-mutated AML. *J. Hematol. Oncol.* **2014**, *7*, 55. [CrossRef] [PubMed]

25. Wouters, B.J.; Löwenberg, B.; Erpelinck-Verschueren, C.A.; van Putten, W.L.; Valk, P.J.; Delwel, R. Double *CEBPA* mutations, but not single *CEBPA* mutations, define a subgroup of acute myeloid leukemia with a distinctive gene expression profile that is uniquely associated with a favorable outcome. *Blood* **2009**, *113*, 3088–3091. [CrossRef] [PubMed]

26. Mueller, B.U.; Pabst, T. C/EBPalpha and the pathophysiology of acute myeloid leukemia. *Curr. Opin. Hematol.* **2006**, *13*, 7–14. [CrossRef] [PubMed]

27. Nerlov, C. C/EBPalpha mutations in acute myeloid leukaemias. *Nat. Rev. Cancer* **2004**, *4*, 394–400. [CrossRef] [PubMed]

28. Pabst, T.; Mueller, B.U.; Zhang, P.; Radomska, H.S.; Narravula, S.; Schnittger, S.; Behre, G.; Hiddemann, W.; Tenen, D.G. Dominant-negative mutations of *CEBPA*, encoding CCAAT/enhancer binding protein-alpha (c/EBPalpha), in acute myeloid leukemia. *Nat. Genet.* **2001**, *27*, 263–270. [CrossRef] [PubMed]

29. Patel, J.P.; Gönen, M.; Figueroa, M.E.; Fernandez, H.; Sun, Z.; Racevskis, J.; Van Vlierberghe, P.; Dolgalev, I.; Thomas, S.; Aminova, O.; *et al.* Prognostic relevance of integrated genetic profiling in acute myeloid leukemia. *N. Engl. J. Med.* **2012**, *366*, 1079–1089. [CrossRef] [PubMed]

30. Shen, Y.; Zhu, Y.M.; Fan, X.; Shi, J.Y.; Wang, Q.R.; Yan, X.J.; Gu, Z.H.; Wang, Y.Y.; Chen, B.; Jiang, C.L.; *et al.* Gene mutation patterns and their prognostic impact in a cohort of 1185 patients with acute myeloid leukemia. *Blood* **2011**, *118*, 5593–5603. [CrossRef] [PubMed]

31. Tian, X.; Xu, Y.; Yin, J.; Tian, H.; Chen, S.; Wu, D.; Sun, A. *TET2* gene mutation is unfavorable prognostic factor in cytogenetically normal acute myeloid leukemia patients with *NPM1*⁺ and *FLT3*-ITD⁻ mutations. *Int. J. Hematol.* **2014**, *100*, 96–104. [CrossRef] [PubMed]

32. Care, R.S.; Valk, P.J.; Goodeve, A.C.; Abu-Duhier, F.M.; Geertsma-Kleinekoort, W.M.; Wilson, G.A.; Gari, M.A.; Peake, I.R.; Löwenberg, B.; Reilly, J.T. Incidence and prognosis of c-*KIT* and *FLT3* mutations in core binding factor (CBF) acute myeloid leukaemias. *Br. J. Haematol.* **2003**, *121*, 775–777. [CrossRef] [PubMed]

33. Beghini, A.; Ripamonti, C.B.; Cairoli, R.; Cazzaniga, G.; Colapietro, P.; Elice, F.; Nadali, G.; Grillo, G.; Haas, O.A.; Biondi, A.; *et al.* *KIT* activating mutations: Incidence in adult and pediatric acute myeloid leukemia, and identification of an internal tandem duplication. *Haematologica* **2004**, *89*, 920–925. [PubMed]

34. Mrózek, K.; Marcucci, G.; Paschka, P.; Bloomfield, C.D. Advances in molecular genetics and treatment of core-binding factor acute myeloid leukemia. *Curr. Opin. Oncol.* **2008**, *20*, 711–718. [CrossRef] [PubMed]

35. Paschka, P.; Marcucci, G.; Ruppert, A.S.; Mrózek, K.; Chen, H.; Kittles, R.A.; Vukosavljevic, T.; Perrotti, D.; Vardiman, J.W.; Carroll, A.J.; *et al.* Adverse prognostic significance of *KIT* mutations in adult acute myeloid leukemia with inv(16) and t(8;21): A cancer and leukemia group B study. *J. Clin. Oncol.* **2006**, *24*, 3904–3911. [CrossRef] [PubMed]

36. Cairoli, R.; Beghini, A.; Grillo, G.; Nadali, G.; Elice, F.; Ripamonti, C.B.; Colapietro, P.; Nichelatti, M.; Pezzetti, L.; Lunghi, M.; *et al.* Prognostic impact of c-*KIT* mutations in core binding factor leukemias: An Italian retrospective study. *Blood* **2006**, *107*, 3463–3468. [CrossRef] [PubMed]

37. Park, S.H.; Chi, H.S.; Min, S.K.; Park, B.G.; Jang, S.; Park, C.J. Prognostic impact of c-*KIT* mutations in core binding factor acute myeloid leukemia. *Leuk. Res.* **2011**, *35*, 1376–1383. [CrossRef] [PubMed]

38. Boissel, N.; Leroy, H.; Brethon, B.; Philippe, N.; de Botton, S.; Auvrignon, A.; Raffoux, E.; Leblanc, T.; Thomas, X.; Hermine, O.; *et al.* Incidence and prognostic impact of c-*KIT*, *FLT3*, and *RAS* gene mutations in core binding factor acute myeloid leukemia (CBF-AML). *Leukemia* **2006**, *20*, 965–970. [CrossRef] [PubMed]

39. Jourdan, E.; Boissel, N.; Chevret, S.; Delabesse, E.; Renneville, A.; Cornillet, P.; Blanchet, O.; Cayuela, J.M.; Recher, C.; Raffoux, E.; *et al.* Prospective evaluation of gene mutations and minimal residual disease in patients with core binding factor acute myeloid leukemia. *Blood* **2013**, *121*, 2213–2223. [CrossRef] [PubMed]

40. Cairoli, R.; Beghini, A.; Turrini, M.; Bertani, G.; Nadali, G.; Rodeghiero, F.; Castagnola, C.; Lazzaroni, F.; Nichelatti, M.; Ferrara, F.; *et al.* Old and new prognostic factors in acute myeloid leukemia with deranged core-binding factor beta. *Am. J. Hematol.* **2013**, *88*, 594–600. [CrossRef] [PubMed]

41. Döhner, H.; Estey, E.H.; Amadori, S.; Appelbaum, F.R.; Büchner, T.; Burnett, A.K.; Dombret, H.; Fenaux, P.; Grimwade, D.; Larson, R.A.; *et al.* Diagnosis and management of acute myeloid leukemia in adults: Recommendations from an international expert panel, on behalf of the european leukemianet. *Blood* **2010**, *115*, 453–474. [CrossRef] [PubMed]

42. Devillier, R.; Gelsi-Boyer, V.; Brecqueville, M.; Carbuccia, N.; Murati, A.; Vey, N.; Birnbaum, D.; Mozziconacci, M.J. Acute myeloid leukemia with myelodysplasia-related changes are characterized by a specific molecular pattern with high frequency of *ASXL1* mutations. *Am. J. Hematol.* **2012**, *87*, 659–662. [CrossRef] [PubMed]

43. Fernandez-Mercado, M.; Yip, B.H.; Pellagatti, A.; Davies, C.; Larrayoz, M.J.; Kondo, T.; Pérez, C.; Killick, S.; McDonald, E.J.; Odero, M.D.; *et al.* Mutation patterns of 16 genes in primary and secondary acute myeloid leukemia (AML) with normal cytogenetics. *PLoS One* **2012**, *7*, e42334. [CrossRef] [PubMed]

44. Metzeler, K.H.; Becker, H.; Maharry, K.; Radmacher, M.D.; Kohlschmidt, J.; Mrózek, K.; Nicolet, D.; Whitman, S.P.; Wu, Y.Z.; Schwind, S.; *et al.* *ASXL1* mutations identify a high-risk subgroup of older patients with primary cytogenetically normal aml within the eln favorable genetic category. *Blood* **2011**, *118*, 6920–6929. [CrossRef] [PubMed]

45. Grossmann, V.; Tiacci, E.; Holmes, A.B.; Kohlmann, A.; Martelli, M.P.; Kern, W.; Spanhol-Rosseto, A.; Klein, H.U.; Dugas, M.; Schindela, S.; *et al.* Whole-exome sequencing identifies somatic mutations of *BCOR* in acute myeloid leukemia with normal karyotype. *Blood* **2011**, *118*, 6153–6163. [CrossRef] [PubMed]

46. Paschka, P.; Schlenk, R.F.; Gaidzik, V.I.; Habdank, M.; Krönke, J.; Bullinger, L.; Späth, D.; Kayser, S.; Zucknick, M.; Götze, K.; *et al. IDH1* and *IDH2* mutations are frequent genetic alterations in acute myeloid leukemia and confer adverse prognosis in cytogenetically normal acute myeloid leukemia with *NPM1* mutation without *FLT3* internal tandem duplication. *J. Clin. Oncol.* **2010**, *28*, 3636–3643. [CrossRef] [PubMed]

47. Marcucci, G.; Maharry, K.; Wu, Y.Z.; Radmacher, M.D.; Mrózek, K.; Margeson, D.; Holland, K.B.; Whitman, S.P.; Becker, H.; Schwind, S.; *et al. IDH1* and *IDH2* gene mutations identify novel molecular subsets within de novo cytogenetically normal acute myeloid leukemia: A cancer and leukemia group Bstudy. *J. Clin. Oncol.* **2010**, *28*, 2348–2355. [CrossRef] [PubMed]

48. Thol, F.; Damm, F.; Wagner, K.; Göhring, G.; Schlegelberger, B.; Hoelzer, D.; Lübbert, M.; Heit, W.; Kanz, L.; Schlimok, G.; *et al.* Prognostic impact of *IDH2* mutations in cytogenetically normal acute myeloid leukemia. *Blood* **2010**, *116*, 614–616. [CrossRef] [PubMed]

49. Abbas, S.; Lugthart, S.; Kavelaars, F.G.; Schelen, A.; Koenders, J.E.; Zeilemaker, A.; van Putten, W.J.; Rijneveld, A.W.; Löwenberg, B.; Valk, P.J. Acquired mutations in the genes encoding *IDH1* and *IDH2* both are recurrent aberrations in acute myeloid leukemia: Prevalence and prognostic value. *Blood* **2010**, *116*, 2122–2126. [CrossRef] [PubMed]

50. Berman, J.N.; Gerbing, R.B.; Alonzo, T.A.; Ho, P.A.; Miller, K.; Hurwitz, C.; Heerema, N.A.; Hirsch, B.; Raimondi, S.C.; Lange, B.; *et al.* Prevalence and clinical implications of *NRAS* mutations in childhood AML: A report from the children's oncology group. *Leukemia* **2011**, *25*, 1039–1042. [CrossRef] [PubMed]

51. Bacher, U.; Haferlach, T.; Schoch, C.; Kern, W.; Schnittger, S. Implications of *NRAS* mutations in AML: A study of 2502 patients. *Blood* **2006**, *107*, 3847–3853. [CrossRef] [PubMed]

52. Bowen, D.T.; Frew, M.E.; Hills, R.; Gale, R.E.; Wheatley, K.; Groves, M.J.; Langabeer, S.E.; Kottaridis, P.D.; Moorman, A.V.; Burnett, A.K.; *et al. RAS* mutation in acute myeloid leukemia is associated with distinct cytogenetic subgroups but does not influence outcome in patients younger than 60 years. *Blood* **2005**, *106*, 2113–2119. [CrossRef] [PubMed]

53. Gaidzik, V.I.; Bullinger, L.; Schlenk, R.F.; Zimmermann, A.S.; Röck, J.; Paschka, P.; Corbacioglu, A.; Krauter, J.; Schlegelberger, B.; Ganser, A.; *et al. RUNX1* mutations in acute myeloid leukemia: Results from a comprehensive genetic and clinical analysis from the AML study group. *J. Clin. Oncol.* **2011**, *29*, 1364–1372. [CrossRef] [PubMed]

54. Gaidzik, V.I.; Paschka, P.; Späth, D.; Habdank, M.; Köhne, C.H.; Germing, U.; von Lilienfeld-Toal, M.; Held, G.; Horst, H.A.; Haase, D.; *et al. TET2* mutations in acute myeloid leukemia (AML): Results from a comprehensive genetic and clinical analysis of the AML study group. *J. Clin. Oncol.* **2012**, *30*, 1350–1357. [CrossRef] [PubMed]

55. Metzeler, K.H.; Maharry, K.; Radmacher, M.D.; Mrózek, K.; Margeson, D.; Becker, H.; Curfman, J.; Holland, K.B.; Schwind, S.; Whitman, S.P.; *et al. TET2* mutations improve the new European leukemianet risk classification of acute myeloid leukemia: A cancer and leukemia group B study. *J. Clin. Oncol.* **2011**, *29*, 1373–1381. [CrossRef] [PubMed]

56. Krauth, M.T.; Alpermann, T.; Bacher, U.; Eder, C.; Dicker, F.; Ulke, M.; Kuznia, S.; Nadarajah, N.; Kern, W.; Haferlach, C.; *et al. WT1* mutations are secondary events in AML, show varying frequencies and impact on prognosis between genetic subgroups. *Leukemia* **2014**.

57. Sano, H.; Shimada, A.; Tabuchi, K.; Taki, T.; Murata, C.; Park, M.J.; Ohki, K.; Sotomatsu, M.; Adachi, S.; Tawa, A.; *et al. WT1* mutation in pediatric patients with acute myeloid leukemia: A report from the Japanese childhood AML cooperative study group. *Int. J. Hematol.* **2013**, *98*, 437–445. [CrossRef] [PubMed]

58. Schnittger, S.; Eder, C.; Jeromin, S.; Alpermann, T.; Fasan, A.; Grossmann, V.; Kohlmann, A.; Illig, T.; Klopp, N.; Wichmann, H.E.; *et al. ASXL1* exon 12 mutations are frequent in AML with intermediate risk karyotype and are independently associated with an adverse outcome. *Leukemia* **2013**, *27*, 82–91. [CrossRef] [PubMed]

59. Liang, D.C.; Liu, H.C.; Yang, C.P.; Jaing, T.H.; Hung, I.J.; Yeh, T.C.; Chen, S.H.; Hou, J.Y.; Huang, Y.J.; Shih, Y.S.; *et al.* Cooperating gene mutations in childhood acute myeloid leukemia with special reference on mutations of *ASXL1, TET2, IDH1, IDH2,* and *DNMT3A. Blood* **2013**, *121*, 2988–2995. [CrossRef] [PubMed]

60. El-Sharkawi, D.; Ali, A.; Evans, C.M.; Hills, R.K.; Burnett, A.K.; Linch, D.C.; Gale, R.E. *ASXL1* mutations are infrequent in young patients with primary acute myeloid leukemia and their detection has a limited role in therapeutic risk stratification. *Leuk. Lymphoma* **2014**, *55*, 1326–1331. [CrossRef] [PubMed]

61. Chou, W.C.; Huang, H.H.; Hou, H.A.; Chen, C.Y.; Tang, J.L.; Yao, M.; Tsay, W.; Ko, B.S.; Wu, S.J.; Huang, S.Y.; *et al.* Distinct clinical and biological features of *de novo* acute myeloid leukemia with additional sex comb-like 1 (*ASXL1*) mutations. *Blood* **2010**, *116*, 4086–4094. [CrossRef] [PubMed]

62. Huynh, K.D.; Fischle, W.; Verdin, E.; Bardwell, V.J. *BCOR*, a novel corepressor involved in BCL-6 repression. *Genes Dev.* **2000**, *14*, 1810–1823. [PubMed]

63. Herold, T.; Metzeler, K.H.; Vosberg, S.; Hartmann, L.; Röllig, C.; Stölzel, F.; Schneider, S.; Hubmann, M.; Zellmeier, E.; Ksienzyk, B.; *et al.* Isolated trisomy 13 defines a homogeneous aml subgroup with high frequency of mutations in spliceosome genes and poor prognosis. *Blood* **2014**, *124*, 1304–1311. [CrossRef] [PubMed]

64. Thota, S.; Viny, A.D.; Makishima, H.; Spitzer, B.; Radivoyevitch, T.; Przychodzen, B.; Sekeres, M.A.; Levine, R.L.; Maciejewski, J.P. Genetic alterations of the cohesin complex genes in myeloid malignancies. *Blood* **2014**, *124*, 1790–1798. [CrossRef] [PubMed]

65. Ibrahem, L.; Mahfouz, R.; Elhelw, L.; Abdsalam, E.M.; Soliman, R. Prognostic significance of *DNMT3A* mutations in patients with acute myeloid leukemia. *Blood Cells Mol. Dis.* **2015**, *54*, 84–89. [CrossRef] [PubMed]

66. Lu, C.; Ward, P.S.; Kapoor, G.S.; Rohle, D.; Turcan, S.; Abdel-Wahab, O.; Edwards, C.R.; Khanin, R.; Figueroa, M.E.; Melnick, A.; *et al.* *IDH* mutation impairs histone demethylation and results in a block to cell differentiation. *Nature* **2012**, *483*, 474–478. [CrossRef] [PubMed]

67. Ward, P.S.; Cross, J.R.; Lu, C.; Weigert, O.; Abel-Wahab, O.; Levine, R.L.; Weinstock, D.M.; Sharp, K.A.; Thompson, C.B. Identification of additional *IDH* mutations associated with oncometabolite r(-)-2-hydroxyglutarate production. *Oncogene* **2012**, *31*, 2491–2498. [CrossRef] [PubMed]

68. Green, C.L.; Evans, C.M.; Hills, R.K.; Burnett, A.K.; Linch, D.C.; Gale, R.E. The prognostic significance of *IDH1* mutations in younger adult patients with acute myeloid leukemia is dependent on *FLT3*/ITD status. *Blood* **2010**, *116*, 2779–2782. [CrossRef] [PubMed]

69. Ho, P.A.; Kutny, M.A.; Alonzo, T.A.; Gerbing, R.B.; Joaquin, J.; Raimondi, S.C.; Gamis, A.S.; Meshinchi, S. Leukemic mutations in the methylation-associated genes *DNMT3A* and *IDH2* are rare events in pediatric AML: A report from the children's oncology group. *Pediatr. Blood Cancer* **2011**, *57*, 204–209. [CrossRef] [PubMed]

70. Green, C.L.; Evans, C.M.; Zhao, L.; Hills, R.K.; Burnett, A.K.; Linch, D.C.; Gale, R.E. The prognostic significance of *IDH2* mutations in AML depends on the location of the mutation. *Blood* **2011**, *118*, 409–412. [CrossRef] [PubMed]

71. Burmeister, T.; Meyer, C.; Schwartz, S.; Hofmann, J.; Molkentin, M.; Kowarz, E.; Schneider, B.; Raff, T.; Reinhardt, R.; Gökbuget, N.; *et al.* The *MLL* recombinome of adult CD10-negative B-cell precursor acute lymphoblastic leukemia: Results from the gmall study group. *Blood* **2009**, *113*, 4011–4015. [CrossRef] [PubMed]

72. Goemans, B.F.; Zwaan, C.M.; Miller, M.; Zimmermann, M.; Harlow, A.; Meshinchi, S.; Loonen, A.H.; Hählen, K.; Reinhardt, D.; Creutzig, U.; *et al.* Mutations in *KIT* and *RAS* are frequent events in pediatric core-binding factor acute myeloid leukemia. *Leukemia* **2005**, *19*, 1536–1542. [CrossRef] [PubMed]

73. Todd, M.A.; Picketts, D.J. *PHF6* interacts with the nucleosome remodeling and deacetylation (NuRD) complex. *J. Proteome Res.* **2012**, *11*, 4326–4337. [CrossRef] [PubMed]

74. Lower, K.M.; Turner, G.; Kerr, B.A.; Mathews, K.D.; Shaw, M.A.; Gedeon, A.K.; Schelley, S.; Hoyme, H.E.; White, S.M.; Delatycki, M.B.; *et al.* Mutations in *PHF6* are associated with Börjeson-Forssman-Lehmann syndrome. *Nat. Genet.* **2002**, *32*, 661–665. [CrossRef] [PubMed]

75. Yoo, N.J.; Kim, Y.R.; Lee, S.H. Somatic mutation of *PHF6* gene in T-cell acute lymphoblatic leukemia, acute myelogenous leukemia and hepatocellular carcinoma. *Acta Oncol.* **2012**, *51*, 107–111. [CrossRef] [PubMed]

76. Van Vlierberghe, P.; Patel, J.; Abdel-Wahab, O.; Lobry, C.; Hedvat, C.V.; Balbin, M.; Nicolas, C.; Payer, A.R.; Fernandez, H.F.; Tallman, M.S.; *et al.* *PHF6* mutations in adult acute myeloid leukemia. *Leukemia* **2011**, *25*, 130–134. [CrossRef] [PubMed]

77. Preudhomme, C.; Renneville, A.; Bourdon, V.; Philippe, N.; Roche-Lestienne, C.; Boissel, N.; Dhedin, N.; André, J.M.; Cornillet-Lefebvre, P.; Baruchel, A.; *et al.* High frequency of *RUNX1* biallelic alteration in acute myeloid leukemia secondary to familial platelet disorder. *Blood* **2009**, *113*, 5583–5587. [CrossRef] [PubMed]

78. Aslanyan, M.G.; Kroeze, L.I.; Langemeijer, S.M.; Koorenhof-Scheele, T.N.; Massop, M.; van Hoogen, P.; Stevens-Linders, E.; van de Locht, L.T.; Tönnissen, E.; van der Heijden, A.; *et al.* Clinical and biological impact of *TET2* mutations and expression in younger adult AML patients treated within the EORTC/GIMEMA AML-12 clinical trial. *Ann. Hematol.* **2014**, *93*, 1401–1412. [PubMed]

79. Langemeijer, S.M.; Jansen, J.H.; Hooijer, J.; van Hoogen, P.; Stevens-Linders, E.; Massop, M.; Waanders, E.; van Reijmersdal, S.V.; Stevens-Kroef, M.J.; Zwaan, C.M.; *et al.* *TET2* mutations in childhood leukemia. *Leukemia* **2011**, *25*, 189–192. [CrossRef] [PubMed]

80. Busque, L.; Patel, J.P.; Figueroa, M.E.; Vasanthakumar, A.; Provost, S.; Hamilou, Z.; Mollica, L.; Li, J.; Viale, A.; Heguy, A.; *et al.* Recurrent somatic *TET2* mutations in normal elderly individuals with clonal hematopoiesis. *Nat. Genet.* **2012**, *44*, 1179–1181. [CrossRef] [PubMed]

81. Yang, L.; Han, Y.; Suarez Saiz, F.; Saurez Saiz, F.; Minden, M.D. A tumor suppressor and oncogene: The *WT1* story. *Leukemia* **2007**, *21*, 868–876. [PubMed]

82. Lyu, X.; Xin, Y.; Mi, R.; Ding, J.; Wang, X.; Hu, J.; Fan, R.; Wei, X.; Song, Y.; Zhao, R.Y. Overexpression of wilms tumor 1 gene as a negative prognostic indicator in acute myeloid leukemia. *PLoS One* **2014**, *9*, e92470. [CrossRef] [PubMed]

83. Woehlecke, C.; Wittig, S.; Arndt, C.; Gruhn, B. Prognostic impact of *WT1* expression prior to hematopoietic stem cell transplantation in children with malignant hematological diseases. *J. Cancer Res. Clin. Oncol.* **2014**.

84. Rossi, G.; Carella, A.M.; Minervini, M.M.; Savino, L.; Fontana, A.; Pellegrini, F.; Greco, M.M.; Merla, E.; Quarta, G.; Loseto, G.; *et al.* Minimal residual disease after allogeneic stem cell transplant: A comparison among multiparametric flow cytometry, wilms tumor 1 expression and chimerism status (complete chimerism *versus* low level mixed chimerism) in acute leukemia. *Leuk. Lymphoma* **2013**, *54*, 2660–2666. [CrossRef] [PubMed]

85. Yoon, J.H.; Kim, H.J.; Shin, S.H.; Yahng, S.A.; Lee, S.E.; Cho, B.S.; Eom, K.S.; Kim, Y.J.; Lee, S.; Min, C.K.; *et al.* Serial measurement of *WT1* expression and decrement ratio until hematopoietic cell transplantation as a marker of residual disease in patients with cytogenetically normal acute myelogenous leukemia. *Biol. Blood Marrow Transpl.* **2013**, *19*, 958–966. [CrossRef]

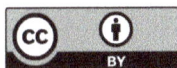

Journal of
Clinical Medicine

MDPI

Review

Intracranial CNS Manifestations of Myeloid Sarcoma in Patients with Acute Myeloid Leukemia: Review of the Literature and Three Case Reports from the Author's Institution

Gustavo M. Cervantes * and Zuzan Cayci *

Department of Neuroradiology, University of Minnesota, Minneapolis, MN 55455, USA;
cerva039@umn.edu (G.M.C.); cayci001@umn.edu (Z.C.); Tel.: +1-612-626-5566; Fax: +1-612-626-5505

Academic Editors: Celalettin Ustun and Lucy A. Godley
Received: 18 December 2014; Accepted: 5 May 2015; Published: 21 May 2015

Abstract: Myeloid sarcoma (MS) of the central nervous system (CNS) is a rare presentation of leukemic mass infiltration outside of the bone marrow. It may involve the subperiosteum and dura mater and, on rare occasions, can also invade the brain parenchyma. The disease is most commonly seen in children or young adults; however, it has been described in multiple age groups. MS can be seen in patients with acute myeloid leukemia (AML), chronic myeloid leukemia and other myeloproliferative disorders. This entity has the potential to be underdiagnosed if the MS appearance precedes the first diagnosis of leukemia. The main reason is that their appearance on CT and MRI has a broad differential diagnosis, and proper diagnosis of MS can only be made if the imaging findings are correlated with the clinical history and laboratory findings. Herein, we describe the intracranial CNS manifestations of MS in patients with AML on CT and MRI involving the brain and/or meninges. This study is based on a systematic review of the literature. In addition, three case reports from the author's institution with AML and intracranial involvement of MS are included. Our aim is to enhance the awareness of this entity among both clinicians and radiologists.

Keywords: AML; acute myeloid leukemia; leukemia; myeloid sarcoma; extramedullary disease; chloroma; intracranial; central nervous system; brain; spine

---

1. Introduction

Central nervous system (CNS) myeloid sarcoma (MS), a rare manifestation of acute myeloid leukemia (AML), chronic myeloid leukemia and other myeloproliferative disorders were first described by Burns in 1811 [1] by the term chloroma. MS can develop when the immature myeloblast groups form solid tumors outside the bone marrow. Intracranially, myeloid sarcomas are often continuous with the meninges or the ependyma. Nevertheless, on rare occasions, myeloid sarcoma may invade the brain parenchyma and, thus, may appear as intra-axial masses.

According to Audouin *et al.*, [2], there are four different patterns of myeloid sarcoma development in AML patients:

(1)   They may develop during the active phase of leukemia;
(2)   They may develop concurrently with known chronic myeloproliferative disorders;
(3)   They may manifest as a relapse after months or years after clinical remission of AML, particularly after bone marrow transplantation;
(4)   They may precede the AML diagnosis and may be detected in previously healthy patients who have a normal peripheral blood cell count and who have no blast infiltration in the bone marrow (0.6% of cases as described by Krause [3]). In this group of patients, most of the patients develop

myeloid leukemia blast infiltration an average of 10.5 months following the diagnosis of a myeloid sarcoma [4]. In a large population-based cohort study from Denmark, the prevalence of myeloid sarcoma among 2261 patients with AML was 9.7%; however, CNS involvement by myeloid sarcoma was only present in 0.4% of these patients [5].

In this review of the literature, we have identified 21 reported cases of myeloid sarcoma in patients with AML and describe the diagnostic and imaging findings pertinent to the brain parenchyma and/or meninges. In addition, three patients from our institution with AML and positive intracranial involvement were included.

2. Literature Review

A PubMed database search using the descriptors chloroma, myeloid sarcoma, myeloid sarcoma and brain, intracranial, central nervous system and cranial nerves retrieved 56 relevant citations from 1971 to 2014. Reviewing the literature, 21 reported cases of myeloid sarcoma with a sufficient description of the diagnosis and imaging findings related to the brain and/or meninges were identified. Leukemic conditions other than AML, such as chronic myeloid leukemia and myeloproliferative disorders, were not included. Only articles in English that were available on the PubMed central publishing platform were considered.

3. Results

CT and MRI were the most commonly utilized imaging modalities for assessment of CNS myeloid sarcoma. Solely MR imaging was used in 11 reported cases, and solely CT was used in four case reports. Combined MR and CT were utilized in six reported cases. Intracranial CNS imaging manifestations of myeloid sarcomas were reviewed in regards to their anatomic site, intra-axial *versus* extra-axial location, single *versus* multiple lesions and CT and/or MR imaging characteristics (Table 1).

A total of 21 reported patients (ten male and ten female) with AML and CNS myeloid sarcoma were included in this review. Gender was not available for one case report [6]. Nineteen patients included were adults, one a three-year-old child and another a 16-year-old adolescent. Patients' ages ranged between three and 58 years old. Mean age at the time of diagnosis of intracranial myeloid sarcoma was 35 years. Out of the 21 reported cases, 13 patients (61%) had preexisting AML, either in remission or in acute bone marrow relapse at the time of the first neurologic symptoms. Eight patients (38%) presented with CNS symptoms preceding their AML diagnosis.

Out of the 21 patients, a total of 24 intracranial myeloid sarcoma lesions were described. Of those, 13 lesions (54%) were described in the intra-axial compartment of the brain and 11 lesions (45%) in the extra-axial brain compartment. One patient had sequential lesions develop in more than one anatomic site in the brain [7]. Another patient had concurrent intra-axial lesions described in the left occipital lobe, right temporal lobe and left cerebellum [8].

Overall, the sites of intracranial myeloid sarcomas included the temporal lobe ($n = 6$), frontal lobe ($n = 4$), cerebellum ($n = 4$), parietal lobe ($n = 3$), occipital lobe ($n = 3$), cerebellopontine angle cistern ($n = 1$), corpus callosum ($n = 1$), basal ganglia ($n = 1$) and subdural space ($n = 1$). Six patients described also showed either concurrent or sequential lesions in locations outside the brain. These extra-cranial locations included the temporal bone ($n = 1$), both kidneys ($n = 1$), multiple bones ($n = 1$), nasopharynx ($n = 1$), cervical and lumbar spine ($n = 1$), thoracic and sacral spine ($n = 1$), scalp tissues ($n = 2$) and infratemporal fossa ($n = 2$). One intracranial vascular lesion involving the superior sagittal sinus was described in one patient ($n = 1$).

Twelve out of a total of 24 lesions were assessed with CT. Among these, 11 lesions (91%) appeared hyperdense on noncontrast CT. Out of all 11 hyperdense lesions, six lesions were intra-axial and five extra-axial. Twenty-two lesions (91%) exhibited avid homogeneous enhancement. One lesion demonstrated inhomogeneous thick peripheral enhancement, indistinguishable from a brain abscess [9]. In another patient, a lesion described in the right temporal lobe demonstrated avid enhancement with a central core of hypoenhancement, suggestive of necrosis [8].

Seven intra-axial MS lesions were assessed with brain MRI. MS demonstrated either a hyper, iso- or hypo-intense signal on T2-weighted images. T2 hyperintensity was described in four lesions, while T2 iso- or hypo-intensity was described in three lesions. Nine extra-axial MS lesions were assessed with MRI. T2 hyperintensity was described in two extra-axial lesions; however, T2 signal findings were not described for the remaining seven extra-axial reported lesions assessed with MRI. Primary bone destruction was evident in one patient, resulting in erosion of the petrous portion of the temporal bone and subsequent intraparenchymal involvement of the right temporal lobe [10].

Vasogenic edema surrounding the enhancing leukemic masses was identifiable on both CT and MRI. This was seen in 11 lesions (45%). Among these, six lesions were in the extra-axial and five in the intra-axial compartment of the brain.

Table 1. Summary of clinical findings, CT and MR features of intracranial myeloid sarcomas (MS) in 21 reported cases presenting with acute myeloid leukemia.

Authors, Year	Age (Years), Gender	AML Diagnosis	Single vs. Multiple	CNS Anatomic Location (s)	Intra- or Extra-Axial	CT and/or MR Characteristics
Yang et al., 2014 [11]	27, male	preceding AML diagnosis	single	occipital lobe (1), spine (2)	extra-axial	meningioma-like, vasogenic edema
Cho et al., 2013 [12]	27, female	AML relapse, 10 months in CR	single	right cerebellopontine angle	extra-axial	meningioma-like, vasogenic edema
Murakami et al., 2011 [10]	52, male	AML relapse, 5 years in CR	multiple	right temporal bone and right temporal lobe	extra-axial	meningioma-like, vasogenic edema
Akhaddar et al., 2011 [6]	27, n/a	preceding AML diagnosis	single	right frontal lobe	intra-axial	intraparenchymal, vasogenic edema
Eom et al., 2011 [7]	49, male	AML relapse, 2 years in CR	multiple	left cerebellum, right frontal lobe and cervical and lumbar spine	intra-axial	intraparenchymal
Cho et al., 2010 [13]	44, male	AML relapse, 2 years in CR	single	corpus callosum	intra-axial	meningioma-like
Grier et al., 2008 [14]	41, female	preceding AML diagnosis	multiple	left temporal lobe, infratemporal extension	extra-axial	meningioma-like
Widhalm et al., 2006 [5]	35, female	preceding AML diagnosis	multiple	right parietal lobe and subgaleal (1), spine (2)	extra-axial	meningioma-like
Smidt et al., 2005 [16]	45, male	AML relapse, 16 years in CR	single	left cerebral hemisphere subdural location	extra-axial	hemispheric subdural mass, C+, mass effect
Best-Aguilera et al., 2005 [17]	37, male	preceding AML diagnosis	multiple	right occipital lobe, mediastinum, retroperitoneum, liver, rectum	extra-axial	meningioma-like, vasogenic edema
Nishimura et al., 2004 [18]	30, female	AML relapse, 16 months in CR	single	right frontal lobe, subgaleal and superior sag. sinus extension	extra-axial	meningioma-like, vasogenic edema
Suzer et al., 2004 [19]	58, female	AML relapse, 6–12 months in CR	single	left cerebellar hemisphere	intra-axial	Intraparenchymal
Park et al., 2003 [20]	3, female	preceding AML diagnosis	multiple	right temporal lobe, infratemporal extension, kidneys, bones	extra-axial	meningioma-like
Nikolic et al., 2003 [21]	45, male	AML relapse, indeterminate CR	single	left frontal lobe	extra-axial	meningioma-like, vasogenic edema
Guermazi et al., 2002 [22]	28, female	AML relapse, 8 months in CR	single	left parietal lobe	intra-axial	intraparenchymal, vasogenic edema
Guermazi et al., 2002 [22]	58, female	preceding AML diagnosis	single	right basal ganglia	intra-axial	intraparenchymal, vasogenic edema
Ooi et al., 2001 [9]	32, male	AML relapse, 18 months in CR	multiple	right temporal lobe, nasopharynx	intra-axial	intraparenchymal, mimicking abscess
Yamamoto et al., 1999 [23]	38, male	AML relapse, 2 years in CR	single	left temporal lobe	intra-axial	intraparenchymal, vasogenic edema
Parker et al., 2005 [24]	29, female	AML relapse, 6 months in CR	single	cerebellar vermis	intra-axial	intraparenchymal
Yoon et al., 1987 [25]	16, female	preceding AML diagnosis	single	left parietal lobe	extra-axial	meningioma-like
Barnett, Zussman 1986 [8] *	34, male	AML relapse, 13 months in CR	multiple	left occipital and left cerebellum	intra-axial (2)	intraparenchymal lesions intraparenchymal,
Barnett, Zussman 1986 [8] *	34, male	AML relapse, 13 months in CR	multiple	right temporal lobe	intra-axial (1)	hypodense lesion, core of necrosis

Asterisks (*) represent a case report from the literature with three concurrent lesions described, which were separated into two paragraphs, because of the peculiar imaging findings of the right temporal lobe lesion; numbers in parentheses represent numerical values of the lesions described; n/a, not available.

4. Authors' Institution Case Reports

CT and MR imaging characteristics of three patients from our institution presenting with acute myeloid leukemia and intracranial CNS manifestations of myeloid sarcoma are described. Case 3 was previously reported in the literature by one of the authors [26].

Case 1: A 69-year-old female patient with a recent history of worsening headaches and flu-like symptoms diagnosed with AML and more than 90% myeloid cells in the blood count during her first admission (Figure 1).

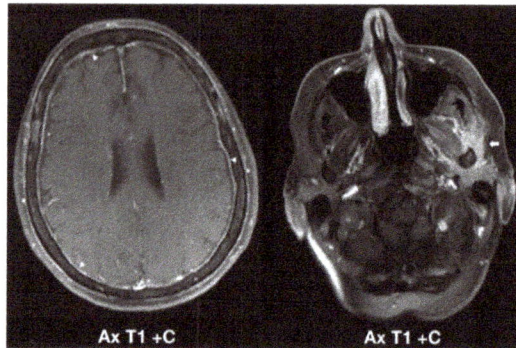

Figure 1. Meningeal infiltration related to AML in a previously healthy 69-year-old woman. Axial post-contrast T1-weighted images with fat saturation (**left image**) demonstrate marked pachymeningeal enhancement (arrowheads), most consistent with leukemic infiltration of the brain meninges. Note the marked ill-defined enhancement of the left infratemporal fossa (**right image**) surrounding the left masticator and deep parotid spaces (arrow), corresponding to extra-cranial leukemic myeloid sarcoma of the soft tissues of the left neck. Complete resolution of the leukemic infiltration within the deep left neck was observed after successful AML induction chemotherapy on follow-up imaging (not shown). Ax, axial; C+, post-contrast.

Case 2: A 56-year-old female patient with acute myelomonocytic leukemia, French-American-British (FAB) classification M4, developed a first relapse of AML with 26% blasts in the blood count during admission. She underwent double umbilical cord blood stem cell transplantation during the remission phase after being successfully treated with induction chemotherapy for her first relapse. On Day 39 of the post-transplant period, she presented with persistent headaches, muscle weakness, falls at home and the onset of leukemia cutis with new skin lesions (Figure 2).

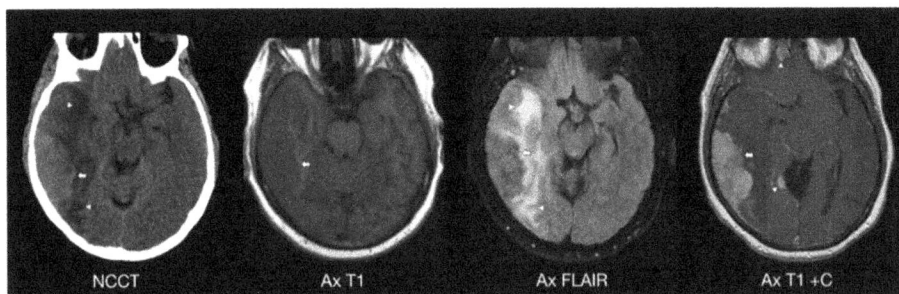

Figure 2. AML relapse in the form of a myeloid sarcoma mass lesion involving the right temporal lobe of a 56-year-old woman 39 days after umbilical cord blood stem cell transplantation. Noncontrast CT images demonstrate a large hyperdense dural-based mass lesion involving the right temporal lobe (NCCT, arrow) with surrounding edema (NCCT, arrowheads), mass effect and midline shift. On MRI, a large ill-defined avidly enhancing dural-based mass lesion involving the posterior aspect of the right temporal lobe (Ax T1 C+, arrow) with surrounding vasogenic edema (Ax FLAIR, arrowheads) was noted. This infiltrating mass revealed hypointense signal intensity on T1 (Ax T1, arrow) and T2-weighted images relative to the adjacent gray-matter. Diffusion weighted images (not shown) demonstrated restricted diffusion in the posterolateral aspect of the right temporal lobe mass consistent with increased cellularity. Additional pachymeningeal foci of nodular enhancement were noted within the gyrus rectus of the right inferior frontal lobe and within the medial aspect of the right inferior temporal lobe (Ax T1 C+, arrowheads). Diffuse right hemispheric pachymeningeal enhancement was also noted (Ax T1 C+, partially shown). Ax, axial; Sag, sagittal; FS, fat saturation; C+, post-contrast; DWI, diffusion-weighted images; ADC, apparent diffusion coefficient.

Case 3: A 53-year-old man with a three-month history of polydipsia and polyuria and indication of myelodysplastic syndrome (MDS) presented with refractory anemia and 16% blast cells in the bone marrow biopsy suggesting a diagnosis of refractory anemia with excess of blasts (RAEB). Diabetes insipidus was confirmed by inappropriately low urine osmolality and low antidiuretic hormone (ADH) levels. AML induction chemotherapy (seven days of cytarabine and three days of idarubicin) along with intrathecal methotrexate after cerebrospinal fluid (CSF) analysis was initiated (Figure 3).

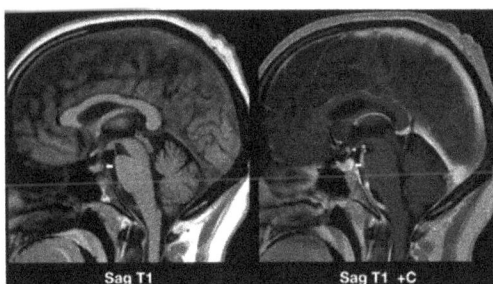

Figure 3. Leukemic infiltration of the neurohypophysis and pituitary stalk in a patient with myelodysplastic syndrome presenting with diabetes insipidus. The sagittal T1-weighted image without contrast administration (**left image**) demonstrates the absence of the neurohypophysis (arrow), confirming the diagnosis of diabetes insipidus. Normally, the neurohypophysis is identified as a bright signal spot on T1-weighted images in the posterior pituitary gland. The sagittal T1-weighted image after contrast administration (**right image**) reveals a 2-mm enhancing nodular lesion in the superior aspect of the pituitary stalk (arrowhead) and curvilinear enhancement along the posterior aspect of the pituitary gland in the expected region of the neurohypophysis (arrow). Sag, sagittal; C+, post-contrast.

21

5. Discussion

CNS leukemic infiltration may present in one or more of the following intracranial forms: (1) meningeal disease, as "carcinomatous meningitis"; (2) intravascular tumor aggregates throughout the brain, as "carcinomatous encephalitis"; or (3) focal tumor masses, as "myeloid sarcomas". When AML manifests as a solid tumor outside the bone marrow, *i.e.*, myeloid sarcoma, the imaging features can be mistaken for some conditions other than the myeloid sarcoma. Myeloid sarcoma seen in leukemic patients may involve any part of the body. The most common sites for myeloid sarcoma deposits are the bones, soft tissues, lymph nodes and the skin. Rarely, they may manifest as single or multiple intracranial lesions [4], most commonly seen within the calvaria and orbits [27]. In our review, out of 24 intracranial MS lesions reviewed from the literature, 13 lesions (48%) have presented as focal tumor masses within the intraparenchymal compartment of the brain.

Myeloid sarcoma can occur at variable ages (1–81 years old), often after the diagnosis of AML. However, in approximately 25% of the patients, MS appears before the initial diagnosis of AML by months or years [28]. According to Neiman *et al.*, of a total of 61 biopsied proven myeloid sarcomas, twenty-two lesions were seen in 15 patients with no known history of acute myeloid leukemia [4]. Most of these patients developed acute leukemia on an average of 10.5 months after the biopsy. In this review, eight out of 21 reported cases (38%) had intracranial CNS imaging manifestations of myeloid sarcoma preceding the diagnosis of AML.

Radiologically, intracranial MS in patients with acute myeloid leukemia most commonly presents as an extra-axial hyperdense mass on noncontrast CT scan. In this review of the literature, all 24 intracranial lesions, except for one, appear as hyperdense masses on the noncontrast CT studies. The differential diagnosis of hyperdense intracranial masses is broad and includes meningioma, B-cell lymphoma and intracranial metastasis. Interestingly, myeloid sarcomas can express B-cell antigens (e.g., CD19, CD79a) and, thus, potentially lead to a histologic misdiagnosis of CNS lymphoma, if no immunohistochemistry or flow cytometry analysis is available [14]. Other less common diagnostic considerations considered are metastatic neuroblastoma (in the pediatric age group), Ewing's sarcoma, hemangiopericytoma and subdural hematoma. A second pattern of presentation is patchy and/or leptomeningeal enhancement seen in patients with acute myeloid leukemia. In this situation, the differential diagnosis to consider is: primary meningeal tumor infiltration by leukemia, secondary leptomeningeal carcinomatosis, viral or bacterial meningitis, neurosarcoidosis, dural sinus thrombosis, intracranial hypotension or postoperative changes.

Vasogenic edema was present on either CT or MR in 11 lesions (45%) out of the 24 intracranial myeloid sarcomas that were included in this review. Further characterization of other CT and/or MR imaging features should be used to distinguish the intracranial MS lesions from other commonly-found intracranial lesions, such as meningioma, lymphoma or brain metastasis, which also commonly show vasogenic edema and can potentially occur concurrently with myeloid sarcoma in patients with acute myeloid leukemia.

Leukemic cell infiltrates are capable of migration from the bone marrow of the periosteum and dura mater into the underlying brain parenchyma once there is disruption of the pial-glial barrier. Despite the close involvement of the extra-cranial and intra-cranial tissues, destructive bony changes are not commonly seen with myeloid sarcomas. Only one patient showed apparent bone destruction of the temporal bone and concomitant involvement of the adjacent right temporal lobe parenchyma [10].

One of the limitations of this study is the small sample of the reported cases available in the literature, since we exclusively included AML patients with intracranial MS lesions. Other forms of acute or chronic leukemias and myeloproliferative disorders could also present with intracranial MS lesions and were not included in this study. Potential selection bias of the study population is another limitation, since the majority of patients included were young adults. Since only one pediatric patient with AML and intracranial CNS myeloid sarcoma was present in our systematic review, our findings cannot be generalized to all age groups.

6. Conclusions

Myeloid sarcoma of the intracranial CNS is a rare presentation of AML. This can be detected before the diagnosis of leukemia or any time throughout the course of the disease during routine neuroimaging studies. Proper CT and MR imaging interpretation in conjunction with relevant clinical information, including the age at the time of diagnosis, symptomatology, such as the presence of headaches, seizures, focal neurological deficits and/or cranial nerve palsy (-ies), a history of hematologic malignancies, prior bone marrow or solid organ transplantation status and immune system status, can help to narrow the clinical diagnosis of intracranial MS. Finally, prompt clinical and laboratory evaluation for acute myeloid leukemia relapse is necessary in patients with a known history of leukemia presenting with meningeal and/or parenchymal lesions.

Author Contributions: The authors contributed equally to the manuscript.

Conflicts of Interest: The authors declare no conflict of interest.

References

1. Burns, A. Observations of surgical anatomy. In *Head and Neck*; Royce: London, UK, 1811; p. 364.
2. Audouin, J.; Comperat, E.; le Tourneau, A.; Camilleri-Broët, S.; Adida, C.; Molina, T.; Diebold, J. Myeloid sarcoma: Clinical and morphologic criteria useful for diagnosis. *Int. J. Surg. Pathol.* 2003, 11, 271–282. [CrossRef] [PubMed]
3. Krause, J.R. Myeloid sarcoma preceding acute leukemia: A report of six cases. *Cancer* 1979, 44, 1017–1021. [CrossRef] [PubMed]
4. Neiman, R.S.; Barcos, M.; Berard, C.; Bonner, H.; Mann, R.; Rydell, R.E.; Bennett, J.M. Myeloid sarcoma: A clinicopathologic study of 61 biopsied cases. *Cancer* 1981, 48, 1426–1437. [CrossRef] [PubMed]
5. Østgaard, L.S.G.; Sengeløv, H.; Holm, M.S.; Johnsen, H.E.; Severinsen, M.T.; Kjeldsen, E.; Bergmann, O.J.; Friis, L.S.; Jensen, M.K.; Nielsen, O.J.; *et al.* Extramedullary Leukemia and Myeloid Sarcoma in AML: New Clues to an Old Issue. Results of a Retrospective Population-Based Registry-Study of 2261 patients. In Annals of 53rd American Society of Hematology Annual Meeting and Exposition, San Diego, CA, USA, 10–13 December 2011.
6. Akhaddar, A.; Zyani, M.; Mikdame, M.; Boucetta, M. Acute myeloid leukemia with brain involvement (chloroma). *Intern. Med.* 2011, 50, 535–536. [CrossRef] [PubMed]
7. Eom, K.S.; Kim, T.Y. Intraparenchymal myeloid sarcoma and subsequent spinal myeloid sarcoma for acute myeloblastic leukemia. *J. Korean Neurosurg. Soc.* 2011, 49, 171–174. [CrossRef] [PubMed]
8. Barnett, M J.; Zussman, W.V. Granulocytic sarcoma of the brain: a case report and review of the literature. *Radiology* 1986, 160, 223–225. [CrossRef] [PubMed]
9. Ooi, G.C.; Chim, C.S.; Khong, P.L.; Au, W.Y.; Lie, A.K.; Tsang, K.W.; Kwong, Y.L. Radiologic manifestations of myeloid sarcoma in adult leukemia. *AJR Am. J. Roentgenol.* 2001, 176, 1427–1431. [CrossRef] [PubMed]
10. Murakami, M.; Uno, T.; Nakaguchi, H.; Yamada, S.M.; Hoya, K.; Yamazaki, K.; Ishida, Y.; Matsuno, A. Isolated recurrence of intracranial and temporal bone myeloid sarcoma—Case report. *Neurol. Med. Chir. Tokyo* 2011, 51, 850–854. [CrossRef] [PubMed]
11. Yang, C.; Liu, Y.; Li, G.; Bai, J.; Qian, J.; Xu, Y. Multifocal myeloid sarcoma in the central nervous system without leukemia. *Clin. Neurol. Neurosurg.* 2014, 120, 99–102. [CrossRef] [PubMed]
12. Cho, S.F.; Liu, T.C.; Chang, C.S. Isolated central nervous system relapse presenting as myeloid sarcoma of acute myeloid leukemia after allogeneic peripheral blood stem cell transplantation. *Ann. Hematol.* 2013, 92, 133–135. [CrossRef] [PubMed]
13. Cho, W.H.; Choi, Y.J.; Choi, B.K.; Cha, S.H. Isolated recurrence of intracranial granulocytic sarcoma mimicking a falx meningioma in acute myeloblastic leukemia. *J. Korean Neurosurg. Soc.* 2010, 47, 385–388. [CrossRef] [PubMed]
14. Grier, D.D.; Al-Quran, S.Z.; Gray, B.; Li, Y.; Braylan, R. Intracranial myeloid sarcoma. *Br. J. Haematol.* 2008, 142, 681. [CrossRef] [PubMed]

15. Widhalm, G.; Dietrich, W.; Müllauer, L.; Streubel, B.; Rabitsch, W.; Kotter, M.R.; Knosp, E.; Roessler, K. Myeloid sarcoma with multiple lesions of the central nervous system in a patient without leukemia. Case report. *J. Neurosurg.* **2006**, *105*, 916–919. [CrossRef] [PubMed]
16. Smidt, M.H.; de Bruin, H.G.; van't Veer, M.B.; van den Bent, M.J. Intracranial granulocytic sarcoma (chloroma) may mimic a subdural hematoma. *J. Neurol.* **2005**, *252*, 498–499. [CrossRef] [PubMed]
17. Best-Aguilera, C.R.; Vazquez-Del Mercado, M.; Muñoz-Valle, J.F.; Herrera-Zarate, L.; Bonilla, G.M.; Navarro-Hernandez, R.E.; Martin-Marquez, B.T.; Oregon-Romero, E.; Ruiz-Quezada, S.; Lomeli-Guerrero, A. Massive myeloid sarcoma affecting the central nervous system, mediastinum, retroperitoneum, liver, and rectum associated with acute myeloblastic leukaemia: A case report. *J. Clin. Pathol.* **2005**, *58*, 325–357. [CrossRef] [PubMed]
18. Nishimura, S.; Kyuma, Y.; Kamijo, A.; Maruta, A. Isolated recurrence of granulocytic sarcoma manifesting as extra- and intracranial masses—Case report. *Neurol. Med. Chir. Tokyo* **2004**, *44*, 311–316. [CrossRef] [PubMed]
19. Suzer, T.; Colakoglu, N.; Cirak, B.; Keskin, A.; Coskun, E.; Tahta, K. Intracerebellar granulocytic sarcoma complicating acute myelogenous leukemia: A case report and review of the literature. *J. Clin. Neurosci.* **2004**, *11*, 914–917. [CrossRef] [PubMed]
20. Park, H.J.; Jeong, D.H.; Song, H.G.; Lee, G.K.; Han, G.S.; Cha, S.H.; Ha, T.S. Myeloid sarcoma of both kidneys, the brain, and multiple bones in a nonleukemic child. *Yonsei Med. J.* **2003**, *44*, 740–743. [CrossRef] [PubMed]
21. Nikolic, B.; Feigenbaum, F.; Abbara, S.; Martuza, R.L.; Schellinger, D. CT changes of an intracranial granulocytic sarcoma on short-term follow-up. *AJR Am. J. Roentgenol.* **2003**, *180*, 78–80. [CrossRef] [PubMed]
22. Guermazi, A.; Feger, C.; Rousselot, P.; Merad, M.; Benchaib, N.; Bourrier, P.; Mariette, X.; Frija, J.; de Kerviler, E. Granulocytic sarcoma (chloroma): Imaging findings in adults and children. *AJR Am. J. Roentgenol.* **2002**, *178*, 319–325. [CrossRef] [PubMed]
23. Yamamoto, K.; Hamaguchi, H.; Nagata, K.; Hara, M.; Tone, O.; Tomita, H.; Ito, U. Isolated recurrence of granulocytic sarcoma of the brain: Successful treatment with surgical resection, intrathecal injection, irradiation and prophylactic systemic chemotherapy. *Jpn. J. Clin. Oncol.* **1999**, *29*, 214–218. [CrossRef] [PubMed]
24. Parker, K.; Hardjasudarma, M.; McClellan, R.L.; Fowler, M.R.; Milner, J.W. MR features of an intracerebellar chloroma. *AJNR Am. J. Neuroradiol.* **1996**, *17*, 1592–1594. [PubMed]
25. Yoon, D.H.; Cho, K.J.; Suh, Y.L.; Kim, C.W.; Chi, J.G.; Han, D.H.; Bang, Y.J.; Kim, B.K.; Kim, N.K.; Cho, H.I. Intracranial granulocytic sarcoma (chloroma) in a nonleukemic patient. *J. Korean. Med. Sci.* **1987**, *2*, 173–178. [CrossRef] [PubMed]
26. Chuang, C.; Parnerkar, V.; Radulescu, A.; Hunt, M.A.; Cayci, Z.; Ustun, C. Diabetes insipidus in myelodysplastic syndrome: What we learnt from a case regarding its diagnosis, pathophysiology and management. *Leuk. Lymphoma* **2014**, *20*, 1–3.
27. Osborn, A.G. Lymphomas, hematopoietic and histiocytic tumors. In *Osborn's Brain: Imaging, Pathology and Anatomy*; AMIRSYS Publishing: Salt Lake City, UT, USA, 2013; pp. 668–671.
28. Avni, B.; Koren-Michowitz, M. Myeloid sarcoma: Current approach and therapeutic options. *Adv. Hematol.* **2011**, *2*, 309–316. [CrossRef]

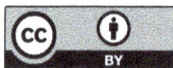

Journal of
Clinical Medicine

MDPI

Review

The Potential of Vitamin D-Regulated Intracellular Signaling Pathways as Targets for Myeloid Leukemia Therapy

Elzbieta Gocek [1] and George P. Studzinski [2,*]

[1] Faculty of Biotechnology, University of Wroclaw, Joliot-Curie 14a, Wroclaw 50-383, Poland;
    elzbieta.gocek@uni.wroc.pl
[2] Department of Pathology, New Jersey Medical School, Rutgers, The State University of New Jersey,
    185 South Orange Ave., Newark, NJ 17101, USA
* Author to whom correspondence should be addressed; studzins@njms.rutgers.edu;
    Tel.: +1-973-972-5869; Fax: +1-973-972-7293.

Academic Editor: Lucy A. Godley
Received: 20 September 2014; Accepted: 6 March 2015; Published: 25 March 2015

Abstract: The current standard regimens for the treatment of acute myeloid leukemia (AML) are curative in less than half of patients; therefore, there is a great need for innovative new approaches to this problem. One approach is to target new treatments to the pathways that are instrumental to cell growth and survival with drugs that are less harmful to normal cells than to neoplastic cells. In this review, we focus on the MAPK family of signaling pathways and those that are known to, or potentially can, interact with MAPKs, such as PI3K/AKT/FOXO and JAK/STAT. We exemplify the recent studies in this field with specific relevance to vitamin D and its derivatives, since they have featured prominently in recent scientific literature as having anti-cancer properties. Since microRNAs also are known to be regulated by activated vitamin D, this is also briefly discussed here, as are the implications of the emerging acquisition of transcriptosome data and potentiation of the biological effects of vitamin D by other compounds. While there are ongoing clinical trials of various compounds that affect signaling pathways, more studies are needed to establish the clinical utility of vitamin D in the treatment of cancer.

Keywords: acute myeloid leukemia; targeted therapy; differentiation; 1,25-dihydroxyvitamin D_3; mitogen-activated kinases

1. Introduction

Cytotoxic therapy can be quite successful in the control of the growth and dissemination of many human malignant diseases, but the established treatment regimens appear to have reached a plateau in their potential for improvement. Therefore, encouraged by the success of Imatinib mesylate, also known as Gleevec, in producing long-lasting remissions of CML by targeting the fusion gene Bcr-Abl with tyrosine kinase activity [1–4] and of ATRA, which targets a fusion TF PML-RARα in acute promyelocytic subtype M3 of AML (APL) [5–10], the search is on for similar targeting of other neoplastic diseases. Derivatives of vitamin D (VDD) have been suggested to have anti-neoplastic properties, but the translation of the results of epidemiological and laboratory studies to the clinic has so far not been successful [11–14]. In this review, we discuss the background for seeking molecular targets related to signaling pathways that current knowledge suggests have the potential for the exploration of their clinical usefulness in subtypes of AML other than CML and APL. While several excellent reviews have been published recently that overlap with this one [15–18], our aim is to update this knowledge, as well as to focus on several selected aspects of the vitamin D and human leukemia field that we feel deserve additional emphasis.

2. Signaling Pathways Studied in Hematopoietic and Myeloid Cells

AML is a predominant acute leukemia among adults and constitutes a very heterogeneous group of blood and bone marrow neoplasms [19–21]. AML is an aggressive disease characterized by over 20% of myeloblasts circulating in the blood or/and bone marrow [20,22–24]. Blast cells are characterized by inhibited differentiation, as well as increased proliferation. Moreover, AML have specific cytogenetic and molecular abnormalities [25]. There are more than two hundred described chromosomal aberrations in leukemic cells of patients with AML [26,27], but also a large group of AMLs without detectable cytogenetic abnormalities [20,28].

Despite significant improvements in chemotherapeutic regimens, poor responsiveness and relapse are still problems in a significant number of patients diagnosed with AML. The clinical outcome with chemotherapy alone is still abysmal for many myeloid leukemia patients, so the development of precision therapy, also called "targeted" therapy, for AML patients based on the molecular features remains an essential aim. Therefore, there is a great need for new therapies with better tolerability and effectiveness than the current treatments. As mentioned above, APL was the first hematological malignancy in which targeted therapy with ATRA has been successfully introduced into clinical practice and induces cell differentiation and death of blast cells [29–31]. Another compound capable of inducing differentiation of AML cells is 1,25-dihydroxyvitamin D_3 (1,25D), which induces monocyte/macrophage-like differentiation and cell cycle arrest [32–36]. The importance of understanding the signaling pathways disturbed in AML cells may improve current treatments and may supplement the conventional therapeutic regimens.

2.1. MAP Kinase Signaling

The MAPKs constitute a family of serine-threonine kinases regulating the proliferation and differentiation of normal and malignant hematopoietic cells [37,38]. MAPKs signal by four main cascades: the ERK1/2, the JNKs, the p38 kinases and ERK5 kinase [37,39] (Figure 1). There are multiple interactions between these pathways, including cooperation and cross-talk between various components, in order to transmit specific signals to the cell [40–43].

MAPKs transduce signals into the cell through a three-tiered cascade, from MAP3Ks (such as Raf1, Cot1, MTK/DLK or ASK1/TAK1/PTK1) through MAP2Ks (such as MEK1/2, MEK5, MKK7/MEK4 or MEK3/6) to MAPKs (ERK1/2, ERK5, JNKs, p38 kinases). Terminally, MAPKs activate several TFs (like c-Fos, c-Jun, PU.1, MEF2, ATF2, c-Myc and Sp1), activating genes responsible for proliferation, differentiation and cell death.

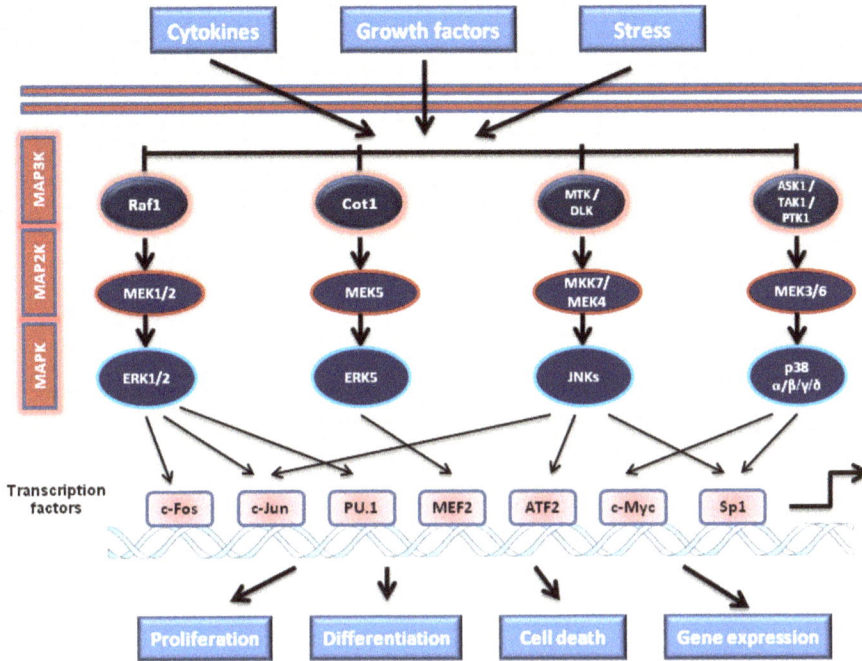

Figure 1. MAPK signaling pathways.

2.1.1. MEK1/2-ERK1/2 Pathway

The ERK1/2 cascade is activated by several reactions initiated by extracellular signals and transmitted by growth factor receptors and cytokine receptors to the small G-coupled protein Ras1 [44], which can sequentially activate Raf1, MEK1/2 and, then, ERK1/2 kinases (Figure 1). When activated by MEK 1/2 phosphorylation, ERK1 and ERK2 are translocated to the nucleus and, in turn, phosphorylate transcription factors crucial for myeloid differentiation, such as C/EBPα, C/EBPβ or PU.1 [45–47]. Kinase suppressor of Ras 1 and 2 (KSR1 and KSR2), considered to be scaffold proteins that bring Ras1, Raf1 and MEK1/2 together, facilitate signaling through pathways mediated by ERK1/2 [48–51]. ERK1/2 have been shown to phosphorylate several different substrates, including ribosomal S6 kinase p90^{RSK} [52]. The Ras1-Raf1-MEK1/2-ERK1/2 pathway is an important positive regulator of monocytic and granulocytic differentiation [38,53,54].

2.1.2. JNKs Pathway

The JNKs family is made up of three members: JNK1, JNK2 and JNK3 [55–57]. These kinases are activated by external stress, apoptotic stimuli and cytokines and are also known as SAPK (stress-activated protein kinases). These signals lead to their phosphorylation by upstream kinases (MEK4, MKK7) [58]. Although JNK1 and JNK2 have somewhat different actions on AML, in general, JNKs phosphorylate TFs, such as c-Jun, ATF-2, p53 and Elk-1, which, in turn, regulate the expression of specific genes to mediate cell proliferation, differentiation or apoptosis [59,60] (Figure 1). C-Jun is essential for monocytic differentiation of human AML cells, as a part of the AP1 TF [53,61].

2.1.3. p38 Kinases Pathway

The p38 MAPKs are activated in cells by environmental stresses and pro-inflammatory cytokines, less often by growth factors. There are four members of the p38 MAPKs family, α, β, γ and δ, which display tissue-specific patterns of expression [62]. p38α and β, the "classical" isoforms, are ubiquitously expressed among tissues, whereas the expression of p38γ and δ appears to be more tissue restricted and, in 1,25D-treated AML cells, have positive effects of differentiation, unlike the classical isoforms [41,63–66]. The p38 kinases share about 40% sequence identity with other MAPKs, but they share only about 60% identity among themselves, which suggests highly diverse functions [67–69]. The p38 MAPKs are activated by phosphorylation by upstream kinases MKK3 and MKK6, although MKK4, the main activator of JNKs, has also been shown to activate p38 MAPKs [70]. Upon activation, p38 proteins translocate from the cytosol to the nucleus, where they orchestrate cellular responses by mediating phosphorylation of downstream targets that regulate apoptosis, cell cycle arrest, cell growth inhibition and differentiation [41,71,72] (Figure 1). Besides transcription factors, p38 kinases downstream targets are other kinases, such as MAPKAPK3 or MAPKAPK5 [65,73].

2.1.4. MEK5-ERK5-MEF2C Pathway

Like the other branches of the MAPK family, the MEK5/ERK5 pathway has been implicated in cell survival, anti-apoptotic signaling, angiogenesis, cell motility, proliferation and cell differentiation [74]. However, ERK5 signaling can have both overlapping and distinct effects from the other MAPKs [75].

The principal activator of ERK5 is MEK5, which can be activated by MAP2Ks, such as MEKK2 and MEKK3 [76,77]. It has been shown that MEKK3 induces activation of the MEK5/ERK5 pathways through growth factor-induced cellular stimulation and oxidative stress [76,78] (Figure 1). ERK5 is activated by two phosphorylations: first, on the N-terminal TEY sequence, usually by MEK5 [79], and then by autophosphorylation on the ERK5 C-terminal transcriptional activation domain [80,81], which allows it to be translocated into the nucleus and to activate several TFs, including MEF2, Sap1, c-Fos and c-Myc [79,82–84]. The auto-phosphorylation of the ERK5 C-terminus may also be required for transcriptional activation [85]. The Cot1 oncogene can activate ERK5 [86,87] and can repress KSR1/2 [42,87].

2.2. PI3 Kinase-Akt1-mTOR Signaling

PI3Ks control the growth, motility, survival and differentiation of many normal and cancer cells [88–90]. The PI3Ks family is composed of heterodimeric proteins grouped into three main classes: I (IA and IB), II and III. Class IA enzymes are composed of three distinct catalytic subunits (p110α, p110β or p110δ), which associate with one of the regulatory subunits (p85α, p85β, p55α, p55γ or p50α) [91,92]. Class IB enzymes encompass one catalytic subunits (p110 γ) and two regulatory subunits (p101 or p87) [93]. Notably, p110α and p110β are ubiquitously expressed in most types of cells, whilst p110δ and p110γ are exclusively expressed in hematopoietic cells [92,94,95]. RTKs, non-RTKs, GPCRs and Ras1 are direct activators of class IA PI3Ks, whereas class IB enzymes are activated only by GPCRs and Ras1 [96,97]. Upon activation, the regulatory subunit mediates binding to the receptor, whereas the catalytic subunit phosphorylates PIP_2 to yield PIP_3. PIP_3 initiates downstream signaling, such as the PDK1, Akt1, mTOR or FOXO family of TFs [98–101] (Figure 2). Direct constitutive activation of PI3K/Akt1/mTOR signaling occurs in the majority of leukemias, such as AML and ALL, Hodgkin's lymphoma, lymphoproliferative disorders or myeloproliferative neoplasms [102–104].

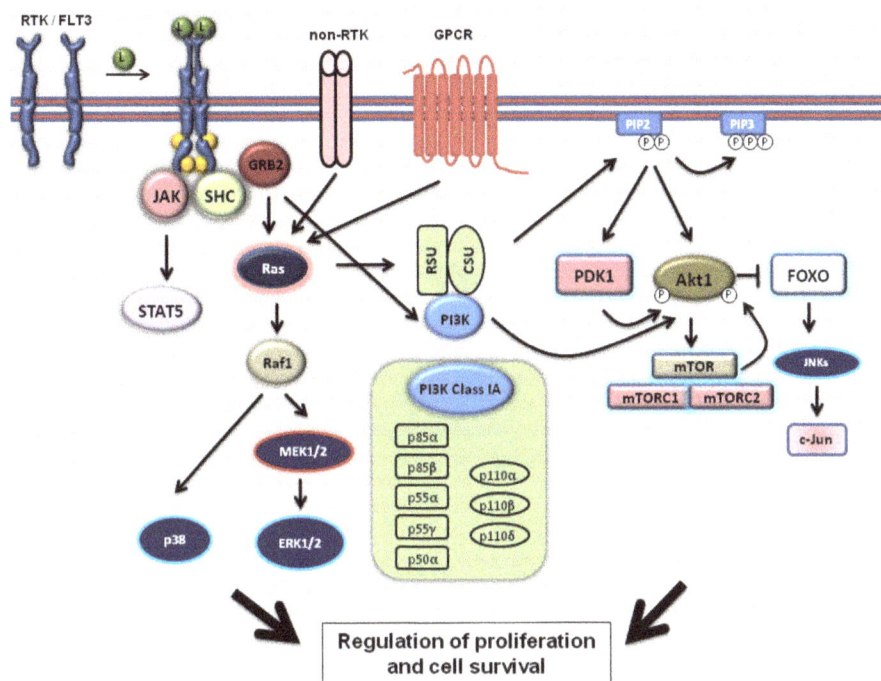

Figure 2. FLT3/PI3 kinase/Akt1/mTOR signaling pathways.

After ligand (L) binding, FLT3 is phosphorylated (yellow circles), at TKD, and activates downstream pathways, such as PI3K/Akt1, MAPKs (MEK1/2, ERK 1/2) and STAT5. Two major classes of activating FLT3 mutations have been identified in AML patients: ITD and TKD point mutations. Mutations cause constitutive activation of FLT3 and aberrant activation of downstream signaling pathways and factor-independent growth. PI3K is activated downstream of RTKs, non-RTKs or GPCRs. Ras1 is a direct activator of class IA of PI3Ks, upon activation regulatory subunit (RSU) mediating the binding to the receptor, whereas the catalytic subunit (CSU) phosphorylates PIP_2 to PIP_3. PIP_3 initiates downstream signaling, PDK1, Akt1, mTOR or FOXO.

2.3. FLT3 Signaling

FLT3 is encoded by a gene located on chromosome 13 and plays an important role in early hematopoiesis and development of myeloid precursors [105,106]. This transmembrane kinase belongs to the class III receptor tyrosine kinase family and is the most commonly mutated in AML [107–109]. The oncogenic mutations in FLT3 (ITD, internal tandem duplication in the juxtamembrane region or point mutation in the catalytic domain) cause ligand-independent dimerization of the FLT3 and its constitutive activation. Thus, the mutated FLT3 receptor activates downstream signaling pathways, such as PI3K, ERK1/2 and p38, LYN and STAT5 kinases, leading to the cytokine-independent proliferation (Figure 2) [109–112].

2.4. C/EBPα Signaling

The C/EBPα belongs to the family of basic leucine zipper TFs, which participate in the differentiation of several cell types, including myeloid progenitor cells from multipotent precursors [113–115]. There are two distinct isoforms of C/EBPα protein, full-length p42 and truncated p30, which lacks two N-terminal trans-activation domains [116]. Only the p42 isoform of C/EBPα can inhibit cell proliferation, while the p30 isoform can support the formation of granulocyte-macrophage progenitors in mice and can lead to the development of AML in the absence of p42 [117]. The relative levels of p42 and p30 in the cell can be regulated through mTOR signaling to control the transition of cell fate [118]. A genetic knockout of C/EBPα results in a complete block in the transition from common myeloid progenitors to the granulocyte/monocyte progenitor stage of differentiation [119]. Mutations in CEBPα occur in approximately 5% to 10% of *de novo* AML and is most common in cytogenetically normal AMLs [114,120].

2.5. Targeting by MicroRNAs

MicroRNAs are small, noncoding and highly conserved RNA molecules that regulate the expression of genes post-transcriptionally by binding to the 3'-UTR regions of the mRNA [121–123]. Several microRNAs are widely expressed in hematopoietic cells (*i.e.*, 106a, 128a, 146, 150, 155, 181a, 221, 222, 223), and their altered expression (e.g., by chromosomal translocations) has been correlated with leukemia [124]. Several studies have shown that specific patterns of microRNA expression are closely associated with cytogenetic and risk/survival predictions in AML patients [125–128]. Importantly, integration of microRNA and mRNA patterns of regulation can reveal the extent of co-regulation, which permits exquisite control of gene expression at the mRNA level [129,130].

2.6. Global Effects of VDDs on AML Cells

Most studies of signaling by VDDs were based on the examination of the expression of a single or a small number of genes. However, powerful new technology is evolving, which, combined with bioinformatics, is poised to transform this field. Therefore, the question can soon be answered of how the perturbations of cellular homeostasis by 1,25D or other VDDs influence the global gene expression. Interesting examples of this approach have recently been published by the Carsten group, which include a genome-wide analysis of VDR binding sites in THP-1 human monocytic leukemia cells. They identified by ChIP-seq 2340 VDR binding locations, of which 1171 occurred uniquely following short exposure to 1,25D and 520 without exposure to 1,25D [131]. Interestingly, it was found that 1,25D binding shifts the locations of VDR occupation to DR3-type response elements that surround its target genes, and there was a large variety of regulatory constellations of VDR binding sites. It is also becoming increasingly clear that VDR binding choices are highly specific for the cell type [130–132]. The biological significance may be derived from microarray analyses following 1,25D treatment, such as that which found that the monocytic marker CD14 and cathelicidin anti-microbial peptide were by far the most markedly upregulated genes in this scenario [131]. Among the genes upregulated early, as shown by the microarray analysis, the monocyte-specific genes and metabolism-related genes are two noticeable groups [132]. The effects of longer exposure to 1,25D include the finding that VDR binding sites are significantly enriched near autoimmune and cancer-associated genes identified from GWA studies [133]. Thus, GWA surveys can lead to deeper understanding of signaling by VDDs.

3. 1,25D as an Important Modifier of Signaling Pathways Disturbed in AML

1,25D is the physiological form of vitamin D that belongs to the family of secosteroid hormones [134,135]. Although the primary function of 1,25D is to maintain calcium and phosphorus metabolism [136], 1,25D is capable of inducing differentiation and inhibiting the proliferation of several types of normal and cancer cells, AML cells among them [137–139]. Exposure of AML cells to 1,25D results in a monocyte-like phenotype, which, upon prolonged exposure to 1,25D, becomes a macrophage-like phenotype, manifested by functional changes (phagocytosis accompanied by monocyte-specific esterase activity and the generation of reactive oxygen species). The phenotypic changes include altered morphology [140,141] and the expression of a receptor for complexes of lipopolysaccharides, CD14, and the adherence protein encoding the subunit of $\alpha_M\beta_2$-integrin, CD11b [142–145].

There are several phases of 1,25D-induced differentiation of AML cells. In the initial phase, the cells continue normal proliferation and cell cycle progression. During this phase, high levels of MEK1/2, ERK1/2, JNKs and p38 kinases are essential [53,146,147]. Latter phases lead to the cell cycle block at the G1/S phase due to the elevated expression of CDK inhibitors, such as p21$^{Cip1/Waf1}$ and p27^{Kip1} [148–150], and anti-apoptotic proteins, including Bcl-XL and Mcl1, which facilitate differentiation by increasing cell survival [151,152].

3.1. Activation of MAPKs by 1,25D

3.1.1. Ras1-Raf1-MEK1/2-ERK1/2

The ERK1/2 signaling pathway maintains cell proliferation during the early stages of 1,25D-induced differentiation of AML cells (24–48 h). ERK1/2 are expressed at a high level and are activated by phosphorylation [53,146]. PD98059, the specific inhibitor of MEK1/2 [153], partially inhibits 1,25D-induced monocytic differentiation of HL60 cells. At the later phase, a high level of phosphorylated ERK1/2 decreases to the basal level, and then, ribosomal S6 kinase p90^{RSK} is activated [53,146,147]. This kinase, in turn, can activate C/EBPβ, the master TF for monocyte/macrophage differentiation [154,155]. C/EBPβ, which can be activated by phosphorylation by ERK1/2 [156], by p90^{RSK} [157] or by ERK5 [141] and can directly interact with the promoter region of CD14, activates its expression [45,156,158].

Raf1 signaling is a requisite for the latter stages of 1,25D-induced differentiation of HL60 cells. Raf1 mediates activation of p90^{RSK}, but independently of the MEK1/2-ERK1/2 module [45]. Moreover, a platform for Raf1 phosphorylation, KSR1 and KSR2 [159] are also upregulated by 1,25D, augmenting the strength of the signal transmitted through Raf1 to downstream targets [49,160,161] (Figure 3). KSR2 knockdown decreases cell survival, which is accompanied by reduced Bcl-2/Bax and Bcl-2/Bad ratios and increased caspase-3 activating cleavage [162].

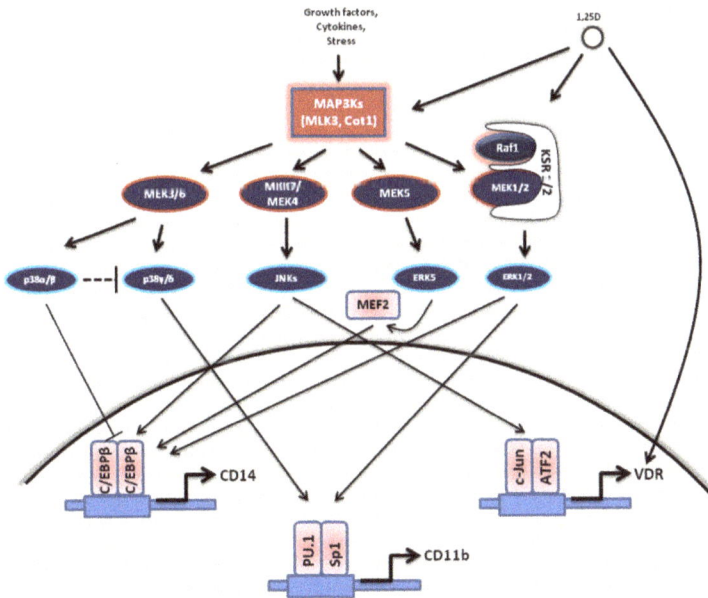

Figure 3. 1,25D's influence on MAPK signaling.

1,25D activates several MAPKs, such as MLK3, Cot1 and MEK1/2. The ERK1/2, ERK5 and JNK (JNK1/2) pathways have positive effects on monocytic differentiation, while the p38 MAPKs pathway may have a dual effect on differentiation. p38α and p38β have an inhibitory effect on monocytic, but not granulocytic differentiation of HL60 cells, while p38γ and δ may positively modulate monocytic differentiation of these cells. 1,25D can amplify the Raf1-MEK1/2-ERK1/2 pathway by direct transcriptional upregulation of KSR1 and KSR2, which act as scaffolds that coordinate signaling along the Ras1/ERK1/2 signaling. Also shown is the potential role of the C/EBPβ, c-Jun/ATF2 and PU.1/Sp1 TFs, which act as positive effectors of 1,25D signals by upregulating the expression of VDR, CD14 and CD11b.

3.1.2. JNKs

During 1,25D-induced differentiation of AML cells, the expression level of JNK1 is highly elevated [147]. JNK1 activates c-Jun and ATF2, two major components of the AP-1 TF complex, as well as C/EBPβ and Jun B [61]. Moreover, the expression level of c-Jun is also elevated in those cells [163], which enhances the differentiation process [164]. Inhibition of JNK1/2 by the specific inhibitor, SP600125 [165], leads to the reduction of c-Jun and ATF2 phosphorylation, as well as to the decreased expression of Egr-1 and c-Fos, which results in the differentiation block [147,166,167]. Importantly, in AML cells resistant to 1,25D, JNK2 antagonizes JNK1 and is considered, at least in part, a negative regulator of the cell proliferation and resistance of those cells [168,169] (Figure 3).

3.1.3. MAPK/p38 Kinases

The p38 kinases are also essential for 1,25D-induced differentiation of AML cells. It was shown that some functions generally attributed to p38 kinases, such as inhibition of 1,25D-induced differentiation [66], are only performed by the classical forms (p38α and p38β), as these, unlike p38γ and δ, are inhibited by SB203580, SB202190 and related compounds [66,170–173]. Because they exert a negative feedback upstream of p38α and p38, the isoforms p38γ and p38δ actually have a positive effect on 1,25D-induced differentiation of human AML cells [66] (Figure 3). Moreover, the inhibition of p38α and p38β leads to an upregulated expression of isoforms p38γ and p38δ in 1,25D-treated AML cell lines and in primary cultures [66].

3.1.4. MEK5-ERK5-MEF2C

1,25D and its analogs upregulate the expression of ERK5, which positively regulates the early-stage monocytic differentiation of AML cells [75,87,141]. The pharmacological inhibitor of MEK5 (an upstream activator of ERK5), BIX02189 [174] and the inhibitor of ERK5 autophosphorylation, XMD8-92 [175], lead to the reduction of cell surface CD14 and an increase in CD11b expression [141]. ERK5 is a positive regulator of C/EBPβ TF, the direct activator of CD14, but negatively regulates the expression of C/EBPα [141]. MEF2C, a known downstream target of ERK5 [82,141], has recently been shown to be involved in 1,25D-induced AML differentiation and is reported to lie upstream of C/EBPβ and to control the expression of CD14, but not CD11b [176]. Importantly, the enzyme activity of Cot1, an upstream regulator of MEK5-ERK5-MEF2C, increases in AML cells during 1,25D-induced differentiation, as does phosphorylation of MEF2C, a downstream target of ERK5 [42,176] (Figure 3). It is also relevant that FLT3 kinase may activate MEK5 by its phosphorylation, which results in the activation of ERK5 of AML cells that have an internal tandem duplication in FLT3 [177]. As CD11b expression generally suggests terminal differentiation, the dissociation of CD14 and CD11b expression by the MEK5-ERK5-MEF2C signaling cascade implies that the monocytic characteristics of AML cells in the early phase of 1,25D-induced differentiation may just be an associated phenomenon, but is not a necessary component of any potential anti-cancer effect of 1,25D.

3.2. The Effect of 1,25D on the PI3 Kinase-Akt1-mTOR Pathway

Activation of the PI3K/Akt1/mTOR pathway is important for 1,25D-mediated protection against apoptosis, as well as for the induction of the differentiation of AML cells [150,178–181]. Inhibition of PI3K by LY294002 or by Wortmannin accentuates the 1,25D-induced G1 to S phase cell cycle block in HL60 cells and is associated with an increased expression of p27^{Kip1} protein [150]. Moreover, LY294002 inhibits nuclear translocation of VDR and prevents activation of 1,25D target genes triggering monocytic differentiation [173].

3.3. The Influence of 1,25D on AML Cells with Mutated FLT3 Kinase

Only a few reports focus on the susceptibility of AML cells to the combined effects of 1,25D-induced differentiation and FLT3 kinase activating mutations. Studies performed on blast cells isolated from the peripheral blood of patients with diagnosed FLT3 mutations revealed that those cells exhibit resistance to 1,25D and to its "semi-selective" analogs [145,182]. This notwithstanding, AML cell lines with mutated FLT3 kinase, such as MV4-11 or MOLM-13, do respond to 1,25D-induced differentiation [145,183]. Treatment of elderly relapsed AML patients with cytotoxic agents, 1,25D and the FLT3 kinase inhibitor, CEP-701, gave highly variable results [13].

3.4. Effects of 1,25D on C/EBPα

It is well documented that C/EBPα is indispensable for granulocytes to develop, while C/EBPβ regulates the differentiation of monocytic cells [115,184,185]. In HL60 cells exposed to 1,25D, C/EBPα isoforms are transiently upregulated in the early stages (up to 24 h) of the differentiation process, while C/EBPβ isoforms are upregulated in a sustained fashion and parallel to the expression of CD14 and CD11b surface markers [45]. A generally accepted scheme assumes that 1,25D-induced expression of C/EBPβ allows the cells to bypass the granulocytic differentiation block caused by dysregulation of C/EBPα and switches the cells into monocytes [45,156,186].

3.5. The Effect of 1,25D on MicroRNAs

Relatively little is known regarding the influence of 1,25D on microRNA expression in AML cells, but it is postulated that similarly to the other types of cancer, the microRNA expression profile ("signature") may be helpful for AML diagnosis and for the selection of suitable therapy. It was shown that during 1,25D-induced differentiation of AML cells, microRNA-181a and microRNA-181b are downregulated [187]. MicroRNA-181a inhibition by 1,25D results in an increase of p27^{Kip1} mRNA and protein level, which, in turn, leads to G1/S blockade [187–189]. Furthermore, microRNA-302c and microRNA-520c are downregulated by 1,25D in Kasumi-1 and K562 AML cell lines, where they enhance the susceptibility of those cells to natural killer cell-mediated cytotoxicity [190]. Other microRNAs downregulated by 1,25D in AML cells are microRNA-17-5p/20a/106a, microRNA-125b and microRNA-155, which target AML1, VDR and C/EBPβ [191].

1,25D can upregulate microRNA-32, which targets pro-apoptotic protein Bim [192]. Decreased expression of microRNA-32 can sensitize AML cells to the cytotoxic agents, for instance arabinocytosine [192]. Another microRNA upregulated by 1,25D in AML cells is microRNA-26a [193], which targets transcriptional repressor E2F7 [194]. The repression of E2F7 by miR-26a contributes to the increased expression of p21$^{Cip1/Waf1}$ observed during 1,25D-induced monocytic differentiation of AML cells. Moreover, silencing of E2F7 results in inhibition of c-Myc activity and downregulation of its transcriptional target, the oncogenic miR-17-92 cluster [194] (Figure 4).

1,25D down-regulates (⊣) the expression of microRNA-181a, which is a negative regulator of p27^{Kip1}. This causes the block of the negative action of microRNA-181a (

) and elevated expression of p27^{Kip1} (↑). 1,25D also downregulates other microRNAs, such as microRNA-106a, -20a and -155, that target and inhibit the expression of VDR and C/EBPβ. 1,25D can up-regulate (→) microRNA-32, which targets pro-apoptotic protein Bim and inhibits its expression (↓). Furthermore, microRNA-26a is upregulated by 1,25D. MicroRNA-26a inhibits transcriptional repressor E2F7, which, in turn, no longer inhibits p21$^{Cip1/Waf1}$, and its expression is elevated. Regulation of microRNA expression by 1,25D leads to the augmented differentiation, inhibition of apoptosis and cell cycle arrest in the G1/S phase.

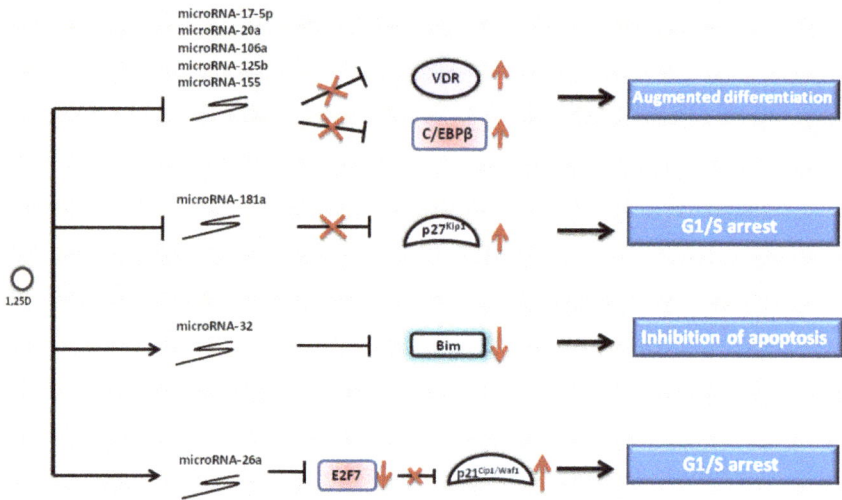

Figure 4. Regulation of microRNA expression by 1,25D in AML cells.

4. Potentiators of 1,25D-Induced Differentiation of AML Cells

1,25D-induced differentiation of AML cells may be augmented by several natural and chemical compounds (Table 1). One such compound is carnosic acid (CA), the plant-derived polyphenolic antioxidant. CA alone is weakly cytostatic to AML cells, but in combination with 1,25D, increases differentiation and upregulates the expression of ERK5, c-Jun and AP1 [87,166,169,195–197]. Moreover, CA together with a 1,25D analog, doxercalciferol, decreases the expression level of microRNA-181a [189]. Similarly to CA, other plant antioxidants, curcumin and silibinin, can inhibit AML cell growth when used alone, but show synergistic or additive effects on differentiation when combined with VDDs [195,198–200].

It was also shown that an inhibitor of the Akt1/mTOR pathway, RAD001 (Everolimus), potentiates 1,25D-induced growth arrest and differentiation of AML cells, due to the enhancement of 1,25D-mediated transcriptional activation of p21$^{Cip1/Waf1}$ in association with increased level of the acetylated forms of histone H3 and VDR bound to the p21$^{Cip1/Waf1}$ promoter [201].

A large number of compounds can potentiate 1,25D-induced differentiation of AML cells [198,202]. Natural compounds include plant polyphenols, carnosic acid, curcumin or silibinin [195,198,203]. Other compounds, such as iron chelators [204] or chemical inhibitors [205], are also capable of enhancing 1,25D action.

Table 1. Examples of potentiators of 1,25D-induced differentiation of AML cells.

Compound	Characteristic	Mode of Action with 1,25D	Citations
Nutlin 3a	*cis*-imidazoline analog, inhibits interaction between Mdm2 and p53	• downregulation of Bcl-2, MDMX, KSR2, phospho-ERK2 • upregulation of PIG-6	[152]
Carnosic acid	natural benzenediol abietane diterpene from rosemary	• upregulation of ERK5, c-Jun and AP1 • downregulation of microRNA-181a expression	[189,196,197]
Curcumin	diarylheptanoid, natural phenol from turmeric	• activation of caspase-3, -8 and -9	[195]
Silibinin	flavonolignan from the milk thistle seeds	• upregulation of c-Jun and C/EBP•	[199,200]
Everolimus	40-O-(2-hydroxyethyl) derivative of sirolimus	• inhibition of Akt/mTOR	[201]
Deferasirox	iron chelator	• induction of VDR expression and phosphorylation	[204,207]
Q-VD-OPh	pan-caspase inhibitor	• upregulation of HPK1 and c-Jun	[205]
Indomethacin	non-steroid inhibitor of cyclooxygenase	• inhibition of phospho-Raf1	[206]

Other compounds that can enhance 1,25D-induced differentiation of AML cells are COX1 and COX2 inhibitors [206]. It was found that a combination treatment with 1,25D and non-specific COX inhibitors acetyl salicylic acid (ASA) or indomethacin can robustly potentiate the differentiation of several AML cell lines and that ASA ± 1,25D is effective in enhanced differentiation of primary AML cultures. Increased cell differentiation is paralleled by arrest of the cells in the G1 phase of the cell cycle and by increased phosphorylation of Raf1 and p90^{RSK1} proteins [206].

Iron chelating agents, such as deferasirox, also turned out to be an effective enhancer of 1,25D-induced differentiation of AML cells [204]. This compound induces expression and phosphorylation of the VDR. The combination of iron-chelating agents and 1,25D resulted in the reversal of pancytopenia and in blast differentiation, suggesting that iron availability modulates myeloid cell commitment and that targeting this cellular differentiation pathway together with the conventional differentiating agents can provide a therapeutic benefit for an AML patient [204]. This conclusion is reinforced by the subsequent retrospective study, which showed that the combination of deferasirox and vitamin D improves overall survival in elderly patients with AML after demethylating agent failure [207]. In accordance with these feasibility studies, a phase 1 and 2 clinical trial (NCT01718366) of combined deferasirox, vitamin D, and azacitidine in high risk MDS is in progress.

5. Clinical Trials with VDDs Targeting Signaling Pathways in AML

Poor responsiveness to standard chemotherapy is still a problem for a significant number of patients with neoplastic diseases. While the current focus in the field is on individualized therapy based on molecular features of the disease, the great heterogeneity of mutations in AML makes this a remote aim. Thus, the possibility that a differentiation-based approach can be used for a large subset of AML patients has been attractive. However, the attempts to utilize the differentiation properties of VDDs have had so far minimal success, possibly due, at least in part, to the variable levels of vitamin D receptors in the malignant cells [18].

A recent review by Kim *et al.* [15] includes a list of clinical trials mainly conducted in the early 1990s, which seem to have mostly "fizzled out", that have not led to any major advances in the treatment of AML. Harrison and Bershadskiy [16] describe these clinical trials in depth and list two more trials in patients with MDS, often a pre-leukemic disease, but neither trial led to dramatic or promising results. More recently, several other trials of VDDs have been conducted in MDS patients; however, the results of those have not yet appeared in the literature, and the only phase 3 trial that could be found at this time (NCT00804050) has been terminated, reportedly due to "difficulties in enrollment". Thus, there remains substantial uncertainty as to whether VDDs, with or without potentiators that were used in the majority of experiments reported to date, will have a significant therapeutic effect in AML. It would appear that at least part of the problem is that the potentiators/enhancers so far used with VDDs had no clearly defined mechanism of potentiation of their combined actions. These have included new cytotoxic agents and their combinations with cell cycle, histone deacetylase inhibitors, monoclonal antibodies, FLT3 kinase inhibitors and hypomethylating agents currently used as enhancers of cytotoxic therapy (Table 2). Such agents do have a clearly defined basis of action as single agents, but the rationales of the potentiation of the differentiation agents are not clear. Most relevant to this topic are phase I/II trials of MEK inhibitors AS703026 3 (pimasertib) and GSK1120212 (trametinib). These trials investigate the safety, pharmacokinetics, pharmacodynamics and clinical activity of these compounds in AML patients with all subtypes, except FAB M3 [208–210]. Further problems in drawing conclusions regarding the efficacy of VDDs in AML based on the clinical trials reported to date are the great heterogeneity of the patient populations studied and the variability in the dose and schedule of the VDDs used to date.

It is proposed that a better understanding of the signaling pathways underlying VDD actions may stimulate the generation of new concepts for clinical trials of VDDs with potentiators. Perhaps a simultaneous, or sequential, targeting of pathways described here by VDDs and enhancers or inhibitors of these pathways will provide conceptually new regimens for clinical trials of VDDs. The importance of optimal sequencing in differentiation therapy is suggested by a recent report that survival of patients with AML/MDS was improved by agents, which included VDDs, administered during the maintenance of remission induced by chemotherapy [211]. Furthermore, in addition to pathway inhibitors, pathway activators should also be considered for the enhancement of VDD therapeutic activity.

Table 2. New agents in AML clinical trials. The recent clinical trials of AML have focused on new cytotoxic drugs, cell cycle and histone deacetylase inhibitors, monoclonal antibodies, FLT3 and MEK kinase inhibitors or hypomethylating agents. These were conducted without VDDs.

Target	Compounds	Phase	Status of the study	Examples of studies
Cell cycle inhibition	rigosertib	I/II	ongoing, recruitment closed	NCT01167166
	volasertib	I	ongoing, recruitment opened	NCT02003573
	clofarabine	I	ongoing, recruitment opened	NCT01289457
Cytotoxicty	sapacitabine	III	ongoing, recruitment opened	NCT01303796
	vosaroxin	I/II	ongoing, recruitment opened	NCT01893320
	azacitidine	II	ongoing, no recruitment	NCT01358734
DNA hypomethylation	decitabine	II	ongoing, recruitment opened	NCT02188706
	SGI-110	II	ongoing, recruitment opened	NCT02096055
	crenolanib	II	ongoing, recur	NCT01657682
FLT3 small-molecule inhibitors	midostaurin	I/II	itment opened	NCT01093573
	sorafenib	II	ongoing, recruitment opened not yet open for recruitment	NCT02196857
	panobinostat	I/II	ongoing, recruitment opened	NCT01451268
Histone deacetylase inhibitors	pracinostat	II	ongoing, recruitment opened	NCT01912274
	vorinostat	I	ongoing, no recruiment	NCT00875745
Monoclonal antibodies	gemtuzumab ozogamicin	III	ongoing, recruitment opened	NCT00893399
	SGN33a	I	ongoing, recruitment opened	NCT01902329
MEK inhibitors	MEK162	I/II	ongoing, recruitment opened	NCT02089230
	trametinib (GSK1120212)	II	ongoing, recruitment opened	NCT01907815

6. Conclusions and Perspectives

It is clear that despite the strong epidemiological evidence that optimal levels of vitamin D reduce overall mortality by at least 7% [212,213], while low vitamin D levels are associated with adverse outcomes in AML [214], translation of this knowledge to cancer prevention or treatment has been disappointingly slow. The early focus on the generation and testing of countless vitamin D analogs for cancer treatment has not led to encouraging results, and combinations of 1,25D or analogs with cytotoxic agents have not led to conclusive results in neoplastic diseases, including AML [215–217]. It appears more likely that the therapeutic regimens for AML will require the addition of small molecule inhibitors, or enhancers of signaling pathways, or entirely new strategies. The latter can capitalize on the known changes in gene expression elicited by 1,25D, summarized here. Although current excitement in the field of cancer therapy is largely directed to targeting specific mutations, found successful for CML and APL, the vast majority of leukemia cases have a highly heterogeneous set of mutations, making targeting not likely in the foreseeable future. Thus, randomized trials with patients with AML other than APL need to be organized, with time to relapse as the main end point, for confirming the findings that MAPKs, and other signaling cascades, present important auxiliary targets that can enhance the effectiveness of the cytotoxic therapy or immunotherapy of cancer.

Acknowledgments: We thank Jonathan Harrison and Ruifang Zheng for valuable comments on the manuscript. The experimental work of the authors was supported by NIH Grant No. R0-1 CA 22744-24 to George P. Studzinski and by the Polish National Science Centre (Grant No. 0351/B/P01/2011/40), as well as the University of Wroclaw Scholarship (Human Capital Program, No. BPZ.506.50.2012.MS) to Elzbieta Gocek.

Author Contributions: The authors equally contributed to the preparation of the manuscript.

Abbreviations

1,25D	1,25-dihydroxyvitamin D_3
Akt1	protein kinase B
ALL	acute lymphoblastic leukemia
AML	acute myeloid leukemia
AP1	activator protein 1
APL	acute promyelocytic leukemia
ATF2	activating transcription factor 2
ATRA	all-trans retinoic acid
CA	carnosic acid
C/EBPs	CCAAT enhancer binding proteins
CML	chronic myelogenous leukemia
Cot1	cancer Osaka thyroid 1
COX	cyclooxygenase
ERK	extracellular signal-regulated protein kinase
FLT3	FMS-like tyrosine kinase 3
GPCRs	G-protein-coupled receptors
GWA	genome-wide association
JNKs	c-Jun N-terminal kinases
KSR	kinase suppressor of Ras
MAPK	mitogen-activated kinase
MAP2K	mitogen-activated kinase kinase
MAP3K	mitogen-activated kinase kinase kinase
MDS	myelodysplastic syndrome
MEF2	myogenic enhancer factor 2
mTOR	mammalian target of rapamycin
non-RTKs	non-receptor tyrosine kinases
PDK1	3-phosphoinositide-dependent kinase 1
PI3K	phosphatidylinositol 3-linase
PIP_2	phosphatidylinositol-4,5-bisphosphate
PIP_3	phosphatidylinositol-3,4,5-trisphosphate
RTKs	receptor tyrosine kinases
TF	transcription factor
TKD	Tyrosine Kinase Domain
VDDs	vitamin D compounds/derivatives
VDR	vitamin D receptor

References

1. Nowell, P.C. Differentiation of human leukemic leukocytes in tissue culture. *Exp. Cell Res.* **1960**, *19*, 267–277. [CrossRef] [PubMed]
2. Lugo, T.G.; Pendergast, A.M.; Muller, A.J.; Witte, O.N. Tyrosine kinase activity and transformation potency of Bcr-Abl oncogene products. *Science* **1990**, *247*, 1079–1082. [CrossRef] [PubMed]
3. Druker, B.J.; Tamura, S.; Buchdunger, E.; Ohno, S.; Segal, G.M.; Fanning, S.; Zimmermann, J.; Lydon, N.B. Effects of a selective inhibitor of the Abl tyrosine kinase on the growth of Bcr-Abl positive cells. *Nat. Med.* **1996**, *2*, 561–566. [CrossRef] [PubMed]
4. Druker, B.J.; Sawyers, C.L.; Kantarjian, H.; Resta, D.J.; Reese, S.F.; Ford, J.M.; Capdeville, R.; Talpaz, M. Activity of a specific inhibitor of the Bcr-Abl tyrosine kinase in the blast crisis of chronic myeloid leukemia and acute lymphoblastic leukemia with the Philadelphia chromosome. *N. Engl. J. Med.* **2001**, *344*, 1038–1042. [CrossRef] [PubMed]
5. Rowley, J.D.; Golomb, H.M.; Dougherty, C. 15/17 translocation, a consistent chromosomal change in acute promyelocytic leukaemia. *Lancet* **1977**, *1*, 549–550. [CrossRef] [PubMed]
6. Borrow, J.; Goddard, A.D.; Sheer, D.; Solomon, E. Molecular analysis of acute promyelocytic leukemia breakpoint cluster region on chromosome 17. *Science* **1990**, *249*, 1577–1580. [CrossRef] [PubMed]
7. Longo, L.; Pandolfi, P.P.; Biondi, A.; Rambaldi, A.; Mencarelli, A.; Lo Coco, F.; Diverio, D.; Pegoraro, L.; Avanzi, G.; Tabilio, A.; *et al.* Rearrangements and aberrant expression of the retinoic acid receptor alpha gene in acute promyelocytic leukemias. *J. Exp. Med.* **1990**, *172*, 1571–1575. [CrossRef] [PubMed]
8. Grignani, F.; De Matteis, S.; Nervi, C.; Tomassoni, L.; Gelmetti, V.; Cioce, M.; Fanelli, M.; Ruthardt, M.; Ferrara, F.F.; Zamir, I.; *et al.* Fusion proteins of the retinoic acid receptor-alpha recruit histone deacetylase in promyelocytic leukaemia. *Nature* **1998**, *391*, 815–818. [CrossRef] [PubMed]
9. Guidez, F.; Ivins, S.; Zhu, J.; Soderstrom, M.; Waxman, S.; Zelent, A. Reduced retinoic acid-sensitivities of nuclear receptor corepressor binding to PML- and PLZF-RARalpha underlie molecular pathogenesis and treatment of acute promyelocytic leukemia. *Blood* **1998**, *91*, 2634–2642. [PubMed]
10. Petrie, K.; Zelent, A.; Waxman, S. Differentiation therapy of acute myeloid leukemia: Past, present and future. *Curr. Opin. Hematol.* **2009**, *16*, 84–91. [CrossRef] [PubMed]
11. Luong, Q.T.; Koeffler, H.P. Vitamin D compounds in leukemia. *J. Steroid Biochem. Mol. Biol.* **2005**, *97*, 195–202. [CrossRef] [PubMed]
12. Yamada, K.; Mizusawa, M.; Harima, A.; Kajiwara, K.; Hamaki, T.; Hoshi, K.; Kozai, Y.; Kodo, H. Induction of remission of relapsed acute myeloid leukemia after unrelated donor cord blood transplantation by concomitant low-dose cytarabine and calcitriol in adults. *Eur. J. Haematol.* **2006**, *77*, 345–348. [CrossRef] [PubMed]
13. Ferrara, F.; Fazi, P.; Venditti, A.; Pagano, L.; Amadori, S.; Mandelli, F. Heterogeneity in the therapeutic approach to relapsed elderly patients with acute myeloid leukaemia: A survey from the Gruppo Italiano Malattie Ematologiche dell' Adulto (GIMEMA) Acute Leukaemia Working Party. *Hematol. Oncol.* **2008**, *26*, 104–107. [CrossRef] [PubMed]
14. Bendik, I.; Friedel, A.; Roos, F.F.; Weber, P.; Eggersdorfer, M. Vitamin D: A critical and essential micronutrient for human health. *Front Physiol* **2014**, *5*, 248. [CrossRef] [PubMed]
15. Kim, M.; Mirandola, L.; Pandey, A.; Nguyen, D.D.; Jenkins, M.R.; Turcel, M.; Cobos, E.; Chiriva-Internati, M. Application of vitamin D and derivatives in hematological malignancies. *Cancer Lett.* **2012**, *319*, 8–22. [CrossRef] [PubMed]
16. Harrison, J.S.; Bershadskiy, A. Clinical experience using vitamin D analogs in the treatment of myelodysplasia and acute myleoid leukemia: A review of the literature. *Leuk. Res. Treat.* **2012**, *2012*. [CrossRef]
17. Hall, A.C.; Juckett, M.B. The role of vitamin D in hematologic disease and stem cell transplantation. *Nutrients* **2013**, *5*, 2206–2221. [CrossRef] [PubMed]
18. Marchwicka, A.; Cebrat, M.; Sampath, P.; Sniezewski, L.; Marcinkowska, E. Perspectives of differentiation therapies of acute myeloid leukemia: The search for the molecular basis of patients' variable responses to 1,25-dihydroxyvitamin D and vitamin D analogs. *Front. Oncol.* **2014**, *4*, 125. [CrossRef] [PubMed]
19. Lowenberg, B. Acute myeloid leukemia: The challenge of capturing disease variety. *Hematol. Am. Soc. Hematol. Educ. Progr.* **2008**, *2008*, 1–11. [CrossRef]

20. Vardiman, J.W. The World Health Organization (WHO) classification of tumors of the hematopoietic and lymphoid tissues: An overview with emphasis on the myeloid neoplasms. *Chem. Biol. Interact.* **2010**, *184*, 16–20. [CrossRef] [PubMed]

21. Hasserjian, R.P. Acute myeloid leukemia: Advances in diagnosis and classification. *Int. J. Lab. Hematol.* **2013**, *35*, 358–366. [CrossRef] [PubMed]

22. Bennett, J.M.; Catovsky, D.; Daniel, M.T.; Flandrin, G.; Galton, D.A.; Gralnick, H.R.; Sultan, C. Proposals for the classification of the acute leukaemias. French-American-British (FAB) co-operative group. *Br. J. Haematol.* **1976**, *33*, 451–458. [CrossRef] [PubMed]

23. Vardiman, J.W.; Harris, N.L.; Brunning, R.D. The World Health Organization (WHO) classification of the myeloid neoplasms. *Blood* **2002**, *100*, 2292–2302. [CrossRef] [PubMed]

24. Bories, P.; Bertoli, S.; Berard, E.; Laurent, J.; Duchayne, E.; Sarry, A.; Delabesse, E.; Beyne-Rauzy, O.; Huguet, F.; Recher, C. Intensive chemotherapy, azacitidine or supportive care in older acute myeloid leukemia patients: An analysis from a regional healthcare network. *Am. J. Hematol.* **2014**, *89*, 244–252. [CrossRef]

25. Sanders, M.A.; Valk, P.J. The evolving molecular genetic landscape in acute myeloid leukaemia. *Curr. Opin. Hematol.* **2013**, *20*, 79–85. [CrossRef] [PubMed]

26. Abdel-Wahab, O.; Levine, R.L. Mutations in epigenetic modifiers in the pathogenesis and therapy of acute myeloid leukemia. *Blood* **2013**, *121*, 3563–3572. [CrossRef] [PubMed]

27. Estey, E.H. Acute myeloid leukemia: 2013 update on risk-stratification and management. *Am. J. Hematol.* **2013**, *88*, 318–327. [CrossRef] [PubMed]

28. Meyer, S.C.; Levine, R.L. Translational implications of somatic genomics in acute myeloid leukaemia. *Lancet Oncol.* **2014**, *15*, e382–e394. [CrossRef] [PubMed]

29. Huang, M.E.; Ye, Y.C.; Chen, S.R.; Chai, J.R.; Lu, J.X.; Zhoa, L.; Gu, L.J.; Wang, Z.Y. Use of all-trans retinoic acid in the treatment of acute promyelocytic leukemia. *Blood* **1988**, *72*, 567–572. [PubMed]

30. Ades, L.; Chevret, S.; Raffoux, E.; Guerci-Bresler, A.; Pigneux, A.; Vey, N.; Lamy, T.; Huguet, F.; Vekhoff, A.; Lambert, J.F.; *et al.* Long-term follow-up of European APL 2000 trial, evaluating the role of cytarabine combined with ATRA and Daunorubicin in the treatment of nonelderly APL patients. *Am. J. Hematol.* **2013**, *88*, 556–559. [CrossRef] [PubMed]

31. Cull, E.H.; Altman, J.K. Contemporary treatment of APL. *Curr. Hematol. Malig. Rep.* **2014**, *9*, 193–201. [CrossRef] [PubMed]

32. Honma, Y.; Hozumi, M.; Abe, E.; Konno, K.; Fukushima, M.; Hata, S.; Nishii, Y.; DeLuca, H.F.; Suda, T. 1 alpha,25-Dihydroxyvitamin D_3 and 1 alpha-hydroxyvitamin D_3 prolong survival time of mice inoculated with myeloid leukemia cells. *Proc. Natl. Acad. Sci. USA* **1983**, *80*, 201–204. [CrossRef] [PubMed]

33. McCarthy, D.M.; San Miguel, J.F.; Freake, H.C.; Green, P.M.; Zola, H.; Catovsky, D.; Goldman, J.M. 1,25-dihydroxyvitamin D_3 inhibits proliferation of human promyelocytic leukaemia (HL60) cells and induces monocyte-macrophage differentiation in HL60 and normal human bone marrow cells. *Leuk. Res.* **1983**, *7*, 51–55. [CrossRef] [PubMed]

34. Studzinski, G.P.; Bhandal, A.K.; Brelvi, Z.S. A system for monocytic differentiation of leukemic cells HL 60 by a short exposure to 1,25-dihydroxycholecalciferol. *Proc. Soc. Exp. Biol. Med.* **1985**, *179*, 288–295. [CrossRef] [PubMed]

35. Studzinski, G.P.; Bhandal, A.K.; Brelvi, Z.S. Cell cycle sensitivity of HL-60 cells to the differentiation-inducing effects of 1-alpha,25-dihydroxyvitamin D_3. *Cancer Res.* **1985**, *45*, 3898–3905. [PubMed]

36. Brelvi, Z.S.; Studzinski, G.P. Changes in the expression of oncogenes encoding nuclear phosphoproteins but not c-Ha-ras have a relationship to monocytic differentiation of HL 60 cells. *J. Cell Biol.* **1986**, *102*, 2234–2243. [CrossRef] [PubMed]

37. Raman, M.; Chen, W.; Cobb, M.H. Differential regulation and properties of MAPKs. *Oncogene* **2007**, *26*, 3100–3112. [CrossRef] [PubMed]

38. Geest, C.R.; Coffer, P.J. MAPK signaling pathways in the regulation of hematopoiesis. *J. Leukoc. Biol.* **2009**, *86*, 237–250. [CrossRef] [PubMed]

39. Zhou, G.; Bao, Z.Q.; Dixon, J.E. Components of a new human protein kinase signal transduction pathway. *J. Biol. Chem.* **1995**, *270*, 12665–12669. [CrossRef] [PubMed]

40. Wang, X.; Rao, J.; Studzinski, G.P. Inhibition of p38 MAP kinase activity up-regulates multiple MAP kinase pathways and potentiates 1,25-dihydroxyvitamin D_3-induced differentiation of human leukemia HL60 cells. *Exp. Cell Res.* **2000**, *258*, 425–437. [CrossRef] [PubMed]

41. Wang, X.; Studzinski, G.P. Inhibition of p38MAP kinase potentiates the JNK/SAPK pathway and AP-1 activity in monocytic but not in macrophage or granulocytic differentiation of HL60 cells. *J. Cell. Biochem.* **2001**, *82*, 68–77. [CrossRef] [PubMed]

42. Wang, X.; Studzinski, G.P. Oncoprotein Cot1 represses kinase suppressors of Ras1/2 and 1,25-dihydroxyvitamin D_3-induced differentiation of human acute myeloid leukemia cells. *J. Cell. Physiol.* **2011**, *226*, 1232–1240. [CrossRef] [PubMed]

43. Jin, W.; Lu, Y.; Li, Q.; Wang, J.; Zhang, H.; Chang, G.; Lin, Y.; Pang, T. Down-regulation of the P-glycoprotein relevant for multidrug resistance by intracellular acidification through the crosstalk of MAPK signaling pathways. *Int. J. Biochem. Cell Biol.* **2014**, *54*, 111–121. [CrossRef] [PubMed]

44. Chang, F.; Steelman, L.S.; Lee, J.T.; Shelton, J.G.; Navolanic, P.M.; Blalock, W.L.; Franklin, R.A.; McCubrey, J.A. Signal transduction mediated by the Ras/Raf/MEK/ERK pathway from cytokine receptors to transcription factors: Potential targeting for therapeutic intervention. *Leukemia* **2003**, *17*, 1263–1293. [CrossRef] [PubMed]

45. Marcinkowska, E.; Garay, E.; Gocek, E.; Chrobak, A.; Wang, X.; Studzinski, G.P. Regulation of C/EBPbeta isoforms by MAPK pathways in HL60 cells induced to differentiate by 1,25-dihydroxyvitamin D_3. *Exp. Cell Res.* **2006**, *312*, 2054–2065. [CrossRef] [PubMed]

46. Miranda, M.B.; Xu, H.; Torchia, J.A.; Johnson, D.E. Cytokine-induced myeloid differentiation is dependent on activation of the MEK/ERK pathway. *Leuk. Res.* **2005**, *29*, 1293–1306. [CrossRef] [PubMed]

47. Ross, S.E.; Radomska, H.S.; Wu, B.; Zhang, P.; Winnay, J.N.; Bajnok, L.; Wright, W.S.; Schaufele, F.; Tenen, D.G.; MacDougald, O.A. Phosphorylation of C/EBPalpha inhibits granulopoiesis. *Mol. Cell. Biol.* **2004**, *24*, 675–686. [CrossRef] [PubMed]

48. Morrison, D.K. KSR: A MAPK scaffold of the Ras pathway? *J. Cell Sci.* **2001**, *114*, 1609–1612. [PubMed]

49. Wang, X.; Studzinski, G.P. Kinase suppressor of RAS (KSR) amplifies the differentiation signal provided by low concentrations 1,25-dihydroxyvitamin D_3. *J. Cell. Physiol.* **2004**, *198*, 333–342. [CrossRef] [PubMed]

50. McKay, M.M.; Ritt, D.A.; Morrison, D.K. Signaling dynamics of the KSR1 scaffold complex. *Proc. Natl. Acad. Sci. USA* **2009**, *106*, 11022–11027. [CrossRef] [PubMed]

51. Zhang, H.; Koo, C.Y.; Stebbing, J.; Giamas, G. The dual function of KSR1: A pseudokinase and beyond. *Biochem. Soc. Trans.* **2013**, *41*, 1078–1082. [CrossRef] [PubMed]

52. Zhao, Y.; Bjorbaek, C.; Moller, D.E. Regulation and interaction of p90 (Rsk) isoforms with mitogen-activated protein kinases. *J. Biol. Chem.* **1996**, *271*, 29773–29779. [CrossRef] [PubMed]

53. Wang, X.; Studzinski, G.P. Activation of extracellular signal-regulated kinases (ERKs) defines the first phase of 1,25-dihydroxyvitamin D_3-induced differentiation of HL60 cells. *J. Cell. Biochem.* **2001**, *80*, 471–482. [CrossRef] [PubMed]

54. Wang, X.; Studzinski, G.P. Raf-1 signaling is required for the later stages of 1,25-dihydroxyvitamin D_3-induced differentiation of HL60 cells but is not mediated by the MEK/ERK module. *J. Cell. Physiol.* **2006**, *209*, 253–260. [CrossRef] [PubMed]

55. Hibi, M.; Lin, A.; Smeal, T.; Minden, A.; Karin, M. Identification of an oncoprotein- and UV-responsive protein kinase that binds and potentiates the c-Jun activation domain. *Genes Dev.* **1993**, *7*, 2135–2148. [CrossRef] [PubMed]

56. Sluss, H.K.; Barrett, T.; Derijard, B.; Davis, R.J. Signal transduction by tumor necrosis factor mediated by JNK protein kinases. *Mol. Cell. Biol.* **1994**, *14*, 8376–8384. [PubMed]

57. Karin, M.; Gallagher, E. From JNK to pay dirt: Jun kinases, their biochemistry, physiology and clinical importance. *IUBMB Life* **2005**, *57*, 283–295. [CrossRef] [PubMed]

58. Tournier, C.; Whitmarsh, A.J.; Cavanagh, J.; Barrett, T.; Davis, R.J. The MKK7 gene encodes a group of c-Jun NH2-terminal kinase kinases. *Mol. Cell. Biol.* **1999**, *19*, 1569–1581. [PubMed]

59. Kyriakis, J.M.; Banerjee, P.; Nikolakaki, E.; Dai, T.; Rubie, E.A.; Ahmad, M.F.; Avruch, J.; Woodgett, J.R. The stress-activated protein kinase subfamily of c-Jun kinases. *Nature* **1994**, *369*, 156–160. [CrossRef] [PubMed]

60. Lee, Y.H.; Giraud, J.; Davis, R.J.; White, M.F. c-Jun N-terminal kinase (JNK) mediates feedback inhibition of the insulin signaling cascade. *J. Biol. Chem.* **2003**, *278*, 2896–2902. [CrossRef] [PubMed]

61. Wang, X.; Studzinski, G.P. The requirement for and changing composition of the activating protein-1 transcription factor during differentiation of human leukemia HL60 cells induced by 1,25-dihydroxyvitamin D_3. *Cancer Res.* **2006**, *66*, 4402–4409. [CrossRef] [PubMed]

62. Krishna, M.; Narang, H. The complexity of mitogen-activated protein kinases (MAPKs) made simple. *Cell. Mol. Life Sci.* **2008**, *65*, 3525–3544. [CrossRef] [PubMed]

63. Hale, K.K.; Trollinger, D.; Rihanek, M.; Manthey, C.L. Differential expression and activation of p38 mitogen-activated protein kinase alpha, beta, gamma, and delta in inflammatory cell lineages. *J. Immunol.* **1999**, *162*, 4246–4252. [PubMed]

64. Uddin, S.; Ah-Kang, J.; Ulaszek, J.; Mahmud, D.; Wickrema, A. Differentiation stage-specific activation of p38 mitogen-activated protein kinase isoforms in primary human erythroid cells. *Proc. Natl. Acad. Sci. USA* **2004**, *101*, 147–152. [CrossRef] [PubMed]

65. Zhang, J.; Posner, G.H.; Danilenko, M.; Studzinski, G.P. Differentiation-inducing potency of the seco-steroid JK-1624F2–2 can be increased by combination with an antioxidant and a p38MAPK inhibitor which upregulates the JNK pathway. *J. Steroid Biochem. Mol. Biol.* **2007**, *105*, 140–149. [CrossRef] [PubMed]

66. Zhang, J.; Harrison, J.S.; Studzinski, G.P. Isoforms of p38MAPK gamma and delta contribute to differentiation of human AML cells induced by 1,25-dihydroxyvitamin D_3. *Exp. Cell Res.* **2011**, *317*, 117–130. [CrossRef] [PubMed]

67. Jiang, Y.; Gram, H.; Zhao, M.; New, L.; Gu, J.; Feng, L.; Di Padova, F.; Ulevitch, R.J.; Han, J. Characterization of the structure and function of the fourth member of p38 group mitogen-activated protein kinases, p38delta. *J. Biol. Chem.* **1997**, *272*, 30122–30128. [CrossRef] [PubMed]

68. Han, S.J.; Choi, K.Y.; Brey, P.T.; Lee, W.J. Molecular cloning and characterization of a Drosophila p38 mitogen-activated protein kinase. *J. Biol. Chem.* **1998**, *273*, 369–374. [CrossRef] [PubMed]

69. Zarubin, T.; Han, J. Activation and signaling of the p38 MAP kinase pathway. *Cell Res.* **2005**, *15*, 11–18. [CrossRef] [PubMed]

70. Brancho, D.; Tanaka, N.; Jaeschke, A.; Ventura, J.J.; Kelkar, N.; Tanaka, Y.; Kyuuma, M.; Takeshita, T.; Flavell, R.A.; Davis, R.J. Mechanism of p38 MAP kinase activation *in vivo*. *Genes Dev.* **2003**, *17*, 1969–1978. [CrossRef] [PubMed]

71. Deacon, K.; Mistry, P.; Chernoff, J.; Blank, J.L.; Patel, R. p38 Mitogen-activated protein kinase mediates cell death and p21-activated kinase mediates cell survival during chemotherapeutic drug-induced mitotic arrest. *Mol. Biol. Cell* **2003**, *14*, 2071–2087. [CrossRef] [PubMed]

72. Cuadrado, A.; Nebreda, A.R. Mechanisms and functions of p38 MAPK signalling. *Biochem. J.* **2010**, *429*, 403–417. [CrossRef] [PubMed]

73. Pritchard, A.L.; Hayward, N.K. Molecular pathways: Mitogen-activated protein kinase pathway mutations and drug resistance. *Clin. Cancer Res.* **2013**, *19*, 2301–2309. [CrossRef] [PubMed]

74. Wang, X.; Tournier, C. Regulation of cellular functions by the ERK5 signalling pathway. *Cell Signal.* **2006**, *18*, 753–760. [CrossRef] [PubMed]

75. Wang, X.; Pesakhov, S.; Harrison, J.S.; Kafka, M.; Danilenko, M.; Studzinski, G.P. The MAPK ERK5, but not ERK1/2, inhibits the progression of monocytic phenotype to the functioning macrophage. *Exp. Cell Res.* **2015**, *330*, 199–211. [CrossRef] [PubMed]

76. Nakamura, K.; Johnson, G.L. PB1 domains of MEKK2 and MEKK3 interact with the MEK5 PB1 domain for activation of the ERK5 pathway. *J. Biol. Chem.* **2003**, *278*, 36989–36992. [CrossRef] [PubMed]

77. Seyfried, J.; Wang, X.; Kharebava, G.; Tournier, C. A novel mitogen-activated protein kinase docking site in the N terminus of MEK5alpha organizes the components of the extracellular signal-regulated kinase 5 signaling pathway. *Mol. Cell. Biol.* **2005**, *25*, 9820–9828. [CrossRef] [PubMed]

78. Lopez-Royuela, N.; Rathore, M.G.; Allende-Vega, N.; Annicotte, J.S.; Fajas, L.; Ramachandran, B.; Gulick, T.; Villalba, M. Extracellular-signal-regulated kinase 5 modulates the antioxidant response by transcriptionally controlling Sirtuin 1 expression in leukemic cells. *Int. J. Biochem. Cell Biol.* **2014**, *53*, 253–261. [CrossRef] [PubMed]

79. Kondoh, K.; Terasawa, K.; Morimoto, H.; Nishida, E. Regulation of nuclear translocation of extracellular signal-regulated kinase 5 by active nuclear import and export mechanisms. *Mol. Cell. Biol.* **2006**, *26*, 1679–1690. [CrossRef] [PubMed]

80. Mody, N.; Campbell, D.G.; Morrice, N.; Peggie, M.; Cohen, P. An analysis of the phosphorylation and activation of extracellular-signal-regulated protein kinase 5 (ERK5) by mitogen-activated protein kinase kinase 5 (MKK5) *in vitro*. *Biochem. J.* **2003**, *372*, 567–575. [CrossRef] [PubMed]

81. Morimoto, H.; Kondoh, K.; Nishimoto, S.; Terasawa, K.; Nishida, E. Activation of a C-terminal transcriptional activation domain of ERK5 by autophosphorylation. *J. Biol. Chem.* **2007**, *282*, 35449–35456. [CrossRef] [PubMed]

82. Kato, Y.; Kravchenko, V.V.; Tapping, R.I.; Han, J.; Ulevitch, R.J.; Lee, J.D. BMK1/ERK5 regulates serum-induced early gene expression through transcription factor MEF2C. *EMBO J.* **1997**, *16*, 7054–7066. [CrossRef] [PubMed]

83. Kamakura, S.; Moriguchi, T.; Nishida, E. Activation of the protein kinase ERK5/BMK1 by receptor tyrosine kinases. Identification and characterization of a signaling pathway to the nucleus. *J. Biol. Chem.* **1999**, *274*, 26563–26571. [CrossRef] [PubMed]

84. Terasawa, K.; Okazaki, K.; Nishida, E. Regulation of c-Fos and Fra-1 by the MEK5-ERK5 pathway. *Genes Cells* **2003**, *8*, 263–273. [CrossRef] [PubMed]

85. Buschbeck, M.; Ullrich, A. The unique C-terminal tail of the mitogen-activated protein kinase ERK5 regulates its activation and nuclear shuttling. *J. Biol. Chem.* **2005**, *280*, 2659–2667. [CrossRef] [PubMed]

86. Chiariello, M.; Marinissen, M.J.; Gutkind, J.S. Multiple mitogen-activated protein kinase signaling pathways connect the Cot oncoprotein to the c-Jun promoter and to cellular transformation. *Mol. Cell. Biol.* **2000**, *20*, 1747–1758. [CrossRef] [PubMed]

87. Wang, X.; Gocek, E.; Novik, V.; Harrison, J.S.; Danilenko, M.; Studzinski, G.P. Inhibition of Cot1/Tlp2 oncogene in AML cells reduces ERK5 activation and up-regulates p27^{Kip1} concomitant with enhancement of differentiation and cell cycle arrest induced by silibinin and 1,25-dihydroxyvitamin D$_3$. *Cell Cycle* **2010**, *9*, 4542–4551. [CrossRef] [PubMed]

88. Katso, R.; Okkenhaug, K.; Ahmadi, K.; White, S.; Timms, J.; Waterfield, M.D. Cellular function of phosphoinositide 3-kinases: Implications for development, homeostasis, and cancer. *Annu. Rev. Cell Dev. Biol.* **2001**, *17*, 615–675. [CrossRef] [PubMed]

89. Ciruelos Gil, E.M. Targeting the PI3K/AKT/mTOR pathway in estrogen receptor-positive breast cancer. *Cancer Treat. Rev.* **2013**, *40*, 862–871. [CrossRef]

90. Jabbour, E.; Ottmann, O.G.; Deininger, M.; Hochhaus, A. Targeting the phosphoinositide 3-kinase pathway in hematologic malignancies. *Haematologica* **2014**, *99*, 7–18. [CrossRef] [PubMed]

91. Yu, J.; Zhang, Y.; McIlroy, J.; Rordorf-Nikolic, T.; Orr, G.A.; Backer, J.M. Regulation of the p85/p110 phosphatidylinositol 3'-kinase: Stabilization and inhibition of the p110alpha catalytic subunit by the p85 regulatory subunit. *Mol. Cell. Biol.* **1998**, *18*, 1379–1387. [PubMed]

92. Hawkins, P.T.; Anderson, K.E.; Davidson, K.; Stephens, L.R. Signalling through Class I PI3Ks in mammalian cells. *Biochem. Soc. Trans.* **2006**, *34*, 647–662. [CrossRef] [PubMed]

93. Krugmann, S.; Hawkins, P.T.; Pryer, N.; Braselmann, S. Characterizing the interactions between the two subunits of the p101/p110gamma phosphoinositide 3-kinase and their role in the activation of this enzyme by G beta gamma subunits. *J. Biol. Chem.* **1999**, *274*, 17152–17158. [CrossRef] [PubMed]

94. Jia, S.; Liu, Z.; Zhang, S.; Liu, P.; Zhang, L.; Lee, S.H.; Zhang, J.; Signoretti, S.; Loda, M.; Roberts, T.M.; *et al.* Essential roles of PI(3)K-p110beta in cell growth, metabolism and tumorigenesis. *Nature* **2008**, *454*, 776–779. [PubMed]

95. Saudemont, A.; Garcon, F.; Yadi, H.; Roche-Molina, M.; Kim, N.; Segonds-Pichon, A.; Martin-Fontecha, A.; Okkenhaug, K.; Colucci, F. p110gamma and p110delta isoforms of phosphoinositide 3-kinase differentially regulate natural killer cell migration in health and disease. *Proc. Natl. Acad. Sci. USA* **2009**, *106*, 5795–5800. [CrossRef] [PubMed]

96. Murga, C.; Laguinge, L.; Wetzker, R.; Cuadrado, A.; Gutkind, J.S. Activation of Akt/protein kinase B by G protein-coupled receptors. A role for alpha and beta gamma subunits of heterotrimeric G proteins acting through phosphatidylinositol-3-OH kinasegamma. *J. Biol. Chem.* **1998**, *273*, 19080–19085. [CrossRef] [PubMed]

97. Kurig, B.; Shymanets, A.; Bohnacker, T.; Prajwal; Brock, C.; Ahmadian, M.R.; Schaefer, M.; Gohla, A.; Harteneck, C.; Wymann, M.P.; *et al.* Ras is an indispensable coregulator of the class IB phosphoinositide 3-kinase p87/p110gamma. *Proc. Natl. Acad. Sci. USA* **2009**, *106*, 20312–20317. [CrossRef] [PubMed]

98. Sarbassov, D.D.; Ali, S.M.; Sengupta, S.; Sheen, J.H.; Hsu, P.P.; Bagley, A.F.; Markhard, A.L.; Sabatini, D.M. Prolonged rapamycin treatment inhibits mTORC2 assembly and Akt/PKB. *Mol. Cell* **2006**, *22*, 159–168. [CrossRef] [PubMed]

99. Bayascas, J.R. Dissecting the role of the 3-phosphoinositide-dependent protein kinase-1 (PDK1) signalling pathways. *Cell Cycle* **2008**, *7*, 2978–2982. [CrossRef] [PubMed]

100. Gutierrez, A.; Sanda, T.; Grebliunaite, R.; Carracedo, A.; Salmena, L.; Ahn, Y.; Dahlberg, S.; Neuberg, D.; Moreau, L.A.; Winter, S.S.; *et al.* High frequency of PTEN, PI3K, and AKT abnormalities in T-cell acute lymphoblastic leukemia. *Blood* **2009**, *114*, 647–650. [CrossRef] [PubMed]

101. Sykes, S.M.; Lane, S.W.; Bullinger, L.; Kalaitzidis, D.; Yusuf, R.; Saez, B.; Ferraro, F.; Mercier, F.; Singh, H.; Brumme, K.M.; *et al.* AKT/FOXO signaling enforces reversible differentiation blockade in myeloid leukemias. *Cell* **2011**, *146*, 697–708. [CrossRef] [PubMed]

102. Tamburini, J.; Chapuis, N.; Bardet, V.; Park, S.; Sujobert, P.; Willems, L.; Ifrah, N.; Dreyfus, F.; Mayeux, P.; Lacombe, C.; *et al.* Mammalian target of rapamycin (mTOR) inhibition activates phosphatidylinositol 3-kinase/Akt by up-regulating insulin-like growth factor-1 receptor signaling in acute myeloid leukemia: Rationale for therapeutic inhibition of both pathways. *Blood* **2008**, *111*, 379–382. [CrossRef] [PubMed]

103. Vu, C.; Fruman, D.A. Target of rapamycin signaling in leukemia and lymphoma. *Clin. Cancer Res.* **2010**, *16*, 5374–5380. [CrossRef] [PubMed]

104. Altman, J.K.; Sassano, A.; Platanias, L.C. Targeting mTOR for the treatment of AML. New agents and new directions. *Oncotarget* **2011**, *2*, 510–517. [PubMed]

105. Rosnet, O.; Birnbaum, D. Hematopoietic receptors of class III receptor-type tyrosine kinases. *Crit. Rev. Oncog.* **1993**, *4*, 595–613. [PubMed]

106. Lyman, S.D. Biology of flt3 ligand and receptor. *Int. J. Hematol.* **1995**, *62*, 63–73. [CrossRef] [PubMed]

107. Schnittger, S.; Schoch, C.; Dugas, M.; Kern, W.; Staib, P.; Wuchter, C.; Loffler, H.; Sauerland, C.M.; Serve, H.; Buchner, T.; *et al.* Analysis of FLT3 length mutations in 1003 patients with acute myeloid leukemia: Correlation to cytogenetics, FAB subtype, and prognosis in the AMLCG study and usefulness as a marker for the detection of minimal residual disease. *Blood* **2002**, *100*, 59–66. [CrossRef] [PubMed]

108. Thiede, C.; Steudel, C.; Mohr, B.; Schaich, M.; Schakel, U.; Platzbecker, U.; Wermke, M.; Bornhauser, M.; Ritter, M.; Neubauer, A.; *et al.* Analysis of FLT3-activating mutations in 979 patients with acute myelogenous leukemia: Association with FAB subtypes and identification of subgroups with poor prognosis. *Blood* **2002**, *99*, 4326–4335. [CrossRef] [PubMed]

109. Janke, H.; Pastore, F.; Schumacher, D.; Herold, T.; Hopfner, K.P.; Schneider, S.; Berdel, W.E.; Buchner, T.; Woermann, B.J.; Subklewe, M.; *et al.* Activating FLT3 mutants show distinct gain-of-function phenotypes *in vitro* and a characteristic signaling pathway profile associated with prognosis in acute myeloid leukemia. *PLoS One* **2014**, *9*, e89560. [CrossRef] [PubMed]

110. Yokota, S.; Kiyoi, H.; Nakao, M.; Iwai, T.; Misawa, S.; Okuda, T.; Sonoda, Y.; Abe, T.; Kahsima, K.; Matsuo, Y.; *et al.* Internal tandem duplication of the FLT3 gene is preferentially seen in acute myeloid leukemia and myelodysplastic syndrome among various hematological malignancies. A study on a large series of patients and cell lines. *Leukemia* **1997**, *11*, 1605–1609. [CrossRef] [PubMed]

111. Choudhary, C.; Muller-Tidow, C.; Berdel, W.E.; Serve, H. Signal transduction of oncogenic Flt3. *Int. J. Hematol.* **2005**, *82*, 93–99. [CrossRef] [PubMed]

112. Takahashi, S. Downstream molecular pathways of FLT3 in the pathogenesis of acute myeloid leukemia: Biology and therapeutic implications. *J. Hematol. Oncol.* **2011**, *4*, 13. [CrossRef] [PubMed]

113. Tenen, D.G.; Hromas, R.; Licht, J.D.; Zhang, D.E. Transcription factors, normal myeloid development, and leukemia. *Blood* **1997**, *90*, 489–519. [PubMed]

114. Pabst, T.; Mueller, B.U.; Zhang, P.; Radomska, H.S.; Narravula, S.; Schnittger, S.; Behre, G.; Hiddemann, W.; Tenen, D.G. Dominant-negative mutations of CEBPA, encoding CCAAT/enhancer binding protein-alpha (C/EBPalpha), in acute myeloid leukemia. *Nat. Genet.* **2001**, *27*, 263–270. [CrossRef] [PubMed]

115. Porse, B.T.; Bryder, D.; Theilgaard-Monch, K.; Hasemann, M.S.; Anderson, K.; Damgaard, I.; Jacobsen, S.E.; Nerlov, C. Loss of C/EBP alpha cell cycle control increases myeloid progenitor proliferation and transforms the neutrophil granulocyte lineage. *J. Exp. Med.* **2005**, *202*, 85–96. [CrossRef] [PubMed]

116. Lin, F.T.; MacDougald, O.A.; Diehl, A.M.; Lane, M.D. A 30-kDa alternative translation product of the CCAAT/enhancer binding protein alpha message: Transcriptional activator lacking antimitotic activity. *Proc. Natl. Acad. Sci. USA* **1993**, *90*, 9606–9610. [CrossRef] [PubMed]

117. Kirstetter, P.; Schuster, M.B.; Bereshchenko, O.; Moore, S.; Dvinge, H.; Kurz, E.; Theilgaard-Monch, K.; Mansson, R.; Pedersen, T.A.; Pabst, T.; *et al.* Modeling of C/EBPalpha mutant acute myeloid leukemia reveals a common expression signature of committed myeloid leukemia-initiating cells. *Cancer Cell* **2008**, *13*, 299–310. [CrossRef] [PubMed]

118. Calkhoven, C.F.; Muller, C.; Leutz, A. Translational control of C/EBPalpha and C/EBPbeta isoform expression. *Genes Dev.* **2000**, *14*, 1920–1932. [PubMed]
119. Zhang, P.; Iwasaki-Arai, J.; Iwasaki, H.; Fenyus, M.L.; Dayaram, T.; Owens, B.M.; Shigematsu, H.; Levantini, E.; Huettner, C.S.; Lekstrom-Himes, J.A.; *et al.* Enhancement of hematopoietic stem cell repopulating capacity and self-renewal in the absence of the transcription factor C/EBP alpha. *Immunity* **2004**, *21*, 853–863. [CrossRef] [PubMed]
120. Schlenk, R.F.; Dohner, K.; Krauter, J.; Frohling, S.; Corbacioglu, A.; Bullinger, L.; Habdank, M.; Spath, D.; Morgan, M.; Benner, A.; *et al.* Mutations and treatment outcome in cytogenetically normal acute myeloid leukemia. *N. Engl. J. Med.* **2008**, *358*, 1909–1918. [CrossRef] [PubMed]
121. Lee, R.C.; Feinbaum, R.L.; Ambros, V. The C. elegans heterochronic gene lin-4 encodes small RNAs with antisense complementarity to lin-14. *Cell* **1993**, *75*, 843–854. [CrossRef] [PubMed]
122. Lagos-Quintana, M.; Rauhut, R.; Lendeckel, W.; Tuschl, T. Identification of novel genes coding for small expressed RNAs. *Science* **2001**, *294*, 853–858. [CrossRef] [PubMed]
123. Bartel, D.P. MicroRNAs: Genomics, biogenesis, mechanism, and function. *Cell* **2004**, *116*, 281–297. [CrossRef] [PubMed]
124. Fabbri, M.; Garzon, R.; Andreeff, M.; Kantarjian, H.M.; Garcia-Manero, G.; Calin, G.A. MicroRNAs and noncoding RNAs in hematological malignancies: Molecular, clinical and therapeutic implications. *Leukemia* **2008**, *22*, 1095–1105. [CrossRef] [PubMed]
125. Marcucci, G.; Radmacher, M.D.; Maharry, K.; Mrozek, K.; Ruppert, A.S.; Paschka, P.; Vukosavljevic, T.; Whitman, S.P.; Baldus, C.D.; Langer, C.; *et al.* MicroRNA expression in cytogenetically normal acute myeloid leukemia. *N. Engl. J. Med.* **2008**, *358*, 1919–1928. [CrossRef] [PubMed]
126. Metzeler, K.H.; Maharry, K.; Kohlschmidt, J.; Volinia, S.; Mrozek, K.; Becker, H.; Nicolet, D.; Whitman, S.P.; Mendler, J.H.; Schwind, S.; *et al.* A stem cell-like gene expression signature associates with inferior outcomes and a distinct microRNA expression profile in adults with primary cytogenetically normal acute myeloid leukemia. *Leukemia* **2013**, *27*, 2023–2031. [CrossRef] [PubMed]
127. Marcucci, G.; Maharry, K.S.; Metzeler, K.H.; Volinia, S.; Wu, Y.Z.; Mrozek, K.; Nicolet, D.; Kohlschmidt, J.; Whitman, S.P.; Mendler, J.H.; *et al.* Clinical role of microRNAs in cytogenetically normal acute myeloid leukemia: MiR-155 upregulation independently identifies high-risk patients. *J. Clin. Oncol.* **2013**, *31*, 2086–2093. [CrossRef] [PubMed]
128. Gimenes-Teixeira, H.L.; Lucena-Araujo, A.R.; Dos Santos, G.A.; Zanette, D.L.; Scheucher, P.S.; Oliveira, L.C.; Dalmazzo, L.F.; Silva-Junior, W.A.; Falcao, R.P.; Rego, E.M. Increased expression of miR-221 is associated with shorter overall survival in T-cell acute lymphoid leukemia. *Exp. Hematol. Oncol.* **2013**, *2*, 10. [CrossRef] [PubMed]
129. Long, M.D.; Sucheston-Campbell, L.E.; Campbell, M.J. Vitamin D Receptor and RXR in the Post-Genomic Era. *J. Cell. Physiol.* **2014**, *230*, 758–766. [CrossRef]
130. Campbell, M.J. Vitamin D and the RNA transcriptome: More than mRNA regulation. *Front. Physiol.* **2014**, *5*, 181. [CrossRef] [PubMed]
131. Heikkinen, S.; Vaisanen, S.; Pehkonen, P.; Seuter, S.; Benes, V.; Carlberg, C. Nuclear hormone 1alpha,25-dihydroxyvitamin D_3 elicits a genome-wide shift in the locations of VDR chromatin occupancy. *Nucleic Acids Res.* **2011**, *39*, 9181–9193. [CrossRef] [PubMed]
132. Ryynanen, J.; Seuter, S.; Campbell, M.J.; Carlberg, C. Gene regulatory scenarios of primary 1,25-dihydroxyvitamin D_3 target genes in a human myeloid leukemia cell line. *Cancers (Basel)* **2013**, *5*, 1221–1241. [CrossRef]
133. Ramagopalan, S.V.; Heger, A.; Berlanga, A.J.; Maugeri, N.J.; Lincoln, M.R.; Burrell, A.; Handunnetthi, L.; Handel, A.E.; Disanto, G.; Orton, S.M.; *et al.* A ChIP-seq defined genome-wide map of vitamin D receptor binding: Associations with disease and evolution. *Genome Res.* **2010**, *20*, 1352–1360. [CrossRef] [PubMed]
134. Moss, G.P. IUPAC-IUB Nomenclature of steroids. Recommendations 1989. *Pure Appl. Chem.* **1989**, *61*, 1783–1822. [CrossRef]
135. Kim, T.K.; Wang, J.; Janjetovic, Z.; Chen, J.; Tuckey, R.C.; Nguyen, M.N.; Tang, E.K.; Miller, D.; Li, W.; Slominski, A.T. Correlation between secosteroid-induced vitamin D receptor activity in melanoma cells and computer-modeled receptor binding strength. *Mol. Cell. Endocrinol.* **2012**, *361*, 143–152. [CrossRef] [PubMed]
136. Morris, H.A. Vitamin D activities for health outcomes. *Ann. Lab. Med.* **2014**, *34*, 181–186. [CrossRef] [PubMed]

137. Gocek, E.; Studzinski, G.P. Vitamin D and differentiation in cancer. *Crit. Rev. Clin. Lab. Sci.* **2009**, *46*, 190–209. [CrossRef] [PubMed]

138. Grober, U.; Spitz, J.; Reichrath, J.; Kisters, K.; Holick, M.F. Vitamin D: Update 2013: From rickets prophylaxis to general preventive healthcare. *Dermatoendocrinology* **2013**, *5*, 331–347. [CrossRef]

139. Feldman, D.; Krishnan, A.V.; Swami, S.; Giovannucci, E.; Feldman, B.J. The role of vitamin D in reducing cancer risk and progression. *Nat. Rev. Cancer* **2014**, *14*, 342–357. [CrossRef] [PubMed]

140. Gutsch, R.; Kandemir, J.D.; Pietsch, D.; Cappello, C.; Meyer, J.; Simanowski, K.; Huber, R.; Brand, K. CCAAT/enhancer-binding protein beta inhibits proliferation in monocytic cells by affecting the retinoblastoma protein/E2F/cyclin E pathway but is not directly required for macrophage morphology. *J. Biol. Chem.* **2011**, *286*, 22716–22729. [CrossRef] [PubMed]

141. Wang, X.; Pesakhov, S.; Harrison, J.S.; Danilenko, M.; Studzinski, G.P. ERK5 pathway regulates transcription factors important for monocytic differentiation of human myeloid leukemia cells. *J. Cell. Physiol.* **2014**, *229*, 856–867. [CrossRef] [PubMed]

142. Hickstein, D.D.; Ozols, J.; Williams, S.A.; Baenziger, J.U.; Locksley, R.M.; Roth, G.J. Isolation and characterization of the receptor on human neutrophils that mediates cellular adherence. *J. Biol. Chem.* **1987**, *262*, 5576–5580. [PubMed]

143. Wright, S.D.; Ramos, R.A.; Tobias, P.S.; Ulevitch, R.J.; Mathison, J.C. CD14, a receptor for complexes of lipopolysaccharide (LPS) and LPS binding protein. *Science* **1990**, *249*, 1431–1433. [CrossRef] [PubMed]

144. Studzinski, G.P.; Rathod, B.; Wang, Q.M.; Rao, J.; Zhang, F. Uncoupling of cell cycle arrest from the expression of monocytic differentiation markers in HL60 cell variants. *Exp. Cell Res.* **1997**, *232*, 376–387. [CrossRef] [PubMed]

145. Gocek, E.; Kielbinski, M.; Baurska, H.; Haus, O.; Kutner, A.; Marcinkowska, E. Different susceptibilities to 1,25-dihydroxyvitamin D$_3$-induced differentiation of AML cells carrying various mutations. *Leuk. Res.* **2010**, *34*, 649–657. [CrossRef] [PubMed]

146. Marcinkowska, E. Evidence that activation of MEK1,2/Erk1,2 signal transduction pathway is necessary for calcitriol-induced differentiation of HL60 cells. *Anticancer Res.* **2001**, *21*, 499–504. [PubMed]

147. Wang, Q.; Wang, X.; Studzinski, G.P. Jun N-terminal kinase pathway enhances signaling of monocytic differentiation of human leukemia cells induced by 1,25-dihydroxyvitamin D$_3$. *J. Cell. Biochem.* **2003**, *89*, 1087–1101. [CrossRef] [PubMed]

148. Wang, Q.M.; Jones, J.B.; Studzinski, G.P. Cyclin-dependent kinase inhibitor p27 as a mediator of the G1/S phase block induced by 1,25-dihydroxyvitamin D$_3$ in HL60 cells. *Cancer Res.* **1996**, *56*, 264–267. [PubMed]

149. Wang, Q.M.; Studzinski, G.P.; Chen, F.; Coffman, F.D.; Harrison, L.E. p53/56(lyn) antisense shifts the 1,25-dihydroxyvitamin D$_3$-induced G1/S block in HL60 cells to S phase. *J. Cell. Physiol.* **2000**, *183*, 238–246. [CrossRef] [PubMed]

150. Zhang, Y.; Zhang, J.; Studzinski, G.P. AKT pathway is activated by 1, 25-dihydroxyvitamin D$_3$ and participates in its anti-apoptotic effect and cell cycle control in differentiating HL60 cells. *Cell Cycle* **2006**, *5*, 447–451. [CrossRef] [PubMed]

151. Xu, H.M.; Tepper, C.G.; Jones, J.B.; Fernandez, C.E.; Studzinski, G.P. 1,25-Dihydroxyvitamin D$_3$ protects HL60 cells against apoptosis but down-regulates the expression of the Bcl-2 gene. *Exp. Cell Res.* **1993**, *209*, 367–374. [CrossRef] [PubMed]

152. Thompson, T.; Andreeff, M.; Studzinski, G.P.; Vassilev, L.T. 1,25-Dihydroxyvitamin D$_3$ enhances the apoptotic activity of MDM2 antagonist nutlin-3a in acute myeloid leukemia cells expressing wild-type p53. *Mol. Cancer Ther.* **2010**, *9*, 1158–1168. [CrossRef] [PubMed]

153. Dudley, D.T.; Pang, L.; Decker, S.J.; Bridges, A.J.; Saltiel, A.R. A synthetic inhibitor of the mitogen-activated protein kinase cascade. *Proc. Natl. Acad. Sci. USA* **1995**, *92*, 7686–7689. [CrossRef] [PubMed]

154. Ramji, D.P.; Foka, P. CCAAT/enhancer-binding proteins: Structure, function and regulation. *Biochem. J.* **2002**, *365*, 561–575. [PubMed]

155. Huber, R.; Pietsch, D.; Panterodt, T.; Brand, K. Regulation of C/EBPbeta and resulting functions in cells of the monocytic lineage. *Cell Signal.* **2012**, *24*, 1287–1296. [CrossRef] [PubMed]

156. Studzinski, G.P.; Wang, X.; Ji, Y.; Wang, Q.; Zhang, Y.; Kutner, A.; Harrison, J.S. The rationale for deltanoids in therapy for myeloid leukemia: Role of KSR-MAPK-C/EBP pathway. *J. Steroid Biochem. Mol. Biol.* **2005**, *97*, 47–55. [CrossRef] [PubMed]

157. Buck, M.; Poli, V.; Hunter, T.; Chojkier, M. C/EBPbeta phosphorylation by RSK creates a functional XEXD caspase inhibitory box critical for cell survival. *Mol. Cell* **2001**, *8*, 807–816. [CrossRef] [PubMed]
158. Pan, Z.; Hetherington, C.J.; Zhang, D.E. CCAAT/enhancer-binding protein activates the CD14 promoter and mediates transforming growth factor beta signaling in monocyte development. *J. Biol. Chem.* **1999**, *274*, 23242–23248. [CrossRef] [PubMed]
159. Michaud, N.R.; Therrien, M.; Cacace, A.; Edsall, L.C.; Spiegel, S.; Rubin, G.M.; Morrison, D.K. KSR stimulates Raf-1 activity in a kinase-independent manner. *Proc. Natl. Acad. Sci. USA* **1997**, *94*, 12792–12796. [CrossRef] [PubMed]
160. Wang, X.; Wang, T.T.; White, J.H.; Studzinski, G.P. Induction of kinase suppressor of RAS-1(KSR-1) gene by 1, alpha25-dihydroxyvitamin D$_3$ in human leukemia HL60 cells through a vitamin D response element in the 5'-flanking region. *Oncogene* **2006**, *25*, 7078–7085. [CrossRef] [PubMed]
161. Wang, X.; Wang, T.T.; White, J.H.; Studzinski, G.P. Expression of human kinase suppressor of Ras 2 (hKSR-2) gene in HL60 leukemia cells is directly upregulated by 1,25-dihydroxyvitamin D$_3$ and is required for optimal cell differentiation. *Exp. Cell Res.* **2007**, *313*, 3034–3045. [CrossRef] [PubMed]
162. Wang, X.; Patel, R.; Studzinski, G.P. hKSR-2, a vitamin D-regulated gene, inhibits apoptosis in arabinocytosine-treated HL60 leukemia cells. *Mol. Cancer Ther.* **2008**, *7*, 2798–2806. [CrossRef] [PubMed]
163. Ito, Y.; Mishra, N.C.; Yoshida, K.; Kharbanda, S.; Saxena, S.; Kufe, D. Mitochondrial targeting of JNK/SAPK in the phorbol ester response of myeloid leukemia cells. *Cell Death Differ.* **2001**, *8*, 794–800. [CrossRef] [PubMed]
164. Szabo, E.; Preis, L.H.; Birrer, M.J. Constitutive cJun expression induces partial macrophage differentiation in U-937 cells. *Cell Growth Differ.* **1994**, *5*, 439–446. [PubMed]
165. Bennett, B.L.; Sasaki, D.T.; Murray, B.W.; O'Leary, E.C.; Sakata, S.T.; Xu, W.; Leisten, J.C.; Motiwala, A.; Pierce, S.; Satoh, Y.; *et al.* SP600125, an anthrapyrazolone inhibitor of Jun N-terminal kinase. *Proc. Natl. Acad. Sci. USA* **2001**, *98*, 13681–13686. [CrossRef] [PubMed]
166. Wang, Q.; Salman, H.; Danilenko, M.; Studzinski, G.P. Cooperation between antioxidants and 1,25-dihydroxyvitamin D$_3$ in induction of leukemia HL60 cell differentiation through the JNK/AP-1/Egr-1 pathway. *J. Cell. Physiol.* **2005**, *204*, 964–974. [CrossRef] [PubMed]
167. Jaeschke, A.; Karasarides, M.; Ventura, J.J.; Ehrhardt, A.; Zhang, C.; Flavell, R.A.; Shokat, K.M.; Davis, R.J. JNK2 is a positive regulator of the cJun transcription factor. *Mol. Cell* **2006**, *23*, 899–911. [CrossRef] [PubMed]
168. Sabapathy, K.; Wagner, E.F. JNK2: A negative regulator of cellular proliferation. *Cell Cycle* **2004**, *3*, 1520–1523. [CrossRef] [PubMed]
169. Chen-Deutsch, X.; Garay, E.; Zhang, J.; Harrison, J.S.; Studzinski, G.P. c-Jun N-terminal kinase 2 (JNK2) antagonizes the signaling of differentiation by JNK1 in human myeloid leukemia cells resistant to vitamin D. *Leuk. Res.* **2009**, *33*, 1372–1378. [CrossRef] [PubMed]
170. Cuenda, A.; Rouse, J.; Doza, Y.N.; Meier, R.; Cohen, P.; Gallagher, T.F.; Young, P.R.; Lee, J.C. SB 203580 is a specific inhibitor of a MAP kinase homologue which is stimulated by cellular stresses and interleukin-1. *FEBS Lett.* **1995**, *364*, 229–233. [CrossRef] [PubMed]
171. Nemoto, S.; Xiang, J.; Huang, S.; Lin, A. Induction of apoptosis by SB202190 through inhibition of p38beta mitogen-activated protein kinase. *J. Biol. Chem.* **1998**, *273*, 16415–16420. [CrossRef] [PubMed]
172. Manthey, C.L.; Wang, S.W.; Kinney, S.D.; Yao, Z. SB202190, a selective inhibitor of p38 mitogen-activated protein kinase, is a powerful regulator of LPS-induced mRNAs in monocytes. *J. Leukoc. Biol.* **1998**, *64*, 409–417. [PubMed]
173. Gocek, E.; Kielbinski, M.; Marcinkowska, E. Activation of intracellular signaling pathways is necessary for an increase in VDR expression and its nuclear translocation. *FEBS Lett.* **2007**, *581*, 1751–1757. [CrossRef] [PubMed]
174. Tatake, R.J.; O'Neill, M.M.; Kennedy, C.A.; Wayne, A.L.; Jakes, S.; Wu, D.; Kugler, S.Z., Jr.; Kashem, M.A.; Kaplita, P.; Snow, R.J. Identification of pharmacological inhibitors of the MEK5/ERK5 pathway. *Biochem. Biophys. Res. Commun.* **2008**, *377*, 120–125. [CrossRef] [PubMed]
175. Yang, Q.; Deng, X.; Lu, B.; Cameron, M.; Fearns, C.; Patricelli, M.P.; Yates, J.R., 3rd; Gray, N.S.; Lee, J.D. Pharmacological inhibition of BMK1 suppresses tumor growth through promyelocytic leukemia protein. *Cancer Cell* **2010**, *18*, 258–267. [CrossRef] [PubMed]

176. Zheng, R.; Wang, X.; Studzinski, G.P. 1,25-Dihydroxyvitamin D₃ induces monocytic differentiation of human myeloid leukemia cells by regulating C/EBPbeta expression through MEF2C. *J. Steroid Biochem. Mol. Biol.* **2014**. [CrossRef]

177. Razumovskaya, E.; Sun, J.; Ronnstrand, L. Inhibition of MEK5 by BIX02188 induces apoptosis in cells expressing the oncogenic mutant FLT3-ITD. *Biochem. Biophys. Res. Commun.* **2011**, *412*, 307–312. [CrossRef] [PubMed]

178. Marcinkowska, E.; Wiedlocha, A.; Radzikowski, C. Evidence that phosphatidylinositol 3-kinase and $p70^{S6K}$ protein are involved in differentiation of HL60 cells induced by calcitriol. *Anticancer Res.* **1998**, *18*, 3507–3514. [PubMed]

179. Hmama, Z.; Nandan, D.; Sly, L.; Knutson, K.L.; Herrera-Velit, P.; Reiner, N.E. 1alpha,25-dihydroxyvitamin D₃-induced myeloid cell differentiation is regulated by a vitamin D receptor-phosphatidylinositol 3-kinase signaling complex. *J. Exp. Med.* **1999**, *190*, 1583–1594. [CrossRef] [PubMed]

180. Marcinkowska, E.; Kutner, A. Side-chain modified vitamin D analogs require activation of both PI3-K and Erk1,2 signal transduction pathways to induce differentiation of human promyelocytic leukemia cells. *Acta Biochim. Pol.* **2002**, *49*, 393–406. [PubMed]

181. Hughes, P.J.; Lee, J.S.; Reiner, N.E.; Brown, G. The vitamin D receptor-mediated activation of phosphatidylinositol 3-kinase (PI3Kalpha) plays a role in the 1alpha,25-dihydroxyvitamin D₃-stimulated increase in steroid sulphatase activity in myeloid leukaemic cell lines. *J. Cell. Biochem.* **2008**, *103*, 1551–1572. [CrossRef] [PubMed]

182. Baurska, H.; Kielbinski, M.; Biecek, P.; Haus, O.; Jazwiec, B.; Kutner, A.; Marcinkowska, E. Monocytic differentiation induced by side-chain modified analogs of vitamin D in *ex vivo* cells from patients with acute myeloid leukemia. *Leuk. Res.* **2014**, *38*, 638–647. [CrossRef] [PubMed]

183. Baurska, H.; Klopot, A.; Kielbinski, M.; Chrobak, A.; Wijas, E.; Kutner, A.; Marcinkowska, E. Structure-function analysis of vitamin D₂ analogs as potential inducers of leukemia differentiation and inhibitors of prostate cancer proliferation. *J. Steroid Biochem. Mol. Biol.* **2011**, *126*, 46–54. [CrossRef] [PubMed]

184. Friedman, A.D. Transcriptional control of granulocyte and monocyte development. *Oncogene* **2007**, *26*, 6816–6828. [CrossRef] [PubMed]

185. Pham, T.H.; Langmann, S.; Schwarzfischer, L.; El Chartouni, C.; Lichtinger, M.; Klug, M.; Krause, S.W.; Rehli, M. CCAAT enhancer-binding protein beta regulates constitutive gene expression during late stages of monocyte to macrophage differentiation. *J. Biol. Chem.* **2007**, *282*, 21924–21933. [CrossRef] [PubMed]

186. Ji, Y.; Studzinski, G.P. Retinoblastoma protein and CCAAT/enhancer-binding protein beta are required for 1,25-dihydroxyvitamin D₃-induced monocytic differentiation of HL60 cells. *Cancer Res.* **2004**, *64*, 370–377. [CrossRef] [PubMed]

187. Wang, X.; Gocek, E.; Liu, C.G.; Studzinski, G.P. MicroRNAs181 regulate the expression of p27Kip1 in human myeloid leukemia cells induced to differentiate by 1,25-dihydroxyvitamin D₃. *Cell Cycle* **2009**, *8*, 736–741. [CrossRef] [PubMed]

188. Cuesta, R.; Martinez-Sanchez, A.; Gebauer, F. miR-181a regulates cap-dependent translation of p27(kip1) mRNA in myeloid cells. *Mol. Cell. Biol.* **2009**, *29*, 2841–2851. [CrossRef] [PubMed]

189. Duggal, J.; Harrison, J.S.; Studzinski, G.P.; Wang, X. Involvement of microRNA181a in differentiation and cell cycle arrest induced by a plant-derived antioxidant carnosic acid and vitamin D analog Doxercalciferol in human leukemia cells. *Microrna* **2012**, *1*, 26–33. [CrossRef] [PubMed]

190. Min, D.; Lv, X.B.; Wang, X.; Zhang, B.; Meng, W.; Yu, F.; Hu, H. Downregulation of miR-302c and miR-520c by 1,25(OH)₂D₃ treatment enhances the susceptibility of tumour cells to natural killer cell-mediated cytotoxicity. *Br. J. Cancer* **2013**, *109*, 723–730. [CrossRef] [PubMed]

191. Iosue, I.; Quaranta, R.; Masciarelli, S.; Fontemaggi, G.; Batassa, E.M.; Bertolami, C.; Ottone, T.; Divona, M.; Salvatori, B.; Padula, F.; *et al.* Argonaute 2 sustains the gene expression program driving human monocytic differentiation of acute myeloid leukemia cells. *Cell Death Dis.* **2013**, *4*, e926. [CrossRef] [PubMed]

192. Gocek, E.; Wang, X.; Liu, X.; Liu, C.G.; Studzinski, G.P. MicroRNA-32 upregulation by 1,25-dihydroxyvitamin D₃ in human myeloid leukemia cells leads to Bim targeting and inhibition of AraC-induced apoptosis. *Cancer Res.* **2012**, *71*, 6230–6239. [CrossRef]

193. Salvatori, B.; Iosue, I.; Djodji Damas, N.; Mangiavacchi, A.; Chiaretti, S.; Messina, M.; Padula, F.; Guarini, A.; Bozzoni, I.; Fazi, F.; *et al.* Critical Role of c-Myc in Acute Myeloid Leukemia Involving Direct Regulation of miR-26a and Histone Methyltransferase EZH2. *Genes Cancer* **2011**, *2*, 585–592. [CrossRef] [PubMed]

194. Salvatori, B.; Iosue, I.; Mangiavacchi, A.; Loddo, G.; Padula, F.; Chiaretti, S.; Peragine, N.; Bozzoni, I.; Fazi, F.; Fatica, A. The microRNA-26a target E2F7 sustains cell proliferation and inhibits monocytic differentiation of acute myeloid leukemia cells. *Cell Death Dis.* **2012**, *3*, e413. [CrossRef] [PubMed]

195. Pesakhov, S.; Khanin, M.; Studzinski, G.P.; Danilenko, M. Distinct combinatorial effects of the plant polyphenols curcumin, carnosic acid, and silibinin on proliferation and apoptosis in acute myeloid leukemia cells. *Nutr. Cancer* **2010**, *62*, 811–824. [CrossRef] [PubMed]

196. Wang, X.; Pesakhov, S.; Weng, A.; Kafka, M.; Gocek, E.; Nguyen, M.; Harrison, J.S.; Danilenko, M.; Studzinski, G.P. ERK 5/MAPK pathway has a major role in 1alpha,25-(OH) vitamin D-induced terminal differentiation of myeloid leukemia cells. *J. Steroid Biochem. Mol. Biol.* **2014**, *144*, 223–227. [CrossRef] [PubMed]

197. Shabtay, A.; Sharabani, H.; Barvish, Z.; Kafka, M.; Amichay, D.; Levy, J.; Sharoni, Y.; Uskokovic, M.R.; Studzinski, G.P.; Danilenko, M. Synergistic antileukemic activity of carnosic acid-rich rosemary extract and the 19-nor Gemini vitamin D analogue in a mouse model of systemic acute myeloid leukemia. *Oncology* **2008**, *75*, 203–214. [CrossRef] [PubMed]

198. Danilenko, M.; Studzinski, G.P. Enhancement by other compounds of the anti-cancer activity of vitamin D_3 and its analogs. *Exp. Cell Res.* **2004**, *298*, 339–358. [CrossRef] [PubMed]

199. Zhang, J.; Harrison, J.S.; Uskokovic, M.; Danilenko, M.; Studzinski, G.P. Silibinin can induce differentiation as well as enhance vitamin D_3-induced differentiation of human AML cells *ex vivo* and regulates the levels of differentiation-related transcription factors. *Hematol. Oncol.* **2010**, *28*, 124–132. [PubMed]

200. Thompson, T.; Danilenko, M.; Vassilev, L.; Studzinski, G.P. Tumor suppressor p53 status does not determine the differentiation-associated G1 cell cycle arrest induced in leukemia cells by 1,25-dihydroxyvitamin D_3 and antioxidants. *Cancer Biol. Ther.* **2010**, *10*, 344–350. [CrossRef] [PubMed]

201. Yang, J.; Ikezoe, T.; Nishioka, C.; Ni, L.; Koeffler, H.P.; Yokoyama, A. Inhibition of mTORC1 by RAD001 (everolimus) potentiates the effects of 1,25-dihydroxyvitamin D_3 to induce growth arrest and differentiation of AML cells *in vitro* and *in vivo*. *Exp. Hematol.* **2010**, *38*, 666–676. [CrossRef] [PubMed]

202. Lainey, E.; Wolfromm, A.; Sukkurwala, A.Q.; Micol, J.B.; Fenaux, P.; Galluzzi, L.; Kepp, O.; Kroemer, G. EGFR inhibitors exacerbate differentiation and cell cycle arrest induced by retinoic acid and vitamin D_3 in acute myeloid leukemia cells. *Cell Cycle* **2013**, *12*, 2978–2991. [CrossRef] [PubMed]

203. Danilenko, M.; Wang, Q.; Wang, X.; Levy, J.; Sharoni, Y.; Studzinski, G.P. Carnosic acid potentiates the antioxidant and prodifferentiation effects of 1alpha,25-dihydroxyvitamin D_3 in leukemia cells but does not promote elevation of basal levels of intracellular calcium. *Cancer Res.* **2003**, *63*, 1325–1332. [PubMed]

204. Callens, C.; Coulon, S.; Naudin, J.; Radford-Weiss, I.; Boissel, N.; Raffoux, E.; Wang, P.H.; Agarwal, S.; Tamouza, H.; Paubelle, E.; *et al.* Targeting iron homeostasis induces cellular differentiation and synergizes with differentiating agents in acute myeloid leukemia. *J. Exp. Med.* **2010**, *207*, 731–750. [CrossRef] [PubMed]

205. Chen-Deutsch, X.; Kutner, A.; Harrison, J.S.; Studzinski, G.P. The pan-caspase inhibitor Q-VD-OPh has anti-leukemia effects and can interact with vitamin D analogs to increase HPK1 signaling in AML cells. *Leuk. Res.* **2012**, *36*, 884–888. [CrossRef] [PubMed]

206. Jamshidi, F.; Zhang, J.; Harrison, J.S.; Wang, X.; Studzinski, G.P. Induction of differentiation of human leukemia cells by combinations of COX inhibitors and 1,25-dihydroxyvitamin D_3 involves Raf1 but not Erk 1/2 signaling. *Cell Cycle* **2008**, *7*, 917–924. [CrossRef] [PubMed]

207. Paubelle, E.; Zylbersztejn, F.; Alkhaeir, S.; Suarez, F.; Callens, C.; Dussiot, M.; Isnard, F.; Rubio, M.T.; Damaj, G.; Gorin, N.C.; *et al.* Deferasirox and vitamin D improves overall survival in elderly patients with acute myeloid leukemia after demethylating agents failure. *PLoS One* **2013**, *8*, e65998. [CrossRef] [PubMed]

208. Clinicaltrials.gov. Available online: http://clinicaltrials.gov/ct2/home (accessed on 12 October 2014).

209. Cancer.gov. Available online: http://www.cancer.gov/clinicaltrials (accessed on 12 October 2014).

210. Leukemia-net.org. Available online: http://www.leukemia-net.org/content/leukemias/aml/aml_trials/database/index_eng (accessed on 12 October 2014).

211. Ferrero, D.; Crisa, E.; Marmont, F.; Audisio, E.; Frairia, C.; Giai, V.; Gatti, T.; Festuccia, M.; Bruno, B.; Riera, L.; *et al.* Survival improvement of poor-prognosis AML/MDS patients by maintenance treatment with low-dose chemotherapy and differentiating agents. *Ann. Hematol.* **2014**, *93*, 1391–1400. [CrossRef] [PubMed]

212. Autier, P.; Gandini, S. Vitamin D supplementation and total mortality: A meta-analysis of randomized controlled trials. *Arch. Intern. Med.* **2007**, *167*, 1730–1737. [CrossRef] [PubMed]

213. Giovannucci, E. Can vitamin D reduce total mortality? *Arch. Intern. Med.* **2007**, *167*, 1709–1710. [CrossRef] [PubMed]

214. Lee, H.J.; Muindi, J.R.; Tan, W.; Hu, Q.; Wang, D.; Liu, S.; Wilding, G.E.; Ford, L.A.; Sait, S.N.; Block, A.W.; *et al.* Low 25(OH) vitamin D$_3$ levels are associated with adverse outcome in newly diagnosed, intensively treated adult acute myeloid leukemia. *Cancer* **2014**, *120*, 521–529. [CrossRef] [PubMed]

215. Ramnath, N.; Daignault-Newton, S.; Dy, G.K.; Muindi, J.R.; Adjei, A.; Elingrod, V.L.; Kalemkerian, G.P.; Cease, K.B.; Stella, P.J.; Brenner, D.E.; *et al.* A phase I/II pharmacokinetic and pharmacogenomic study of calcitriol in combination with cisplatin and docetaxel in advanced non-small-cell lung cancer. *Cancer Chemother. Pharmacol.* **2013**, *71*, 1173–1182. [CrossRef] [PubMed]

216. Ma, J.; Ma, Z.; Li, W.; Ma, Q.; Guo, J.; Hu, A.; Li, R.; Wang, F.; Han, S. The mechanism of calcitriol in cancer prevention and treatment. *Curr. Med. Chem.* **2013**, *20*, 4121–4130. [CrossRef] [PubMed]

217. Mazzaferro, S.; Goldsmith, D.; Larsson, T.E.; Massy, Z.A.; Cozzolino, M. Vitamin D metabolites and/or analogs: Which D for which patient? *Curr. Vasc. Pharmacol.* **2014**, *12*, 339–349. [CrossRef] [PubMed]

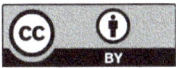

Journal of
Clinical Medicine

MDPI

Review

Targeted Therapy of FLT3 in Treatment of AML—Current Status and Future Directions

Caroline Benedicte Nitter Engen [1], Line Wergeland [1], Jørn Skavland [1] and Bjørn Tore Gjertsen [1,2,*]

[1]   Center for Cancer Biomarkers CCBIO, Department of Clinical Science, University of Bergen, Bergen N-5020, Norway; caroline.engen@k2.uib.no (C.B.N.E.); line@wergeland.jacobsen.net (L.W.); jorn.skavland@k2.uib.no (J.S.)

[2]   Department of Internal Medicine, Hematology Section, Haukeland University Hospital, Bergen N-5021, Norway

*   Author to whom correspondence should be addressed; bjorn.gjertsen@uib.no; Tel.: +47-55-97-29-68; Fax: +47-55-97-29-50.

External Editor: Celalettin Ustun
Received: 21 September 2014; in revised form: 27 November 2014; Accepted: 28 November 2014; Published: 15 December 2014

Abstract: Internal tandem duplications (ITDs) of the gene encoding the Fms-Like Tyrosine kinase-3 (FLT3) receptor are present in approximately 25% of patients with acute myeloid leukemia (AML). The mutation is associated with poor prognosis, and the aberrant protein product has been hypothesized as an attractive therapeutic target. Various tyrosine kinase inhibitors (TKIs) have been developed targeting FLT3, but in spite of initial optimism the first generation TKIs tested in clinical studies generally induce only partial and transient hematological responses. The limited treatment efficacy generally observed may be explained by numerous factors; extensively pretreated and high risk cohorts, suboptimal pharmacodynamic and pharmacokinetic properties of the compounds, acquired TKI resistance, or the possible fact that inhibition of mutated FLT3 alone is not sufficient to avoid disease progression. The second-generation agent quizartinib is showing promising outcomes and seems better tolerated and with less toxic effects than traditional chemotherapeutic agents. Therefore, new generations of TKIs might be feasible for use in combination therapy or in a salvage setting in selected patients. Here, we sum up experiences so far, and we discuss the future outlook of targeting dysregulated FLT3 signaling in the treatment of AML.

Keywords: acute myeloid leukemia; FLT3; tyrosine kinase inhibitors; clinical trials

1. Introduction

1.1. Acute Myeloid Leukemia

Acute myeloid leukemia (AML) is the most frequent acute leukemia in adults [1,2]. It is a heterogeneous clonal disorder of the myeloid precursor cells [3], and although patients today are treated with similar nonspecific treatment regimens that have remained more or less unchanged for decades [4–6], it has for an equally long period been recognized that there is considerable genetic, biological, and clinical heterogeneity in the patient group [7,8]. This variation is clearly reflected in the diverging relapse rate and overall survival in response to standard of care, ranging from 10%–70%, dependent on both patient and disease related factors [9,10]. Current risk stratification at the time of diagnosis usually include age, performance status, white blood cell count, determining if the disease is *de novo*, secondary or therapy related, cytogenetics, and mutation analysis [11]. Several cytogenetic [12,13], molecular genetic (e.g., Fms-Like Tyrosine kinase-3 (FLT3), nucleophosmin 1

(NPM1), CCAAT enhancer-binding protein-α (CEBPA)) [14], and epigenetic changes [15], as well as aberrantly expressed RNA, and microRNA [16] have been identified as prognostic markers for disease outcome, and as shown in other hematological malignancies it is thought that some of these changes represent feasible therapy targets. The challenge we are facing today is to translate this knowledge into tailored treatment for AML, identifying and directing the treatment towards cancer-specific pathways aiming for improved patient outcome.

1.2. Mutations and Signaling Pathways in AML

Normal hematopoiesis is controlled by the microenvironment and external signaling molecules, transmitting signals through intracellular signal transduction pathways via cell surface receptors. These intracellular pathways form a highly complex network of signaling cascades, including receptors, kinases, phosphatases and transcription factors that cross-talk extensively on multiple levels. Changes in this network by cytogenetic abnormalities, mutations or epigenetic alterations may lead to non-functional or hyper-activated pathways, that in turn can lead to anti-apoptosis and increased proliferation of the cells [17,18].

The group of genes most frequently mutated in AML is signaling genes, including genes coding for receptor tyrosine kinases such as FLT3 and KIT, Serine-Threonine kinases, KRAS/NRAS and protein tyrosine phosphatases [19]. Aberrant regulation of intracellular signaling pathways accordingly appears to be an important leukemia promoting mechanism, and like inhibition of Bcr-Abl revolutionized patient outcome in chronic myeloid leukemia [20], targeting signaling onco-proteins seems like a feasible strategy in AML [21].

The one most frequent mutated gene in AML, with mutations detected in up to 35% of the patients, is the Fms-Like Tyrosine kinase-3 (FLT3) gene on chromosome 13q12. Two major classes of FLT3 mutations have been identified: length mutations, predominantly internal tandem duplications (ITD) in the juxtamembrane domain of FLT3, first described by Nakao *et al.* in 1996 [22], and tyrosine kinase domain (TKD) point mutations [23,24]. ITDs are detected in 20%–25% of AML patients, while about 5%–10% of patients have point mutations within the TKD, with a mutation at codon 835 being the most frequent one [22–24].

1.3. Aberrant FLT3 Activation in AML

FLT3 is a member of the tyrosine kinase III family and functions as a membrane bound growth factor receptor, usually expressed by human hematopoietic progenitor cells [25]. Binding of its ligand, FLT3-ligand (FL) induces a conformational change in the protein that causes activation of the intrinsic tyrosine kinase domain. The enzyme phosphorylates intracellular molecules and consequently activates multiple downstream signaling pathways involved in cellular survival, proliferation and differentiation [26]. The expression of FLT3 is normally lost upon differentiation [27,28], but as AML is caused by a block in differentiation and uncontrolled proliferation of the myeloid progenitor cells the expression is frequently "captured" in many AML blasts, and remains highly expressed in most AML cases [29,30]. While overexpression of the receptor has been associated with poor prognosis [31], the presence of FLT3-ITD mutations confers even stronger independent prognostic information as it significantly correlates with an increased risk of relapse and dismal overall survival, in comparison to the TKD mutation where such an associations is absent [32–34]. Although FLT3-ITD positive AML is not considered a distinct entity of AML, FLT3-ITD status has been included in the WHO 2008 guidelines and the European LeukemiaNet recommendations for classification of AML, providing important prognostic information [11,35]. The survival advantage of leukemic blasts driven by mutant FLT3 is to a large extent thought to be explained by a constitutive activation of the receptor causing FL independent autophosphorylation [36], and initiation of two major intracellular pathways essential for growth, survival and proliferation; PI3K/AKT/mTOR and RAS/RAF/MEK/ERK [37]. The signal transducers and activators of transcription (STATs) are usually not regulated via RTKs, but for mutations like FLT3-ITD a constitutive phosphorylation and transcriptional activation of STAT5 also occur [38,39].

   With aberrant signaling appearing as a key component in FLT3-ITD mutated AML the constitutive active surface protein stands out as an attractive target for small molecule receptor inhibitor-based therapy [40,41]. Over the 15 years since the discovery of the mutated receptor and its clinical significance, more than a dozen different tyrosine kinase inhibitors (TKI) have been developed and tested preclinically, and many have shown to selectively induce cell death in FLT3 mutated AML blasts by suppressing FLT3 autophosphorylation and downstream signaling pathways [40–42]. Several of the agents, including the first generation agents lestaurtinib, linifanib, midostaurin, semaxanib, sorafenib, sunitinib, and tandutinib as well as the second generation agent quizartinib, have reached clinical trials where their safety, tolerability, and efficiency have been assessed. In the following section we will discuss and compare the most relevant FLT3 TKIs in clinical trials. Both trials where the TKIs are used as monotherapy and trials where conventional treatment is combined with a TKI will be assessed and summarized, with focus on antileukemic efficacy and side effects (Table 1).

Table 1. Overview of evaluated clinical trials.

Agent	Study Phase	Patient Population	n	Median/Mean Age (years)	FLT3-ITD	FLT3-Point-Mutation Only	Treatment	Dose	Ref.
Lestaurtinib—CEP-701	Phase 1/2	AML, refractory/relapsed	17	61 (18–71)	94.1% (n = 16)	5.9% (n = 1)	Monotherapy	40 mg–80 mg × 2	[43]
	Phase 2	AML, untreated	29	73 (67–82)	6.9% (n = 2)	10.3% (n = 3)	Monotherapy	60 mg–80 mg × 2	[44]
	Phase 2 (Randomized)	AML, first relapse	224	56.5 (20–81)	92% (n = 206)	7.6% (n = 17)	Monotherapy + Mitoxantrone, Etoposide & Cytarabine	80 mg × 2,	[45]
Linifanib—ABT-869	Phase 1	AML, refractory/relapsed	47	56.3 (23–81)	12.8% (n = 6)	10.6% (n = 5)	Monotherapy/+ Cytarabine	5–25 mg	[46]
Midostaurin—PKC412	Phase 2	AML, refractory/relapsed, High risk MDS	20	62 (29–78)	90% (n = 18)	10% (n = 2)	Monotherapy	75 mg × 3	[47]
	Phase 2B	AML, refractory/relapsed, High risk MDS	95	64% ≥ 65 years	27.4% (n = 26)	9.5% (n = 9)	Monotherapy	50 mg–100 mg × 2	[48]
	Phase 1B	AML, untreated	69	48.5	17.4% (n = 12)	8.7% (n = 6)	+ Daunorubicin & Cytarabine	50 mg–100 mg × 2	[49]
Semaxanib—SU5416	Phase 2	AML, refractory or advanced, High risk MDS	33	64 (23–76)	4.5% (n = 1/22)	NA	Monotherapy	145 mg/m², twice weekly	[50]
	Phase 2	AML, advanced, c-kit pos.	43	65 (27–79)	20% (n = 7/35)	NA	Monotherapy	145 mg/m², twice weekly	[51]
	Phase 2	AML refractory, High risk MDS	55	64–66 (22–80)	NA	NA	Monotherapy	145 mg/m², twice weekly	[52]
Sorafanib—BAY 43-9006	Phase 1	AML, refractory/relapsed	16	61.5 (48–81)	43.8% (n = 7)	12.5% (n = 2)	Monotherapy	200 mg–600 mg × 2	[53]
	Phase 1	AML, refractory/relapsed, High risk MDS	42	71.3	33% (n = 9/27)	NA	Monotherapy	100 mg–400 mg × 2	[54]
	Phase 2 (Randomized)	AML, >60 years	197	68 (61–80)	14%	NA	+ Cytarabin and Daunorubicin	400 mg × 2	[55]
	Phase 1	Acute leukemia, refractory/relapsed	12	9.5 (6–17)	41.7% (n = 5)	NA	+ Clofarabine & Cytarabine	150 mg/m²/200 mg/m² × 2	[56]
	Phase 1/2	AML, refractory/relapsed	43	64 (24–87)	93% (n = 40)	NA	+ 5-Azacytidine	400 mg × 2	[57]
Sunitinib—SU11248	Phase 1	AML	25	67 (19–82)	10.3% (n = 3)	6.9% (n = 2)	Monotherapy	50 mg–350 mg as a single dose	[58]
	Phase 1	AML, refractory	15	72 (54–80)	14.3% (n = 2/14)	14.3% (n = 2/14)	Monotherapy	50 mg–75 mg	[59]
Tandutinib—MLN-518	Phase 1	AML, High-risk MDS	40	70.5 (22–90)	20% (n = 8)	2.5% (n = 1)	Monotherapy	50 mg–700 mg × 2	[60]
Quizartinib—AC220	Phase 1	AML	76	60 (23–83)	27% (n = 18/65)	NA	Monotherapy	12–450 mg × 1	[61]
	Phase 2	AML, refractory/relapse	76	53 (19–77)	100% (n = 76)	NA	Monotherapy	30–60 mg	[62]
	Phase 2	AML, refractory/relapse, unfit	270	60.4 (19–85)	70.7% (n = 191)	NA	Monotherapy	90–135 mg	[63,64]
	Phase 1	AML, untreated >60 years old	55	69 (62–87)	7.3% (n = 4)	NA	+ Cytarabin, Daunorubicin & Etoposide	40–135 mg	[65]
	Phase 1	AML, MLL-rearranged ALL, >1 month, ≤21 years	22	NA	27.3% (n = 6)	NA	+ Cytarabin & Etoposide	25–60 mg/m²	[66]

2. Evaluation of Selected Small Molecule Inhibitors against FLT3 Used in Clinical Trials

2.1. First Generation TKIs

2.1.1. Lestaurtinib (CEP-701)

Lestaurtinib is an orally bioavailable polyaromatic inolocarbazole alkoid compound that is synthetically derived from the bacterial fermentation product K-252a. It was originally identified as an inhibitor of the neurotropin receptor TrkA, and was initially studied in patients with solid tumors [42]. It has successively been found to be a potent FLT3 inhibitor, and has been investigated in AML patients [43–45]. In a phase 1/2 trial FLT3-mutated patients with advanced AML the drug was found to be generally well tolerated; with observed treatment related toxicities including mild nausea and emesis, and generalized weakness and fatigue. Clinical activity was observed in 29% of the patients during a limited time period, ranging from two weeks to three months. The drug significantly lowered peripheral blood blasts, and some patients had evidence of transient normal hematopoiesis [43]. In a phase 2 trial, lestaurtinib was administered in monotherapy as first-line treatment in 29 older AML patients not considered eligible for intensive chemotherapy. The drug was given for eight weeks, regardless of FLT3-mutation status. Observed toxicities included mild gastrointestinal side effects. No complete or partial remissions were seen, but transient reduction in bone marrow and peripheral-blood blasts was achieved in 60% (3/5) of the FLT3-mutated patients, compared to a 22.7% (5/22) response rate in the FLT3-wild-type group. The clinical response was however of short duration, with a median time to progression of 25 days [44]. In a bigger randomized phase 2 trial, 220 FLT3 mutated AML patients at first relapse received either chemotherapy alone or chemotherapy followed by lestaurtinib. There was no significant difference in the rate of adverse effects in the two groups, however, the seriousness of adverse effects was higher in the lestaurtinib-treated group. Of the patients receiving lestaurtinib 25.9% (29/112) patients achieved complete remission or complete remission with incomplete platelet recovery, compared to 20.5% (23/112) patients attaining equal treatment responses in the control group. There was however no significant difference in overall survival between the two groups, providing no clear benefit to adult AML patients with FLT3 mutations [45].

2.1.2. Linifanib (ABT-869)

Linifanib is an orally available potent inhibitor of FLT3 and VEGFR. Preclinically it has shown antileukemic effects both as monotherapy and in combination with cytarabine in FLT3-mutated human AML xenograft models [67]. In a phase 1 dose-escalation study, relapsed or refractory AML patients were treated either with linifanib alone or linifanib in combination with intermediate-dose cytarabine. Generally linifanib was well tolerated, and the most common side effects related to the treatment were fatigue, gastrointestinal distress and infections. The primary objective in the study did not include efficacy, but antileukemic effects were observed both in patients with FLT3 mutated as well as FLT3 wild-type patients [46].

2.1.3. Midostaurin (PKC412, N-Benzoylstaurosporin)

Midostaurin is a derivate of staurosporine, initially developed as a protein kinase C inhibitor, and extensively used as model agent for the study of apoptosis. It is a multi-targeting TKI, inhibiting tyrosine kinases such as c-Kit and PDGFR as well as FLT3 [68]. In a phase 2 trial FLT3 mutated patients with relapsed or refractory AML or high-risk MDS not considered candidates for chemotherapy, were treated with midostaurin in monotherapy. The drug was generally well tolerated with the most frequent treatment related adverse effect being nausea and vomiting. The drug showed some transient clinical activity, reducing the amount of peripheral blasts by 50% in 70% (14/20) of the patients, and reducing bone marrow blast counts by 50% in 30% (6/20) of the patients [47,69]. In a larger phase 2B trial 95 AML/high risk MDS patients were randomized to receive either 50 mg or 100 mg of oral midostaurin twice daily, independently of FLT3 mutation status. Midostaturin was generally well tolerated in both concentrations and there were no clear difference in results according to dose regime. Side effects included nausea and vomiting. In the 92 patients, treatment efficiency could be assessed the reduction in peripheral blood or bone marrow blasts by 50% or more was 71% in the FLT3-mutated group compared to 42% in the FLT3-wild-type group. The majority of patients with FLT3-mutations responded with a reduction in blast count. One partial response was seen in a FLT3-ITD positive patient at the 100 mg per day regime. Hematological improvement was seen in 46% of the patients with FLT3-ITD versus 35% of the FLT3-wild-type patients. All therapy naive FLT3-ITD patients had a clear reduction of peripheral blood and bone marrow blasts [48]. In a phase 1B study, 69 younger newly diagnosed AML patients were treated with midostaurin in addition to a standard of care regime consisting of daunorubicin and cytarabine. The treatment cycle run for 28 days with one group getting the inhibitor concomitant starting on day 1–7 and day 15–21 and a second group getting the inhibitor administered sequentially starting on day 8–21 with 14 treatment days per cycle. The first 29 patients received midostaurin 100 mg orally twice daily. This dosage regime was discontinued because of adverse effects and followed by 40 AML patients who received midostaurin 50 mg twice daily. The treatment at the 50 mg twice-daily regime was generally well tolerated. The complete remission rate of the patients in the FLT mutant group (n = 18) and wild-type group (n = 51) was 92% and 74%, respectively [49]. Initial results from a phase 1/2 study of midostaurin and 5-Azacytinine in combination in refractory or relapsed AML demonstrates that it is a feasible alternative with a complete remission rate of 25%, and additionally 20% of patients achieving complete remission with incomplete platelet recovery [70]. An additional phase 1 study of midostaurin, bortezomib and chemotherapy shows promising antileukemic activity in refractory/relapsed AML patients and further investigation is ongoing [71]. A larger placebo controlled phase 3 trial (ClinicalTrials.gov identifier: NCT00651261), comparing midostaurin in addition to standard induction therapy is currently in completion and may indicate the pathway forward for midostaurin in AML treatment.

2.1.4. Semaxanib (SU5416)

Semaxanib is an indolinone derivate that inhibits VEGFR, c-Kit and FLT3. It produces a dose dependent inhibition of tumor progress in a diversity of xenograft models, comprising malignant melanoma, glioma, fibrosarcoma and carcinomas of the lung, breast, prostate, and the skin [72]. In a phase 2 study of 33 patients, either with refractory AML or advanced MDS, the effect of semaxanib in monotherapy was assessed. Semaxanib was infused intravenously twice weekly in a dose of 145 mg/m^2. Objective responses were seen in 18.2% (4/22) of the AML patients; three patients attained a partial response while one patient achieved a hematologic improvement [50]. In a second phase 2 trial, c-Kit positive patients with advanced AML were treated with semaxanib in monotherapy. Observed toxicities included nausea, musculoskeletal pain, headache, insomnia, vomiting, vertigo, fatigue/malaise, abdominal pain, sweating, and arthralgia. Half of the patients included in the study experienced severe adverse effects, with pneumonia and sepsis being the most frequent. Of the 25 patients evaluable for clinical response, no remissions were observed among the FLT3-ITD positive patients (n = 7). One patient achieved a morphologic remission while 28% (7/25) patients experienced a transient partial response with at least 50% reduction in bone marrow and peripheral blood blasts. The mean response duration of all eight responding patients was 1.6 months until disease progression. Patients with AML blasts expressing high levels of VEGF mRNA had a significantly higher response rate compared to the rest of the patient group, indicating that the main antileukemic effect was mediated by semaxanib's antiangiogenic properties rather than direct growth inhibition [51]. In a third phase 2 trial, 55 patients with refractory AML or advanced MDS were treated with semaxanib in monotherapy. Observed toxicities included headache, dyspnea, fatigue, thromboembolic events, bone pain and gastrointestinal events. Objective responses were obtained in 7.3% of the patients; three patients achieved partial responses and one patient experienced a hematologic improvement [52].

2.1.5. Sorafenib (BAY 43-9006)

Sorafenib is an orally available bi-aryl urea that inhibits several kinases, including RAF-kinase, VEGFR-2, c-Kit, and FLT3. It is currently approved for the treatment of metastatic renal cancer and advanced hepatocellular carcinoma [73]. In a phase 1 trial, refractory or relapsed AML patients were treated with sorafenib 200 mg twice daily. A clinical response was seen in 56.3% (9/16) of the patients, including all of the FLT3-ITD positive patients (*n* = 6). Both circulating and bone marrow blasts were strongly reduced in patients with FLT3-ITD mutation, while there was no essential change in the patients without FLT3-ITD [53]. In a randomized phase 1 clinical and biologic study of sorafenib, 42 patients with either AML or MDS were randomized either to continuously administration of the drug, or intermittent. The drug was administered twice daily, and the dose increased during the trial to evaluate dose-limiting toxicity. Of the patients assessed 33% (9/27) were FLT3-ITD positive. Dose-limiting toxicity was prevalent at the 400 mg twice-daily regime. The most seen drug related side effects were of gastrointestinal character, including abdominal pain, nausea, and vomiting. Palmar-plantar dysesthesia among other toxic skin reactions were also seen. Three patients experienced arterial thrombosis; myocardial infarction, brain stem infarction and splenic infarcts. One complete remission, lasting 2.7 months, was observed in a FLT3-ITD positive patient. In 33.3% of the FLT3-ITD positive patients, an improvement in peripheral blood and bone marrow blast counts was observed [54]. Recently, the results from a randomized, placebo-controlled trial concluded that the combination of standard induction treatment with sorafenib as consolidating treatment was of no benefit for AML patients older than 60 years of age compared to standard induction therapy alone. On the contrary, this combination seemed to cause worse outcomes with more adverse effects. Event-free survival and overall survival was not significantly improved, and these results were consistent also in the FLT3-ITD positive subgroup of patients [55]. Initial results from a similar study however indicated that the addition of sorafenib to standard chemotherapy is associated with a high rate of complete remission and an acceptable toxicity profile in FLT3-mutated older AML patients [74]. In a phase 1 pharmacokinetic and pharmacodynamic trial sorafenib was studied in concurrence with the cytotoxic agents clofarabine and cytarabine in pediatric acute myeloid leukemia patients, who all had either relapsed or refractory disease. All patients experienced hand-foot skin reactions and/or rash, which was also the dose-limiting toxicities, with maximum tolerated dose determined to 150 mg/m^2 twice daily. On day 8, sorafenib decreased blast percentages in 83.3% (10/12) of the patients. After combination chemotherapy three of five patients with FLT3-ITD mutations and three FLT3-wild-type patients achieved complete remissions. One additional FLT3-wild-type patient with AML attained a partial remission [56]. A retrospective assessment of FLT3-ITD positive pediatric patients suggested that post-transplant therapy with sorafenib might also improve outcome in patients that have been treated with hematopoietic stem cell transplantation [75]. In a phase 2 trial, 43 AML patients, mainly FLT3-ITD positive (93%), were treated with sorafenib in combination with 5-Azacytidine. Antileukemic efficacy was observed in 46% of the assessable patients, including a 27% complete remission rate [57].

2.1.6. Sunitinib (SU11248)

Sunitinib is an oral multi-targeting TKI, predominantly targeting PDGFR, VEGFR, c-Kit and FLT3. It has been used in treatment for multiple solid malignancies, and is approved for the treatment of metastatic renal cell carcinoma and gastrointestinal stromal tumors [76]. In a phase 1 clinical trial, 29 AML patients were treated with a single dose of sunitinib. The dose was escalated in 50 mg increments from 50 mg to a highest dose of 350 mg. Adverse effects occurred in 31% of patients reported at the 250–350 mg dose levels. The toxicities were mainly of mild gastrointestinal character, like diarrhea and nausea. Determination of clinical response was not a study target and was not assessed thoroughly. Peripheral blood blast counts were however analyzed at 24 and 48 hours after treatment and five patients exhibited a large decrease in blast count. Of these five patients, two had an FLT3-ITD mutation [58]. In a phase 1 study, 15 patients with refractory or resistant AML or patients not amenable for conventional therapy were treated with sunitinib in 4-week cycles at the starting dose of 50 mg, followed by 75 mg. In total, 33.3% of the patients were FLT3-mutated. Treatment related side effects were generally of mild character. At the 50 mg treatment regime three patients experienced grade 2 adverse effects. One patient experienced lower limbs edema and fatigue, a second patient experienced taste disturbances and dry skin, and a third patient experienced fatigue, nausea and vomiting, tenesmus, mouth ulcerations, gingivitis, circulation disorders, hematuria, proteinuria and increased creatinine. Both patients treated with 75 mg experienced dose limiting side effects. Forty percent of the patients experienced transitory morphologic or partial responses with reduction of the percentage of leukemic blasts in peripheral blood and bone marrow, including 100% of the patients within the FLT3-mutated group in comparison with 20% of the FLT3 wild-type patients [59].

2.1.7. Tandutinib (MLN-518)

Tandutinib is a piperazinyl quiazoline type III TKI with very limited inhibition of kinases outside this receptor family of FLT3, PDGFR and KIT [77]. In a phase 1 study, 40 patients were given tandutinib orally in doses ranging from 50 mg to 700 mg twice daily. The patients had either AML, or high-risk MDS. The most frequent toxicities associated with tandutinib treatment were nausea and vomiting, less frequent diarrhea and peripheral and periorbital edema. Muscular weakness and fatigue were the dose limiting toxicities, and were observed at dose levels of 525 mg and 700 mg twice daily. One patient experienced hyperreflexia with clonus. Preclinical evaluation of tandutinib suggested that it might prolong the QT interval, and one patient had a 270 ms increase of QT_c on day 28. The QT interval however returned within normal range during continuous dosing. No complete or partial remissions were seen in this study. However, of the five patients with FLT3-ITD mutations that were assessed for treatment efficacy, antileukemic activity was shown in two patients. They both had a greater than 99% decrease in absolute peripheral blast count and a decrease in bone marrow blast percentage from 91% to 62% and 80% to 15% over the first 28 days of treatment. Within two months however they both experienced disease progression. Four patients without FLT3-ITD mutation sustained steady peripheral blood counts and bone marrow blast counts in periods ranging from 154–190 days [60].

2.2. Second Generation TKIs

Quizartinib (AC220)

Quizartinib is unique among FLT3 inhibitors currently in development, in that it combines high potency and high kinase selectivity with favorable pharmacokinetic properties, and it is currently suggested as the most promising FLT3 targeting TKI [78]. It showed promising results already in a phase 1 study [61], and the optimism has remained high until now. In a phase 2 study, quizartinib was administered as monotherapy in 333 relapsed or refractory AML patients. The most frequent experienced treatment-related adverse events were nausea, anemia, QT interval prolongation, vomiting, febrile neutropenia, diarrhea, and fatigue. Quizartinib seemed to reduce blasts in both FLT3-wild-type as well as FLT3-ITD positive patients, though more efficiently in FLT3-ITD positive patients, and the overall clinical response rates were high, however few complete remissions were seen [63,64]. Results from a phase 2 study assessing quizartinib as monotherapy comparing two different dosing scheduled confirm a high degree of antileukemic activity of quizartinib in FLT3-ITD positive AML patients with half of included patients achieving a hematological response, and as many as 33% of patients were successfully bridged to hematological stem cell transplantation [62]. A pilot establishing that quizartinib safely can be combined with chemotherapy demonstrated a 79% complete remission rate in evaluable patients [65]. Quizartinib in combination with cytarabine and etoposide was also assessed in 18 pediatric AML patients, either with relapsed or refractory disease. Eight of the patients were FLT3-ITD positive and of the six assessed four patients achieved complete remission or complete remission with incomplete platelet recovery [66].

3. Discussion

Current clinically established therapy regimes for AML mainly fail to achieve durable responses due to high relapse rates associated with development of drug resistance. Those patients who harbor a constitutively activating FLT3-ITD mutation have particular poor initial therapy response, high relapse rate, and inferior overall survival. Optimism was substantial when the therapeutic principle based on inhibition of FLT3 emerged, and multiple compounds have been developed and tested. Eight of the TKIs investigated in clinical trials have here been presented and the results of their clinical efficacy compared, including the first-generation agents; lestaurtinib, linifanib, midostaurin, semaxanib, sorafenib, sunitinib and tandutinib, as well as the second-generation TKI quizartinib. Though the various compounds diverge in degree of treatment responses as well as character and seriousness of adverse effects, they are generally well tolerated with less toxic effects than conventional chemotherapy provided in high or intermediate dose levels. However, TKIs seems only to induce modest clinical effects, including partial and transient responses, usually only in peripheral blasts.

There may be several reasons for why AML patients with FLT3-ITD mutations do not respond to treatment as anticipated. In the majority of the clinical trials, the treatment with TKIs were limited to patients with relapsed or refractory disease, or to patients not eligible for conventional treatment. The experience from this selected patient group might not be applicable to the group of newly diagnosed or younger AML patients.

In vivo inhibition of FLT3 autophosphorylation seems to be greatly associated with remission rate, and insufficient prolonged inhibitory drug levels might be another reasons for treatment failure [79]. Clinical response occurred in patients who sustained plasma FLT3 inhibitory activity and had an inherent sensitivity of blasts to the cytotoxic effects of lestaurtinib [44]. Several second generation TKIs, in addition to quizartinib, are under development, offering improved pharmacodynamic and pharmacokinetic properties including increased potency and selectivity towards FLT3-mutated cells [80]. VX-322 [81], BPR1J-097 [82], TT-3002 [83,84], AKN-028 and AKN-032 [85,86] are examples of novel FLT3 inhibitors that are showing promising *in vitro* and *in vivo* antileukemia activities.

Many of the compounds tested in clinical trials gave an initial response but of short duration before relapse, indicating development of resistance. Acquired point mutations in the molecular target of FLT3 in response to TKI treatment, precluding the drug from adequate binding appears to be an important mechanism in this process [87,88]. Aberrant activation of alternate growth and viability pathways is yet another possible mechanism for acquired resistance [89–91].

Unexpectedly, it was not so easy to predict who would benefit from the treatment as assumed. Not all FLT3-ITD positive patients responds to TKI therapy, while on the contrary some FLT3 wild-type patients seem to benefit from TKI treatment. Biomarkers predictive of therapy response are warranted. It is suggested that quizartinib does not induce complete remission, but decrease blast numbers with presence of dysplastic changes in the bone marrow [92]. In a small study of quizartinib-treated AML patients examined by mass spectrometric super-SILAC of phospho-protein, the team of Hubert Serve have indicated that a profile of four proteins may determine responders of quizartinib independent of FLT3-ITD [93]. This proposes phophoprotein profiling in prediction of therapy response, and may be transferred to a clinical diagnostics assay format like flow cytometric analysis of intracellular phosphoproteins [94].

Although FLT3 is a well-characterized oncoprotein in AML, and its role as an important player in AML leukemogenesis established, our knowledge of the normal and pathologic FLT3 signaling network may still be inadequate for identification of the most effective therapeutic approach, as there are many aspects of the mutation we do not fully comprehend.

An initial concern in the study of FLT3 in AML was the heterogeneity of the mutations, both the difference between point mutations and ITDs and within the group of ITDs. The mutation can appear in various lengths in the same patient, either simultaneously or over time, and in response to intensive chemotherapy the mutation can appear in previously FLT3-ITD negative patients, it can disappear or dramatically change at relapse [95–99]. The size of the ITD has been reported as a prognostic marker, with patients with a insertion of 48–60 base pairs seems to have worse outcome compared to patients with shorter or longer insertions in one study [100], and with increasing size as a marker for poor outcome in another [101]. High mutational load measured by a high FLT3-ITD/FLT3wt ratio, indicative of loss of heterozygosity, has been associated with inferior outcome [102,103], as well as the site of the ITD insertion, with insertions within the tyrosine kinase domain-1 conferring unfavorable prognosis [104]. Also, the number of FLT3-ITD mutations affects disease outcome [105].

Methodological advances have recently shed further light to the complex interplay of events that contribute to AML leukemogenesis [106]. In addition to formerly well-characterized frequent cytogenetic lesions, next generation sequencing of AML patient material has revealed 23 recurrently mutated genes probable to be involved in AML pathogenesis. Based on patterns of co-occurring and mutually exclusive genetic lesions probable biological co-operations driving disease progression are emerging [19,107]. Additionally, mapping of variant allele frequencies makes it possible to assess the intra-tumor clonal hierarchy, while temporal assessment of leukemic cell populations makes it achievable to determine the clonal evolution and the sequential order of acquisition of somatic mutation during disease development and progression, from pre-leukemic hematopoietic stem cells to AML blasts [108–110]. Accumulating evidence indicate that mutations in the FLT3 gene are disease promoting rather than disease initiating events [111,112], and that mutant FLT3 cooperates with other oncogenes and aberrantly regulated proteins associated with AML, e.g., NPM1, DNMT3A [19], NUP98/NSD1 [113] DEP-1, PML-RAR and AXL [114–116]. The potency of the TKI alone may consequently not be the best measure for the antileukemic effect, and a multi-targeted therapeutic approach may rather be of potential clinical benefit, combining agents targeting cooperative lesions, inhibitors of alternate pathways, or targeting downstream signaling molecules. The superior efficiency of sorafenib compared to other inhibitors supports this theory, as the effect might be a result of sorafenib's ability to suppress the activity of multiple pathways [53]. The pathways that most frequently are activated, PI3K/AKT/mTOR and RAS/RAF/MEK/ERK, may be feasible to target with a combined inhibitor approach. Effective AKT/mTOR inhibitors and MEK/ERK inhibitors are in clinical trials [117,118]. FLT3-ITD is additionally shown to accumulate in the endoplasmic compartment of the cell [119], and may form intracellular signaling protein complexes that represent a different signaling context compared to transmembrane FLT3 signaling [120], that might also be important to take into consideration.

The nature of internal tandem duplication mimic damages in DNA repair caused by anthracyclines [121,122]. Clinical studies with increasing doses of daunorubicin suggested that this dose escalation was not beneficial in FLT3-ITD patients [123]. Additionally, a retrovirally induced mouse leukemia model comprising FLT3-ITD indicated that the FLT3-ITD responded to cytarabine but not anthracycline in a p53 dependent manner [124]. Additionally, excessive receptor tyrosine kinase activity has been associated with increased endogenous DNA damage [125], and FLT3-ITD is associated with high redox activity in the leukemic cells, also related to increased DNA damage [126]. In the discussion of driver and passenger role for FLT3-ITD, it is difficult to neglect the possibility that leukemia with FLT3-ITD may be created through a fundamental genomic instability. This genomic instability may be targeting the FLT3 gene due to structural DNA features through the myelopoiesis when FLT3 expression is modulated as function of differentiation. This predisposition of FLT3-ITD may make these leukemia cells particularly vulnerable for anthracyline therapy, generating more FLT3-ITD mutations when exposed for this topoisomerase II inhibitor. Together, these observations indicate that FLT3-ITD positive patients does not benefit from anthracycline therapy. If this is correct, a dramatic change in current AML therapy needs to be undertaken, since all current induction therapy include anthracycline.

Together, the proven high relapse rate in FLT3-ITD and the emerging speculations in an underlying mutational vulnerability in the FLT3 gene should spur investigators to develop non-genotoxic therapy in particular for FLT3-ITD positive AML patients.

4. Concluding Remarks

A fundamental question that remains unanswered is whether the fairly modest clinical activity of first generation FLT3 inhibitors can be improved through the second generation of TKIs, offering better pharmacodynamic and pharmacokinetic properties, or if the potential benefits of FLT3 inhibitors are essentially inadequate. We are still awaiting results from ongoing clinical trials investigating various combinations of TKIs in different subgroups of AML patients. The preliminary conclusion concerning the agents investigated is that their therapeutic efficiency is limited when administered in monotherapy. It seems like the FLT3 inhibitors currently in clinical trials will have to be used in conjunction with established treatment or in combination with additional targeted therapeutics to ultimately improve outcomes in AML patients with FLT3-ITD mutations. It is also to be decided in which phase of the treatment is should be used; as part of first line induction therapy, as consolidation or post-remission treatment or in a relapse or refractory setting.

If presence of FLT3-ITD is a marker for less effective anthracycline therapy, we will need to perform a difficult switch to alternative induction regimes in these patients. Future trials should explore targeting of downstream FLT3 signaling, particular signaling unique for FLT3-ITD, and with a clear strategy for blocking bypass mechanisms that may cause TKI resistance. These alternative strategies of signal transduction therapy may be tested in future trials incorporating *in vitro* leukemic resistance screens [127,128] determining the value of functional genomics in individualized therapy strategies [126,127].

Acknowledgments: This study was supported by grants from the Norwegian Cancer Society with Solveig and Ove Lund's legacy.

Author Contributions: Caroline Benedicte Nitter Engen performed literature searches and wrote the manuscript. Line Wergeland and Jørn Skavland participated in writing sections of the manuscript. Bjørn Tore Gjertsen conceived, performed literature searches and wrote the manuscript. All authors have edited and approved the final manuscript.

Conflicts of Interest: Bjørn Tore Gjertsen has received consultant honoraria and grant support from Novartis, and received advisory board honoraria from Clavis Pharma AS, Boehringer Ingelheim GmbH, and BerGenBio AS. The remaining authors have no conflicts of interest to declare.

References

1. Sant, M.; Allemani, C.; Tereanu, C.; de Angelis, R.; Capocaccia, R.; Visser, O.; Marcos-Gragera, R.; Maynadie, M.; Simonetti, A.; Lutz, J.M.; *et al.* Incidence of hematologic malignancies in Europe by morphologic subtype: Results of the HAEMACARE project. *Blood* **2010**, *116*, 3724–3734. [CrossRef] [PubMed]
2. Smith, A.; Howell, D.; Patmore, R.; Jack, A.; Roman, E. Incidence of haematological malignancy by sub-type: A report from the Haematological Malignancy Research Network. *Br. J. Cancer* **2011**, *105*, 1684–1692. [CrossRef] [PubMed]
3. Estey, E.; Dohner, H. Acute myeloid leukaemia. *Lancet* **2006**, *368*, 1894–1907. [CrossRef] [PubMed]
4. Roboz, G.J. Current treatment of acute myeloid leukemia. *Curr. Opin. Oncol.* **2012**, *24*, 711–719. [CrossRef] [PubMed]
5. Dombret, H. Optimal acute myeloid leukemia therapy in 2012. *Hematol. Educ.: Educ. Program Annu. Congr. Eur. Hematol. Assoc.* **2012**, *6*, 41–48.
6. Estey, E.H. Acute myeloid leukemia: 2013 update on risk-stratification and management. *Am. J. Hematol.* **2013**, *88*, 318–327. [CrossRef] [PubMed]
7. Patel, J.P.; Gonen, M.; Figueroa, M.E.; Fernandez, H.; Sun, Z.; Racevskis, J.; van Vlierberghe, P.; Dolgalev, I.; Thomas, S.; Aminova, O.; *et al.* Prognostic relevance of integrated genetic profiling in acute myeloid leukemia. *N. Engl. J. Med.* **2012**, *366*, 1079–1089. [CrossRef] [PubMed]
8. Schlenk, R.F.; Dohner, K.; Krauter, J.; Frohling, S.; Corbacioglu, A.; Bullinger, L.; Habdank, M.; Spath, D.; Morgan, M.; Benner, A.; *et al.* Mutations and treatment outcome in cytogenetically normal acute myeloid leukemia. *N. Engl. J. Med.* **2008**, *358*, 1909–1918. [CrossRef] [PubMed]
9. Foran, J.M. New prognostic markers in acute myeloid leukemia: Perspective from the clinic. *Hematol. Am. Soc. Hematol. Educ. Program.* **2010**, *2010*, 47–55. [CrossRef]

10. Marcucci, G.; Haferlach, T.; Dohner, H. Molecular genetics of adult acute myeloid leukemia: Prognostic and therapeutic implications. *J. Clin. Oncol.* **2011**, *29*, 475–486. [CrossRef] [PubMed]
11. Dohner, H.; Estey, E.H.; Amadori, S.; Appelbaum, F.R.; Buchner, T.; Burnett, A.K.; Dombret, H.; Fenaux, P.; Grimwade, D.; Larson, R.A.; *et al.* Diagnosis and management of acute myeloid leukemia in adults: Recommendations from an international expert panel, on behalf of the European LeukemiaNet. *Blood* **2010**, *115*, 453–474. [CrossRef] [PubMed]
12. Grimwade, D. The clinical significance of cytogenetic abnormalities in acute myeloid leukaemia. *Best Pract. Res. Clin. Haematol.* **2001**, *14*, 497–529. [CrossRef] [PubMed]
13. Grimwade, D.; Hills, R.K.; Moorman, A.V.; Walker, H.; Chatters, S.; Goldstone, A.H.; Wheatley, K.; Harrison, C.J.; Burnett, A.K.; National Cancer Research Institute Adult Leukaemia Working Group. Refinement of cytogenetic classification in acute myeloid leukemia: Determination of prognostic significance of rare recurring chromosomal abnormalities among 5876 younger adult patients treated in the United Kingdom Medical Research Council trials. *Blood* **2010**, *116*, 354–365. [CrossRef] [PubMed]
14. Port, M.; Bottcher, M.; Thol, F.; Ganser, A.; Schlenk, R.; Wasem, J.; Neumann, A.; Pouryamout, L. Prognostic significance of FLT3 internal tandem duplication, nucleophosmin 1, and CEBPA gene mutations for acute myeloid leukemia patients with normal karyotype and younger than 60 years: A systematic review and meta-analysis. *Ann. Hematol.* **2014**, *93*, 1279–1286. [CrossRef] [PubMed]
15. Gutierrez, S.E.; Romero-Oliva, F.A. Epigenetic changes: A common theme in acute myelogenous leukemogenesis. *J. Hematol. Oncol.* **2013**, *6*, 57. [CrossRef] [PubMed]
16. Shivarov, V.; Bullinger, L. Expression profiling of leukemia patients: Key lessons and future directions. *Exp. Hematol.* **2014**, *42*, 651–660. [CrossRef] [PubMed]
17. Raaijmakers, M.H. Niche contributions to oncogenesis: Emerging concepts and implications for the hematopoietic system. *Haematologica* **2011**, *96*, 1041–1048. [CrossRef] [PubMed]
18. Whichard, Z.L.; Sarkar, C.A.; Kimmel, M.; Corey, S.J. Hematopoiesis and its disorders: A systems biology approach. *Blood* **2010**, *115*, 2339–2347. [CrossRef] [PubMed]
19. The Cancer Genome Atlas Research Network. Genomic and epigenomic landscapes of adult *de novo* acute myeloid leukemia. *N. Engl. J. Med.* **2013**, *368*, 2059–2074.
20. Deininger, M.; Buchdunger, E.; Druker, B.J. The development of imatinib as a therapeutic agent for chronic myeloid leukemia. *Blood* **2005**, *105*, 2640–2653. [CrossRef] [PubMed]
21. Daver, N.; Cortes, J. Molecular targeted therapy in acute myeloid leukemia. *Hematology* **2012**, *17* (Suppl 1), 59–62. [PubMed]
22. Nakao, M.; Yokota, S.; Iwai, T.; Kaneko, H.; Horiike, S.; Kashima, K.; Sonoda, Y.; Fujimoto, T.; Misawa, S. Internal tandem duplication of the flt3 gene found in acute myeloid leukemia. *Leukemia* **1996**, *10*, 1911–1918. [PubMed]
23. Matsuno, N.; Nanri, T.; Kawakita, T.; Mitsuya, H.; Asou, N. A novel FLT3 activation loop mutation N841K in acute myeloblastic leukemia. *Leukemia* **2005**, *19*, 480–481. [CrossRef] [PubMed]
24. Yamamoto, Y.; Kiyoi, H.; Nakano, Y.; Suzuki, R.; Kodera, Y.; Miyawaki, S.; Asou, N.; Kuriyama, K.; Yagasaki, F.; Shimazaki, C.; *et al.* Activating mutation of D835 within the activation loop of FLT3 in human hematologic malignancies. *Blood* **2001**, *97*, 2434–2439. [CrossRef] [PubMed]
25. Brasel, K.; Escobar, S.; Anderberg, R.; de Vries, P.; Gruss, H.J.; Lyman, S.D. Expression of the flt3 receptor and its ligand on hematopoietic cells. *Leukemia* **1995**, *9*, 1212–1218. [PubMed]
26. Piacibello, W.; Fubini, L.; Sanavio, F.; Brizzi, M.F.; Severino, A.; Garetto, L.; Stacchini, A.; Pegoraro, L.; Aglietta, M. Effects of human FLT3 ligand on myeloid leukemia cell growth: Heterogeneity in response and synergy with other hematopoietic growth factors. *Blood* **1995**, *86*, 4105–4114. [PubMed]
27. Drexler, H.G.; Quentmeier, H. FLT3: Receptor and ligand. *Growth Factors* **2004**, *22*, 71–73. [CrossRef] [PubMed]
28. Gotze, K.S.; Ramirez, M.; Tabor, K.; Small, D.; Matthews, W.; Civin, C.I. Flt3high and Flt3low CD34+ progenitor cells isolated from human bone marrow are functionally distinct. *Blood* **1998**, *91*, 1947–1958. [PubMed]
29. Birg, F.; Courcoul, M.; Rosnet, O.; Bardin, F.; Pebusque, M.J.; Marchetto, S.; Tabilio, A.; Mannoni, P.; Birnbaum, D. Expression of the FMS/KIT-like gene FLT3 in human acute leukemias of the myeloid and lymphoid lineages. *Blood* **1992**, *80*, 2584–2593. [PubMed]

30.   Carow, C.E.; Levenstein, M.; Kaufmann, S.H.; Chen, J.; Amin, S.; Rockwell, P.; Witte, L.; Borowitz, M.J.; Civin, C.I.; Small, D. Expression of the hematopoietic growth factor receptor FLT3 (STK-1/Flk2) in human leukemias. *Blood* **1996**, *87*, 1089–1096. [PubMed]

31.   Ozeki, K.; Kiyoi, H.; Hirose, Y.; Iwai, M.; Ninomiya, M.; Kodera, Y.; Miyawaki, S.; Kuriyama, K.; Shimazaki, C.; Akiyama, H.; *et al.* Biologic and clinical significance of the FLT3 transcript level in acute myeloid leukemia. *Blood* **2004**, *103*, 1901–1908. [CrossRef] [PubMed]

32.   Kiyoi, H.; Naoe, T.; Nakano, Y.; Yokota, S.; Minami, S.; Miyawaki, S.; Asou, N.; Kuriyama, K.; Jinnai, I.; Shimazaki, C.; *et al.* Prognostic implication of FLT3 and N-RAS gene mutations in acute myeloid leukemia. *Blood* **1999**, *93*, 3074–3080. [PubMed]

33.   Abu-Duhier, F.M.; Goodeve, A.C.; Wilson, G.A.; Gari, M.A.; Peake, I.R.; Rees, D.C.; Vandenberghe, E.A.; Winship, P.R.; Reilly, J.T. FLT3 internal tandem duplication mutations in adult acute myeloid leukaemia define a high-risk group. *Br. J. Haematol.* **2000**, *111*, 190–195. [CrossRef] [PubMed]

34.   Kottaridis, P.D.; Gale, R.E.; Frew, M.E.; Harrison, G.; Langabeer, S.E.; Belton, A.A.; Walker, H.; Wheatley, K.; Bowen, D.T.; Burnett, A.K.; *et al.* The presence of a FLT3 internal tandem duplication in patients with acute myeloid leukemia (AML) adds important prognostic information to cytogenetic risk group and response to the first cycle of chemotherapy: Analysis of 854 patients from the United Kingdom Medical Research Council AML 10 and 12 trials. *Blood* **2001**, *98*, 1752–1759. [CrossRef] [PubMed]

35.   Vardiman, J.W.; Thiele, J.; Arber, D.A.; Brunning, R.D.; Borowitz, M.J.; Porwit, A.; Harris, N.L.; le Beau, M.M.; Hellstrom-Lindberg, E.; Tefferi, A.; *et al.* The 2008 revision of the World Health Organization (WHO) classification of myeloid neoplasms and acute leukemia: Rationale and important changes. *Blood* **2009**, *114*, 937–951. [CrossRef] [PubMed]

36.   Kiyoi, H.; Towatari, M.; Yokota, S.; Hamaguchi, M.; Ohno, R.; Saito, H.; Naoe, T. Internal tandem duplication of the FLT3 gene is a novel modality of elongation mutation which causes constitutive activation of the product. *Leukemia* **1998**, *12*, 1333–1337. [CrossRef] [PubMed]

37.   Kornblau, S.M.; Womble, M.; Qiu, Y.H.; Jackson, C.E.; Chen, W.; Konopleva, M.; Estey, E.H.; Andreeff, M. Simultaneous activation of multiple signal transduction pathways confers poor prognosis in acute myelogenous leukemia. *Blood* **2006**, *108*, 2358–2365. [CrossRef] [PubMed]

38.   Toffalini, F.; Demoulin, J.B. New insights into the mechanisms of hematopoietic cell transformation by activated receptor tyrosine kinases. *Blood* **2010**, *116*, 2429–2437. [CrossRef] [PubMed]

39.   Choudhary, C.; Brandts, C.; Schwable, J.; Tickenbrock, L.; Sargin, B.; Ueker, A.; Bohmer, F.D.; Berdel, W.E.; Muller-Tidow, C.; Serve, H. Activation mechanisms of STAT5 by oncogenic Flt3-ITD. *Blood* **2007**, *110*, 370–374. [CrossRef] [PubMed]

40.   Tse, K.F.; Novelli, E.; Civin, C.I.; Bohmer, F.D.; Small, D. Inhibition of FLT3-mediated transformation by use of a tyrosine kinase inhibitor. *Leukemia* **2001**, *15*, 1001–1010. [CrossRef] [PubMed]

41.   Levis, M.; Tse, K.F.; Smith, B.D.; Garrett, E.; Small, D. A FLT3 tyrosine kinase inhibitor is selectively cytotoxic to acute myeloid leukemia blasts harboring FLT3 internal tandem duplication mutations. *Blood* **2001**, *98*, 885–887. [CrossRef] [PubMed]

42.   Levis, M.; Allebach, J.; Tse, K.F.; Zheng, R.; Baldwin, B.R.; Smith, B.D.; Jones-Bolin, S.; Ruggeri, B.; Dionne, C.; Small, D. A FLT3-targeted tyrosine kinase inhibitor is cytotoxic to leukemia cells *in vitro* and *in vivo*. *Blood* **2002**, *99*, 3885–3891. [CrossRef] [PubMed]

43.   Smith, B.D.; Levis, M.; Beran, M.; Giles, F.; Kantarjian, H.; Berg, K.; Murphy, K.M.; Dauses, T.; Allebach, J.; Small, D. Single-agent CEP-701, a novel FLT3 inhibitor, shows biologic and clinical activity in patients with relapsed or refractory acute myeloid leukemia. *Blood* **2004**, *103*, 3669–3676. [CrossRef] [PubMed]

44.   Knapper, S.; Burnett, A.K.; Littlewood, T.; Kell, W.J.; Agrawal, S.; Chopra, R.; Clark, R.; Levis, M.J.; Small, D. A phase 2 trial of the FLT3 inhibitor lestaurtinib (CEP701) as first-line treatment for older patients with acute myeloid leukemia not considered fit for intensive chemotherapy. *Blood* **2006**, *108*, 3262–3270. [CrossRef] [PubMed]

45.   Levis, M.; Ravandi, F.; Wang, E.S.; Baer, M.R.; Perl, A.; Coutre, S.; Erba, H.; Stuart, R.K.; Baccarani, M.; Cripe, L.D.; *et al.* Results from a randomized trial of salvage chemotherapy followed by lestaurtinib for patients with FLT3 mutant AML in first relapse. *Blood* **2011**, *117*, 3294–3301. [CrossRef] [PubMed]

46.   Wang, E.S.; Yee, K.; Koh, L.P.; Hogge, D.; Enschede, S.; Carlson, D.M.; Dudley, M.; Glaser, K.; McKeegan, E.; Albert, D.H.; *et al.* Phase 1 trial of linifanib (ABT-869) in patients with refractory or relapsed acute myeloid leukemia. *Leuk Lymphoma* **2012**, *53*, 1543–1551. [CrossRef] [PubMed]

47. Stone, R.M.; DeAngelo, D.J.; Klimek, V.; Galinsky, I.; Estey, E.; Nimer, S.D.; Grandin, W.; Lebwohl, D.; Wang, Y.; Cohen, P.; *et al.* Patients with acute myeloid leukemia and an activating mutation in FLT3 respond to a small-molecule FLT3 tyrosine kinase inhibitor, PKC412. *Blood* **2005**, *105*, 54–60. [CrossRef] [PubMed]
48. Fischer, T.; Stone, R.M.; Deangelo, D.J.; Galinsky, I.; Estey, E.; Lanza, C.; Fox, E.; Ehninger, G.; Feldman, E.J.; Schiller, G.J.; *et al.* Phase IIB trial of oral Midostaurin (PKC412), the FMS-like tyrosine kinase 3 receptor (FLT3) and multi-targeted kinase inhibitor, in patients with acute myeloid leukemia and high-risk myelodysplastic syndrome with either wild-type or mutated FLT3. *J. Clin. Oncol.* **2010**, *28*, 4339–4345. [CrossRef] [PubMed]
49. Stone, R.M.; Fischer, T.; Paquette, R.; Schiller, G.; Schiffer, C.A.; Ehninger, G.; Cortes, J.; Kantarjian, H.M.; DeAngelo, D.J.; Huntsman-Labed, A.; *et al.* Phase IB study of the FLT3 kinase inhibitor midostaurin with chemotherapy in younger newly diagnosed adult patients with acute myeloid leukemia. *Leukemia* **2012**, *26*, 2061–2068. [CrossRef] [PubMed]
50. O'Farrell, A.M.; Yuen, H.A.; Smolich, B.; Hannah, A.L.; Louie, S.G.; Hong, W.; Stopeck, A.T.; Silverman, L.R.; Lancet, J.E.; Karp, J.E.; *et al.* Effects of SU5416, a small molecule tyrosine kinase receptor inhibitor, on FLT3 expression and phosphorylation in patients with refractory acute myeloid leukemia. *Leuk. Res.* **2004**, *28*, 679–689. [CrossRef] [PubMed]
51. Fiedler, W.; Mesters, R.; Tinnefeld, H.; Loges, S.; Staib, P.; Duhrsen, U.; Flasshove, M.; Ottmann, O.G.; Jung, W.; Cavalli, F.; *et al.* A phase 2 clinical study of SU5416 in patients with refractory acute myeloid leukemia. *Blood* **2003**, *102*, 2763–2767. [CrossRef] [PubMed]
52. Giles, F.J.; Stopeck, A.T.; Silverman, L.R.; Lancet, J.E.; Cooper, M.A.; Hannah, A.L.; Cherrington, J.M.; O'Farrell, A.M.; Yuen, H.A.; Louie, S.G.; *et al.* SU5416, a small molecule tyrosine kinase receptor inhibitor, has biologic activity in patients with refractory acute myeloid leukemia or myelodysplastic syndromes. *Blood* **2003**, *102*, 795–801. [CrossRef] [PubMed]
53. Zhang, W.; Konopleva, M.; Shi, Y.X.; McQueen, T.; Harris, D.; Ling, X.; Estrov, Z.; Quintas-Cardama, A.; Small, D.; Cortes, J.; *et al.* Mutant FLT3: A direct target of sorafenib in acute myelogenous leukemia. *J. Natl. Cancer Inst.* **2008**, *100*, 184–198. [CrossRef] [PubMed]
54. Crump, M.; Hedley, D.; Kamel-Reid, S.; Leber, B.; Wells, R.; Brandwein, J.; Buckstein, R.; Kassis, J.; Minden, M.; Matthews, J.; *et al.* A randomized phase I clinical and biologic study of two schedules of sorafenib in patients with myelodysplastic syndrome or acute myeloid leukemia: A NCIC (National Cancer Institute of Canada) Clinical Trials Group Study. *Leuk. Lymphoma* **2010**, *51*, 252–260. [CrossRef] [PubMed]
55. Serve, H.; Krug, U.; Wagner, R.; Sauerland, M.C.; Heinecke, A.; Brunnberg, U.; Schaich, M.; Ottmann, O.; Duyster, J.; Wandt, H.; *et al.* Sorafenib in combination with intensive chemotherapy in elderly patients with acute myeloid leukemia: Results from a randomized, placebo-controlled trial. *J. Clin. Oncol.* **2013**, *31*, 3110–3118. [CrossRef] [PubMed]
56. Inaba, H.; Rubnitz, J.F.; Coustan-Smith, E.; Li, L.; Furmanski, B.D.; Mascara, G.P.; Heym, K.M.; Christensen, R.; Onciu, M.; Shurtleff, S.A.; *et al.* Phase I pharmacokinetic and pharmacodynamic study of the multikinase inhibitor sorafenib in combination with clofarabine and cytarabine in pediatric relapsed/refractory leukemia. *J. Clin. Oncol.* **2011**, *29*, 3293–3300. [CrossRef] [PubMed]
57. Ravandi, F.; Alattar, M.L.; Grunwald, M.R.; Rudek, M.A.; Rajkhowa, T.; Richie, M.A.; Pierce, S.; Daver, N.; Garcia-Manero, G.; Faderl, S.; *et al.* Phase 2 study of azacytidine plus sorafenib in patients with acute myeloid leukemia and FLT-3 internal tandem duplication mutation. *Blood* **2013**, *121*, 4655–4662. [CrossRef] [PubMed]
58. O'Farrell, A.M.; Foran, J.M.; Fiedler, W.; Serve, H.; Paquette, R.L.; Cooper, M.A.; Yuen, H.A.; Louie, S.G.; Kim, H.; Nicholas, S.; et al. An innovative phase I clinical study demonstrates inhibition of FLT3 phosphorylation by SU11248 in acute myeloid leukemia patients. *Clin. Cancer Res.* **2003**, *9*, 5465–5476. [PubMed]
59. Fiedler, W.; Serve, H.; Dohner, H.; Schwittay, M.; Ottmann, O.G.; O'Farrell, A.M.; Bello, C.L.; Allred, R.; Manning, W.C.; Cherrington, J.M.; *et al.* A phase 1 study of SU11248 in the treatment of patients with refractory or resistant acute myeloid leukemia (AML) or not amenable to conventional therapy for the disease. *Blood* **2005**, *105*, 986–993. [CrossRef] [PubMed]
60. DeAngelo, D.J.; Stone, R.M.; Heaney, M.L.; Nimer, S.D.; Paquette, R.L.; Klisovic, R.B.; Caligiuri, M.A.; Cooper, M.R.; Lecerf, J.M.; Karol, M.D.; *et al.* Phase 1 clinical results with tandutinib (MLN518), a novel FLT3 antagonist, in patients with acute myelogenous leukemia or high-risk myelodysplastic syndrome: Safety, pharmacokinetics, and pharmacodynamics. *Blood* **2006**, *108*, 3674–3681. [CrossRef] [PubMed]

61. Cortes, J.; Foran, J.; Ghirdaladze, D.; DeVetten, M.P.; Zodelava, M.; Holman, P.; Levis, M.J.; Kantarjian, H.M.; Borthakur, G.; James, J.; *et al.* AC220, a Potent, Selective, Second Generation FLT3 Receptor Tyrosine Kinase (RTK) Inhibitor, in a First-in-Human (FIH) Phase 1 AML Study. *Blood (ASH Annual Meeting Abstracts)* **2009**, *114*, 636.

62. Cortes, J.E.; Tallman, M.S.; Schiller, G.; Trone, D.; Gammon, G.; Goldberg, S.; Perl, A.E.; Marie, J.P.; Martelli, G.; Levis, M. Results of a Phase 2 Randomized, Open-Label, Study of Lower Doses of Quizartinib (AC220; ASP2689) in Subjects With FLT3-ITD Positive Relapsed or Refractory Acute Myeloid Leukemia (AML). *Blood (ASH Annual Meeting Abstracts)* **2013**, *122*, 494.

63. Levis, M.J.; Perl, A.E.; Dombret, H.; Döhner, H.; Steffen, B.; Rousselot, P.; Martinelli, G.; Estey, E.H.; Burnett, A.K.; Gammon, G.; *et al.* Final Results of a Phase 2 Open-Label, Monotherapy Efficacy and Safety Study of Quizartinib (AC220) in Patients with FLT3-ITD Positive or Negative Relapsed/Refractory Acute Myeloid Leukemia After Second-Line Chemotherapy or Hematopoietic Stem Cell Transplantation. *Blood (ASH Annual Meeting Abstracts)* **2012**, *120*, 673.

64. Cortes, J.E.; Perl, A.E.; Dombret, H.; Kayser, S.; Steffen, B.; Rousselot, P.; Martinelli, G.; Estey, E.H.; Burnett, A.K.; Gammon, G.; *et al.* Final Results of a Phase 2 Open-Label, Monotherapy Efficacy and Safety Study of Quizartinib (AC220) in Patients 60 Years of Age with FLT3 ITD Positive or Negative Relapsed/Refractory Acute Myeloid Leukemia. *Blood (ASH Annual Meeting Abstracts)* **2012**, *120*, 46.

65. Burnett, A.K.; Bowen, D.; Russell, N.; Knapper, S.; Milligan, D.; Hunter, A.E.; Khwaja, A.; Clark, R.E.; Culligan, D.; Clark, H.; *et al.* AC220 (Quizartinib) Can be Safely Combined with Conventional Chemotherapy in Older Patients with Newly Diagnosed Acute Myeloid Leukaemia: Experience from the AML18 Pilot Trial. *Blood* **2013**, *122*, 622. [CrossRef]

66. Cooper, T.M.; Malvar, J.; Cassar, J.; Eckroth, E.; Sposto, R.; Gaynon, P.; Dubois, S.; Gore, L.; Macy, M.E.; August, K. A Phase I Study of AC220 (Quizartinib) in Combination with Cytarabine and Etoposide in Relapsed/Refractory Childhood ALL and AML: A Therapeutic Advances in Childhood Leukemia & Lymphoma (TACL) Study. *Blood* **2013**, *122*, 624. [CrossRef] [PubMed]

67. Shankar, D.B.; Li, J.; Tapang, P.; Owen McCall, J.; Pease, L.J.; Dai, Y.; Wei, R.Q.; Albert, D.H.; Bouska, J.J.; Osterling, D.J.; *et al.* ABT-869, a multitargeted receptor tyrosine kinase inhibitor: Inhibition of FLT3 phosphorylation and signaling in acute myeloid leukemia. *Blood* **2007**, *109*, 3400–3408. [CrossRef] [PubMed]

68. Weisberg, E.; Boulton, C.; Kelly, L.M.; Manley, P.; Fabbro, D.; Meyer, T.; Gilliland, D.G.; Griffin, J.D. Inhibition of mutant FLT3 receptors in leukemia cells by the small molecule tyrosine kinase inhibitor PKC412. *Cancer Cell* **2002**, *1*, 433–443. [CrossRef] [PubMed]

69. Stone, R.M.; de Angelo, J.; Galinsky, I.; Estey, E.; Klimek, V.; Grandin, W.; Lebwohl, D.; Yap, A.; Cohen, P.; Fox, E.; *et al.* PKC 412 FLT3 inhibitor therapy in AML: Results of a phase II trial. *Ann. Hematol.* **2004**, *83* (Suppl 1), 89–90.

70. Strati, P.; Kantarjian, H.M.; Nazha, A.; Borthakur, G.; Daver, N.G.; Kadia, T.M.; Estrov, Z.; Garcia-Manero, G.; Rajkhowa, T.; Ravandi, F.; *et al.* Early Results of a Phase I/II Trial of Midostaurin (PKC412) and 5-Azacytidine (5-AZA) for Patients (Pts) with Acute Myeloid Leukemia and Myelodysplastic Syndrome. *Blood (ASH Annual Meeting Abstracts)* **2013**, *122*, 3949.

71. Walker, A.R.; Wang, H.; Klisovic, R.; Walsh, K.; Vasu, S.; Garzon, R.; Devine, S.M.; Drake, A.; Blum, W.; Marcucci, G. Phase I Study of The Combination of Midostaurin, Bortezomib and Chemotherapy in Relapsed/Refractory Acute Myeloid Leukemia (AML): Targeting Aberrant Tyrosine Kinase Activity. *Blood (ASH Annual Meeting Abstracts)* **2013**, *122*, 3966.

72. Yee, K.W.; O'Farrell, A.M.; Smolich, B.D.; Cherrington, J.M.; McMahon, G.; Wait, C.L.; McGreevey, L.S.; Griffith, D.J.; Heinrich, M.C. SU5416 and SU5614 inhibit kinase activity of wild-type and mutant FLT3 receptor tyrosine kinase. *Blood* **2002**, *100*, 2941–2949. [CrossRef] [PubMed]

73. Auclair, D.; Miller, D.; Yatsula, V.; Pickett, W.; Carter, C.; Chang, Y.; Zhang, X.; Wilkie, D.; Burd, A.; Shi, H.; *et al.* Antitumor activity of sorafenib in FLT3-driven leukemic cells. *Leukemia* **2007**, *21*, 439–445. [CrossRef] [PubMed]

74. Uy, G.L.; Sandford, B.; Marcucci, G.; Zhao, W.; Geyer, S.; Keplin, H.; Powell, B.L.; Baer, M.R.; Stock, W.; Stone, R.; *et al.* Initial Results of a Phase II Trial of Sorafenib Plus Standard Induction in Older Adults With Mutant FLT3 Acute Myeloid Leukemia (AML) (Alliance trial C11001). *Blood (ASH Annual Meeting Abstracts)* **2013**, *122*, 2653.

75. Pollard, J.; Chang, B.H.; Cooper, T.M.; Gross, T.; Gupta, S.; Ho, P.A.; McGlodrick, S.M.; Watt, T.C. Sorafenib Treatment Following Hematopoietic Stem Cell Transplant in Pediatric FLT3/ITD+ AML. *Blood* **2013**, *122*, 3969.

76. O'Farrell, A.M.; Abrams, T.J.; Yuen, H.A.; Ngai, T.J.; Louie, S.G.; Yee, K.W.; Wong, L.M.; Hong, W.; Lee, L.B.; Town, A.; *et al.* SU11248 is a novel FLT3 tyrosine kinase inhibitor with potent activity *in vitro* and *in vivo*. *Blood* **2003**, *101*, 3597–3605. [CrossRef] [PubMed]

77. Griswold, I.J.; Shen, L.J.; la Rosee, P.; Demehri, S.; Heinrich, M.C.; Braziel, R.M.; McGreevey, L.; Haley, A.D.; Giese, N.; Druker, B.J.; *et al.* Effects of MLN518, a dual FLT3 and KIT inhibitor, on normal and malignant hematopoiesis. *Blood* **2004**, *104*, 2912–2918. [CrossRef] [PubMed]

78. Zarrinkar, P.P.; Gunawardane, R.N.; Cramer, M.D.; Gardner, M.F.; Brigham, D.; Belli, B.; Karaman, M.W.; Pratz, K.W.; Pallares, G.; Chao, Q.; *et al.* AC220 is a uniquely potent and selective inhibitor of FLT3 for the treatment of acute myeloid leukemia (AML). *Blood* **2009**, *114*, 2984–2992. [CrossRef] [PubMed]

79. Levis, M.; Brown, P.; Smith, B.D.; Stine, A.; Pham, R.; Stone, R.; Deangelo, D.; Galinsky, I.; Giles, F.; Estey, E.; *et al.* Plasma inhibitory activity (PIA): A pharmacodynamic assay reveals insights into the basis for cytotoxic response to FLT3 inhibitors. *Blood* **2006**, *108*, 3477–3483. [CrossRef]

80. Weisberg, E.; Sattler, M.; Ray, A.; Griffin, J.D. Drug resistance in mutant FLT3-positive AML. *Oncogene* **2010**, *29*, 5120–5134. [CrossRef] [PubMed]

81. Heidary, D.K.; Huang, G.; Boucher, D.; Ma, J.; Forster, C.; Grey, R.; Xu, J.; Arnost, M.; Choquette, D.; Chen, G.; *et al.* VX-322: A novel dual receptor tyrosine kinase inhibitor for the treatment of acute myelogenous leukemia. *J. Med. Chem.* **2012**, *55*, 725–734. [CrossRef] [PubMed]

82. Lin, W.H.; Jiaang, W.T.; Chen, C.W.; Yen, K.J.; Hsieh, S.Y.; Yen, S.C.; Chen, C.P.; Chang, K.Y.; Chang, C.Y.; Chang, T.Y.; *et al.* BPR1J-097, a novel FLT3 kinase inhibitor, exerts potent inhibitory activity against AML. *Br. J. Cancer* **2012**, *106*, 475–481. [CrossRef] [PubMed]

83. Ma, H.S.; Nguyen, B.; Duffield, A.S.; Li, L.; Galanis, A.; Williams, A.B.; Brown, P.A.; Levis, M.J.; Leahy, D.J.; Small, D. FLT3 Kinase Inhibitor TTT-3002 Overcomes both Activating and Drug Resistance Mutations in FLT3 in Acute Myeloid Leukemia. *Cancer Res.* **2014**, *74*, 5206–5217. [CrossRef] [PubMed]

84. Ma, H.; Nguyen, B.; Li, L.; Greenblatt, S.; Williams, A.; Zhao, M.; Levis, M.; Rudek, M.; Duffield, A.; Small, D. TTT-3002 is a novel FLT3 tyrosine kinase inhibitor with activity against FLT3-associated leukemias *in vitro* and *in vivo*. *Blood* **2014**, *123*, 1525–1534. [CrossRef] [PubMed]

85. Eriksson, A.; Hoglund, M.; Lindhagen, E.; Aleskog, A.; Hassan, S.B.; Ekholm, C.; Fholenhag, K.; Jensen, A.J.; Lothgren, A.; Scobie, M.; *et al.* Identification of AKN-032, a novel 2-aminopyrazine tyrosine kinase inhibitor, with significant preclinical activity in acute myeloid leukemia. *Biochem. Pharmacol.* **2010**, *80*, 1507–1516. [CrossRef]

86. Eriksson, A.; Hermanson, M.; Wickstrom, M.; Lindhagen, E.; Ekholm, C.; Jenmalm Jensen, A.; Lothgren, A.; Lehmann, F.; Larsson, R.; Parrow, V.; *et al.* The novel tyrosine kinase inhibitor AKN-028 has significant antileukemic activity in cell lines and primary cultures of acute myeloid leukemia. *Blood Cancer J.* **2012**, *2*, e81. [CrossRef] [PubMed]

87. Alvarado, Y.; Kantarjian, H.M.; Luthra, R.; Ravandi, F.; Borthakur, G.; Garcia-Manero, G.; Konopleva, M.; Estrov, Z.; Andreeff, M.; Cortes, J.E. Treatment with FLT3 inhibitor in patients with FLT3-mutated acute myeloid leukemia is associated with development of secondary FLT3-tyrosine kinase domain mutations. *Cancer* **2014**, *120*, 2142–2149. [CrossRef] [PubMed]

88. Albers, C.; Leischner, H.; Verbeek, M.; Yu, C.; Illert, A.L.; Peschel, C.; von Bubnoff, N.; Duyster, J. The secondary FLT3-ITD F691L mutation induces resistance to AC220 in FLT3-ITD(+) AML but retains *in vitro* sensitivity to PKC412 and Sunitinib. *Leukemia* **2013**. [CrossRef]

89. Knapper, S.; Mills, K.I.; Gilkes, A.F.; Austin, S.J.; Walsh, V.; Burnett, A.K. The effects of lestaurtinib (CEP701) and PKC412 on primary AML blasts: The induction of cytotoxicity varies with dependence on FLT3 signaling in both FLT3-mutated and wild-type cases. *Blood* **2006**, *108*, 3494–3503. [CrossRef] [PubMed]

90. Siendones, E.; Barbarroja, N.; Torres, L.A.; Buendia, P.; Velasco, F.; Dorado, G.; Torres, A.; Lopez-Pedrera, C. Inhibition of Flt3-activating mutations does not prevent constitutive activation of ERK/Akt/STAT pathways in some AML cells: A possible cause for the limited effectiveness of monotherapy with small-molecule inhibitors. *Hematol. Oncol.* **2007**, *25*, 30–37. [CrossRef] [PubMed]

91. Piloto, O.; Wright, M.; Brown, P.; Kim, K.T.; Levis, M.; Small, D. Prolonged exposure to FLT3 inhibitors leads to resistance via activation of parallel signaling pathways. *Blood* **2007**, *109*, 1643–1652. [CrossRef]

92. Nybakken, G.E.; Watt, C.; Morrissette, J.J.D.; Bagg, A.; Carroll, M.; Perl, A.E. Diverse Histopathologic and Molecular Responses of Acute Myeloid Leukemia to the FLT3 Inhibitor Quizartinib (AC220). *Blood (ASH Annual Meeting Abstracts)* **2012**, *120*, 885.

93. Schaab, C.; Oppermann, F.; Pfeifer, H.; Klammer, M.; Tebbe, A.; Oellerich, T.; Krauter, J.; Levis, M.J.; Perl, A.E.; Daub, H.; *et al.* Global Phosphoproteome Analysis of AML Bone Marrow Reveals Predictive Markers for the Treatment with AC220. *Blood (ASH Annual Meeting Abstracts)* **2012**, *120*, 786.

94. Skavland, J.; Jorgensen, K.M.; Hadziavdic, K.; Hovland, R.; Jonassen, I.; Bruserud, O.; Gjertsen, B.T. Specific cellular signal-transduction responses to *in vivo* combination therapy with ATRA, valproic acid and theophylline in acute myeloid leukemia. *Blood Cancer J.* **2011**, *1*, e4. [CrossRef] [PubMed]

95. Hovland, R.; Gjertsen, B.T.; Bruserud, O. Acute myelogenous leukemia with internal tandem duplication of the Flt3 gene appearing or altering at the time of relapse: A report of two cases. *Leuk Lymphoma* **2002**, *43*, 2027–2029. [CrossRef] [PubMed]

96. Nazha, A.; Cortes, J.; Faderl, S.; Pierce, S.; Daver, N.; Kadia, T.; Borthakur, G.; Luthra, R.; Kantarjian, H.; Ravandi, F. Activating internal tandem duplication mutations of the fms-like tyrosine kinase-3 (FLT3-ITD) at complete response and relapse in patients with acute myeloid leukemia. *Haematologica* **2012**, *97*, 1242–1245. [CrossRef] [PubMed]

97. Nakano, Y.; Kiyoi, H.; Miyawaki, S.; Asou, N.; Ohno, R.; Saito, H.; Naoe, T. Molecular evolution of acute myeloid leukaemia in relapse: Unstable N-ras and FLT3 genes compared with p53 gene. *Br. J. Haematol.* **1999**, *104*, 659–664. [CrossRef] [PubMed]

98. Shih, L.Y.; Huang, C.F.; Wu, J.H.; Lin, T.L.; Dunn, P.; Wang, P.N.; Kuo, M.C.; Lai, C.L.; Hsu, H.C. Internal tandem duplication of FLT3 in relapsed acute myeloid leukemia: A comparative analysis of bone marrow samples from 108 adult patients at diagnosis and relapse. *Blood* **2002**, *100*, 2387–2392. [CrossRef] [PubMed]

99. Kottaridis, P.D.; Gale, R.E.; Langabeer, S.E.; Frew, M.E.; Bowen, D.T.; Linch, D.C. Studies of FLT3 mutations in paired presentation and relapse samples from patients with acute myeloid leukemia: Implications for the role of FLT3 mutations in leukemogenesis, minimal residual disease detection, and possible therapy with FLT3 inhibitors. *Blood* **2002**, *100*, 2393–2398. [CrossRef] [PubMed]

100. Koszarska, M.; Meggyesi, N.; Bors, A.; Batai, A.; Csacsovszki, O.; Lehoczky, E.; Adam, E.; Kozma, A.; Lovas, N.; Sipos, A.; *et al.* Medium-sized FLT3 internal tandem duplications confer worse prognosis than short and long duplications in a non-elderly acute myeloid leukemia cohort. *Leuk Lymphoma* **2014**, *55*, 1510–1517. [CrossRef] [PubMed]

101. Stirewalt, D.L.; Kopecky, K.J.; Meshinchi, S.; Engel, J.H.; Pogosova-Agadjanyan, E.L.; Linsley, J.; Slovak, M.L.; Willman, C.L.; Radich, J.P. Size of FLT3 internal tandem duplication has prognostic significance in patients with acute myeloid leukemia. *Blood* **2006**, *107*, 3724–3726. [CrossRef] [PubMed]

102. Gale, R.E.; Green, C.; Allen, C.; Mead, A.J.; Burnett, A.K.; Hills, R.K.; Linch, D.C.; Medical Research Council Adult Leukaemia Working Party. The impact of FLT3 internal tandem duplication mutant level, number, size, and interaction with NPM1 mutations in a large cohort of young adult patients with acute myeloid leukemia. *Blood* **2008**, *111*, 2776–2784. [CrossRef] [PubMed]

103. Whitman, S.P.; Archer, K.J.; Feng, L.; Baldus, C.; Becknell, B.; Carlson, B.D.; Carroll, A.J.; Mrozek, K.; Vardiman, J.W.; George, S.L.; *et al.* Absence of the wild-type allele predicts poor prognosis in adult de novo acute myeloid leukemia with normal cytogenetics and the internal tandem duplication of FLT3: A cancer and leukemia group B study. *Cancer Res.* **2001**, *61*, 7233–7239. [PubMed]

104. Kayser, S.; Schlenk, R.F.; Londono, M.C.; Breitenbuecher, F.; Wittke, K.; Du, J.; Groner, S.; Spath, D.; Krauter, J.; Ganser, A.; *et al.* Insertion of FLT3 internal tandem duplication in the tyrosine kinase domain-1 is associated with resistance to chemotherapy and inferior outcome. *Blood* **2009**, *114*, 2386–2392. [CrossRef] [PubMed]

105. Borthakur, G.; Kantarjian, H.; Patel, K.P.; Ravandi, F.; Qiao, W.; Faderl, S.; Kadia, T.; Luthra, R.; Pierce, S.; Cortes, J.E. Impact of numerical variation in FMS-like tyrosine kinase receptor 3 internal tandem duplications on clinical outcome in normal karyotype acute myelogenous leukemia. *Cancer* **2012**, *118*, 5819–5822. [CrossRef] [PubMed]

106. Ley, T.J.; Mardis, E.R.; Ding, L.; Fulton, B.; McLellan, M.D.; Chen, K.; Dooling, D.; Dunford-Shore, B.H.; McGrath, S.; Hickenbotham, M.; *et al.* DNA sequencing of a cytogenetically normal acute myeloid leukaemia genome. *Nature* **2008**, *456*, 66–72. [CrossRef] [PubMed]

107. Welch, J.S.; Ley, T.J.; Link, D.C.; Miller, C.A.; Larson, D.E.; Koboldt, D.C.; Wartman, L.D.; Lamprecht, T.L.; Liu, F.; Xia, J.; *et al.* The origin and evolution of mutations in acute myeloid leukemia. *Cell* **2012**, *150*, 264–278. [CrossRef] [PubMed]

108. Ding, L.; Ley, T.J.; Larson, D.E.; Miller, C.A.; Koboldt, D.C.; Welch, J.S.; Ritchey, J.K.; Young, M.A.; Lamprecht, T.; McLellan, M.D.; *et al.* Clonal evolution in relapsed acute myeloid leukaemia revealed by whole-genome sequencing. *Nature* **2012**, *481*, 506–510. [CrossRef] [PubMed]

109. Corces-Zimmerman, M.R.; Hong, W.J.; Weissman, I.L.; Medeiros, B.C.; Majeti, R. Preleukemic mutations in human acute myeloid leukemia affect epigenetic regulators and persist in remission. *Proc. Natl. Acad. Sci. USA* **2014**, *111*, 2548–2553. [CrossRef] [PubMed]

110. Shlush, L.I.; Zandi, S.; Mitchell, A.; Chen, W.C.; Brandwein, J.M.; Gupta, V.; Kennedy, J.A.; Schimmer, A.D.; Schuh, A.C.; Yee, K.W.; *et al.* Identification of pre-leukaemic haematopoietic stem cells in acute leukaemia. *Nature* **2014**, *506*, 328–333. [CrossRef] [PubMed]

111. Shih, L.Y.; Huang, C.F.; Wang, P.N.; Wu, J.H.; Lin, T.L.; Dunn, P.; Kuo, M.C. Acquisition of FLT3 or N-ras mutations is frequently associated with progression of myelodysplastic syndrome to acute myeloid leukemia. *Leukemia* **2004**, *18*, 466–475. [CrossRef] [PubMed]

112. Horiike, S.; Yokota, S.; Nakao, M.; Iwai, T.; Sasai, Y.; Kaneko, H.; Taniwaki, M.; Kashima, K.; Fujii, H.; Abe, T.; *et al.* Tandem duplications of the FLT3 receptor gene are associated with leukemic transformation of myelodysplasia. *Leukemia* **1997**, *11*, 1442–1446. [CrossRef] [PubMed]

113. Ostronoff, F.; Othus, M.; Gerbing, R.B.; Loken, M.R.; Raimondi, S.C.; Hirsch, B.A.; Lange, B.J.; Petersdorf, S.; Radich, J.; Appelbaum, F.R.; *et al.* Co-expression of NUP98/NSD1 and FLT3/ITD is more prevalent in younger AML patients and leads to high-risk of induction failure: A COG and SWOG report. *Blood* **2014**, *124*, 2400–2407. [CrossRef] [PubMed]

114. Kelly, L.M.; Kutok, J.L.; Williams, I.R.; Boulton, C.L.; Amaral, S.M.; Curley, D.P.; Ley, T.J.; Gilliland, D.G. PML/RARalpha and FLT3-ITD induce an APL-like disease in a mouse model. *Proc. Natl. Acad. Sci. USA* **2002**, *99*, 8283–8288. [CrossRef] [PubMed]

115. Godfrey, R.; Arora, D.; Bauer, R.; Stopp, S.; Muller, J.P.; Heinrich, T.; Bohmer, S.A.; Dagnell, M.; Schnetzke, U.; Scholl, S.; *et al.* Cell transformation by FLT3 ITD in acute myeloid leukemia involves oxidative inactivation of the tumor suppressor protein-tyrosine phosphatase DEP-1/ PTPRJ. *Blood* **2012**, *119*, 4499–4511. [CrossRef] [PubMed]

116. Park, I.K.; Mishra, A.; Chandler, J.; Whitman, S.P.; Marcucci, G.; Caligiuri, M.A. Inhibition of the receptor tyrosine kinase Axl impedes activation of the FLT3 internal tandem duplication in human acute myeloid leukemia: Implications for Axl as a potential therapeutic target. *Blood* **2013**. [CrossRef]

117. Chapuis, N.; Tamburini, J.; Green, A.S.; Vignon, C.; Bardet, V.; Neyret, A.; Pannetier, M.; Willems, L.; Park, S.; Macone, A.; *et al.* Dual inhibition of PI3K and mTORC1/2 signaling by NVP-BEZ235 as a new therapeutic strategy for acute myeloid leukemia. *Clin. Cancer Res.* **2010**, *16*, 5424–5435. [CrossRef] [PubMed]

118. Ricciardi, M.R.; Scerpa, M.C.; Bergamo, P.; Ciuffreda, L.; Petrucci, M.T.; Chiaretti, S.; Tavolaro, S.; Mascolo, M.G.; Abrams, S.L.; Steelman, L.S.; *et al.* Therapeutic potential of MEK inhibition in acute myelogenous leukemia: Rationale for "vertical" and "lateral" combination strategies. *J Mol Med (Berl)* **2012**, *90*, 1133–1144. [CrossRef]

119. Koch, S.; Jacobi, A.; Ryser, M.; Ehninger, G.; Thiede, C. Abnormal localization and accumulation of FLT3-ITD, a mutant receptor tyrosine kinase involved in leukemogenesis. *Cells Tissues Organs* **2008**, *188*, 225–235. [CrossRef] [PubMed]

120. Schmidt-Arras, D.; Bohmer, S.A.; Koch, S.; Muller, J.P.; Blei, L.; Cornils, H.; Bauer, R.; Korasikha, S.; Thiede, C.; Bohmer, F.D. Anchoring of FLT3 in the endoplasmic reticulum alters signaling quality. *Blood* **2009**, *113*, 3568–3576. [CrossRef] [PubMed]

121. D'Incalci, M.; Capranico, G.; Giaccone, G.; Zunino, F.; Garattini, S. DNA topoisomerase inhibitors. *Cancer Chemother. Biol. Response Modif.* **1993**, *14*, 61–85. [PubMed]

122. Bilardi, R.A.; Kimura, K.I.; Phillips, D.R.; Cutts, S.M. Processing of anthracycline-DNA adducts via DNA replication and interstrand crosslink repair pathways. *Biochem. Pharmacol.* **2012**, *83*, 1241–1250. [CrossRef] [PubMed]

123. Fernandez, H.F.; Sun, Z.; Yao, X.; Litzow, M.R.; Luger, S.M.; Paietta, E.M.; Racevskis, J.; Dewald, G.W.; Ketterling, R.P.; Bennett, J.M.; *et al.* Anthracycline dose intensification in acute myeloid leukemia. *N. Engl. J. Med.* **2009**, *361*, 1249–1259. [CrossRef] [PubMed]

124. Pardee, T.S.; Zuber, J.; Lowe, S.W. Flt3-ITD alters chemotherapy response *in vitro* and *in vivo* in a p53-dependent manner. *Exp. Hematol.* **2011**, *39*, 473–485. [CrossRef] [PubMed]

125. Zhao, R.; Yang, F.T.; Alexander, D.R. An oncogenic tyrosine kinase inhibits DNA repair and DNA-damage-induced Bcl-xL deamidation in T cell transformation. *Cancer Cell* **2004**, *5*, 37–49. [CrossRef] [PubMed]

126. Sallmyr, A.; Fan, J.; Datta, K.; Kim, K.T.; Grosu, D.; Shapiro, P.; Small, D.; Rassool, F. Internal tandem duplication of FLT3 (FLT3/ITD) induces increased ROS production, DNA damage, and misrepair: Implications for poor prognosis in AML. *Blood* **2008**, *111*, 3173–3182. [CrossRef] [PubMed]

127. Heckman, C.A.; Kontro, M.; Pemovska, T.; Eldfors, S.; Edgren, H.; Kulesskiy, E.; Majumder, M.M.; Karjalainen, R.; Yadav, B.; Szwajda, A.; *et al.* High-Throughput *ex Vivo* Drug Sensitivity and Resistance Testing (DSRT) Integrated with Deep Genomic and Molecular Profiling Reveal New Therapy Options with Targeted Drugs in Subgroups of Relapsed Chemorefractory AML. *Blood (ASH Annual Meeting Abstracts)* **2012**, *2012*, 288.

128. Dishing out cancer treatment. *Nat. Biotechnol.* **2013**, *31*, 85.

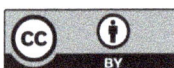

Journal of
Clinical Medicine

MDPI

Review

Clinical Results of Hypomethylating Agents in AML Treatment

Marjan Cruijsen [1], Michael Lübbert [2], Pierre Wijermans [3] and Gerwin Huls [1,*

[1] Department of Hematology, Radboud University Medical Center, PO Box 9191,
6500 HB Nijmegen, The Netherlands; marjan.cruijsen@radboudumc.nl
[2] Department of Medicine, University of Freiburg Medical Center, D-79106, Freiburg, Germany;
michael.luebbert@uniklinik-freiburg.de
[3] Department of Hematology, Haga Hospital, 2545 CH, The Hague, The Netherlands;
p.wijermans@hagaziekenhuis.nl
* Author to whom correspondence should be addressed; gerwin.huls@radboudumc.nl;
Tel.: +31-24-8187384; Fax: +31-24-3542080.

Academic Editor: Celalettin Ustun

Received: 18 September 2014; Accepted: 2 December 2014; Published: 25 December 2014

Abstract: Epigenetic changes play an important role in the development of acute myeloid leukemia (AML). Unlike gene mutations, epigenetic changes are potentially reversible, which makes them attractive for therapeutic intervention. Agents that affect epigenetics are the DNA methyltransferase inhibitors, azacitidine and decitabine. Because of their relatively mild side effects, azacitidine and decitabine are particularly feasible for the treatment of older patients and patients with co-morbidities. Both drugs have remarkable activity against AML blasts with unfavorable cytogenetic characteristics. Recent phase 3 trials have shown the superiority of azacitidine and decitabine compared with conventional care for older AML patients (not eligible for intensive treatment). Results of treatment with modifications of the standard azacitidine (seven days 75 mg/m^2 SC; every four weeks) and decitabine (five days 20 mg/m^2 IV; every four weeks) schedules have been reported. Particularly, the results of the 10-day decitabine schedule are promising, revealing complete remission (CR) rates around 45% (CR + CRi (*i.e.*, CR with incomplete blood count recovery) around 64%) almost comparable with intensive chemotherapy. Application of hypomethylating agents to control AML at the cost of minimal toxicity is a very promising strategy to "bridge" older patients with co-morbidities to the potential curative treatment of allogeneic hematopoietic cell transplantation. In this article, we discuss the role of DNA methyltransferase inhibitors in AML.

Keywords: AML; azacitidine; decitabine; hypomethylating agents; elderly; epigenetics

1. Introduction

Epigenetic changes include, by definition, through mitosis and meiosis, heritable changes in gene expression that are not caused by changes in the primary DNA sequence [1]. Epigenetic changes affect the spatial structure of the DNA that is coiled around histones. The spatial structure determines whether the transcription machinery, which transcribes DNA into RNA, can or cannot bind to the promoter of a gene, in order to initiate transcription. The best-known epigenetic changes are methylation and acetylation of amino acid residues in histones and methylation of cytosine (C) bases in areas of the genome rich in CpG dinucleotides (CpG islands). Methylation of cytosines, mediated by one of the DNA methyltransferases (DNMTs), results in silencing of gene expression. DNMT1 maintains existing methylation patterns following DNA replication, whereas DNMT3A and 3B methylate unmethylated CpGs (*de novo* methylation). It is increasingly clear that epigenetic changes play a role in oncogenesis. Cancer cells generally exhibit genome-wide hypomethylation, resulting in genetic instability, and CpG islands hypermethylation, modifying gene expression (e.g., preventing the expression of tumor suppressor genes) [2]. In contrast to genetic changes, epigenetic changes are considered to be reversible. This makes epigenetic changes an attractive candidate for therapeutic intervention. There is considerable evidence that abnormal methylation plays an important role in the pathogenesis of hematological malignancies, including acute myeloid leukemia (AML). AML blasts have distinct methylation patterns compared with normal CD34+ cells, and various subtypes of AML, e.g., with mutated NPM1, have distinct methylation profiles [3,4]. Recent studies using massively parallel sequencing technologies have identified mutations of *DNMT3A*, *TET2* and *IDH* (1 and 2) in 12%–22%, 7%–23% and 15%–33%, respectively, of the AML patients [5,6]. These genes are involved in DNA methylation, and therefore, their mutated variants may help elucidate the mechanisms of aberrant DNA methylation in AML blasts. Furthermore, translocations (e.g., *MLL* (mixed lineage leukemia gene)) and mutations (e.g., *ASXL1*, *UTX*) in genes affecting histone modifications are frequently observed.

2. DNA Hypomethylating Agents

In the 1960s, 5-azacytidine (further called azacitidine) and 5-aza-2′-deoxycytidine (further called decitabine) were synthesized to develop analogs of cytosine (like cytarabine) for the treatment of AML. Although these drugs clearly had anti-neoplastic activity, they turned out to be extremely toxic at high doses. Renewed interest in azacitidine and decitabine arose after discovering the hypomethylating properties of these drugs. The DNA hypomethylating property of azacitidine and decitabine was traced to their ability to incorporate into DNA, trap DNA methyltransferases (DNMTs) and target these enzymes for degradation [7]. DNA synthesis in the absence of these enzymes then results in hypomethylation in the daughter cells and eventually to reactivation of silenced gene expression (Figure 1). It is important to recognize that while inhibiting DNA methylation is a molecularly precise, targeted therapy approach, the downstream effects on neoplastic behavior are quite nonspecific. The trapping of DNMTs onto DNA creates bulky adducts that can inhibit DNA synthesis and eventually result in cell death by cytotoxicity [2,7]. Furthermore, if one considers reactivated genes, these drugs affect multiple pathways, including cell cycle arrest (for example, via p15 activation), apoptosis, differentiation, stem cell renewal, invasion, angiogenesis, immune recognition *etc.* In particular, the pre-clinical data, which suggest that azanucleotides increase the immunogenicity of AML blasts by promoting the expression of silenced antigens (e.g., of melanoma-associated antigens (MAGE)), could become a fruitful lead for future (transplantation) studies [8].

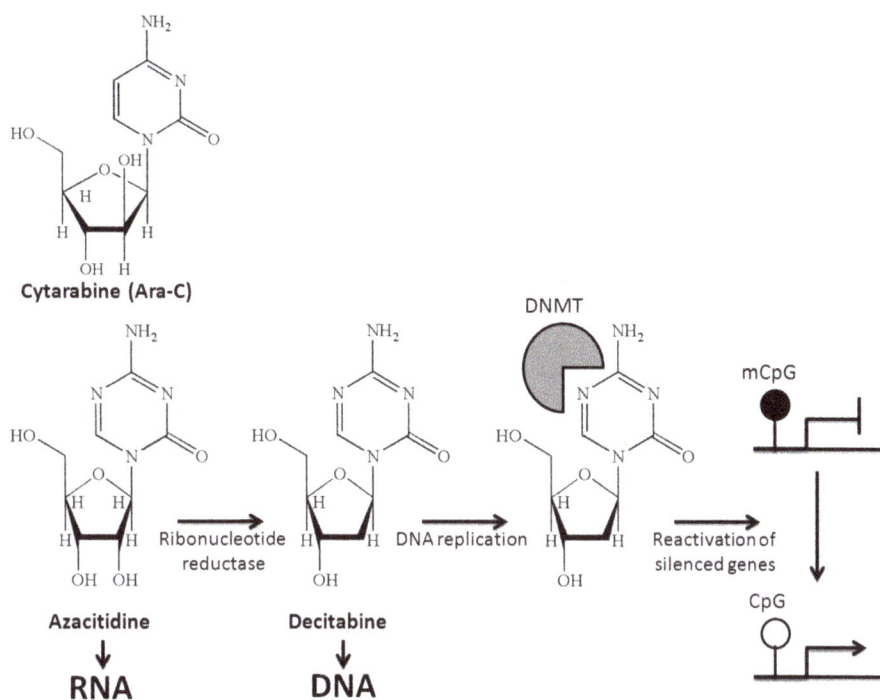

Figure 1. Mechanism of action of hypomethylating agents. (Black circles, methylated CpG; white circles, unmethylated CpG.)

The observation that hypomethylating agents (HMAs) have to be incorporated into DNA to inhibit DNA methylation (and consequently, transcription activation) implies that these agents should be used differently than conventional chemotherapy. HMAs have to be given for at least 3–6 cycles before it can be concluded whether they have activity against the disease (or not). These drugs should be given at a standard dose at fixed times, despite the presence of cytopenias. Further, these drugs can have meaningful clinical activity (e.g., transfusion independency) and improve survival, despite the fact that no CR is achieved. Indeed, the recovery of peripheral blood counts and quality of life are important reasons to continue treatment with HMAs.

3. Azacitidine and AML

Azacitidine was tested in two separate phase 3 studies in myelodysplastic syndromes (MDS) [9,10]. Response rates ranging from 30% to 60% were observed, with documented improved survival compared with either supportive care or cytotoxic chemotherapy. Since some of the included patients would currently be considered as AML patients (according to WHO criteria), this allowed studying the anti-leukemic effect of azacitidine in AML patients. In the Cancer and Leukemia Group B (CALGB) 9221 study, 27 patients with AML were randomly assigned to azacitidine and 12 AML patients were assigned to observation [11]. The median survival time for the treated patients was 19.3 months compared to 12.9 months in the group assigned to observation (*n* = 25; including the control arms of CALGB 8421 and 8921). A post hoc analysis of the pivotal MDS001 trial for older patients who met the WHO criteria for AML (*i.e.*, 20%–30% bone marrow (BM) blasts) showed 18% CR, with a survival benefit in favor of azacitidine (24.5 *vs.* 16 months, *p* = 0.005), including higher two-year OS (38% *vs.* 0%, *p* = 0.01) in patients with adverse cytogenetics [12].

Recently, the data of the AML001 study, a global, multi-center, randomized study, including 488 AML patients 65 years or older, were presented at the EHA (*i.e.*, European Hematology Association) meeting in 2014 in Milano [13]. In this study, older AML patients with newly-diagnosed or secondary AML with >30% bone marrow blasts and white blood cell counts $\leq 15 \times 10^9$/L (prior hydroxyurea allowed) were pre-selected to receive one of three regimens per investigator's choice (*i.e.*, intensive chemotherapy (standard "7 + 3" regimen), low-dose cytarabine (Ara-C) (20 mg twice per day SC for 10 days of each 28-day cycle) or best supportive care only. Patients were then randomized to receive either azacitidine (n = 241) (75 mg/m^2/day for seven days SC of each 28-day cycle) or their preselected treatment (*i.e.*, conventional care regimen (CCR)) (n = 247). Median OS, the primary endpoint of the study, was 10.4 months for patients receiving azacitidine compared to 6.5 months for patients receiving CCR, which did not reach statistical significance (HR = 0.84 (95% CI 0.69–1.02), p = 0.0829). Primarily patients with poor risk cytogenetics (HR = 0.68 (95% CI 0.5–0.94)) and those with AML with dysplasia (HR = 0.69 (95% CI 0.48–0.98)) benefitted from azacitidine compared with CCR. Additionally, a pre-specified sensitivity analysis for OS that censored patients at the start of subsequent AML therapy was conducted. Results of this analysis showed a longer median OS for patients receiving azacitidine (median: 12.1 months) compared to patients receiving CCR (median: 6.9 months) (stratified HR = 0.76 (95% CI 0.60–0.96), p = 0.019). Remarkable was the superior outcome of patients who received azacitidine as the first subsequent therapy after CCR (n = 21) compared with those patients who received a cytarabine-based treatment as the first subsequent therapy after azacitidine upfront treatment (n = 21) (median OS 8.0 *vs.* 3.6 months (p = 0.01)). With the intention to treat analysis, the one-year survival was 47% for patients in the azacitidine arm compared to 34% for patients in the CCR arm.

4. Decitabine and AML

Decitabine has been studied in AML patients in various dosing schedules. In a phase 2 study of decitabine, patients over 60 years old with untreated AML (n = 227; median age 72 years) and ineligible for induction chemotherapy were treated with decitabine [14]. In this study, patients received decitabine 15 mg/m^2 IV for three hours every eight hours for three days (total: 135 mg/m^2), which was repeated every six weeks. A median of two cycles was administered (range, 1–4). Patients who completed four cycles of treatment (n = 52) subsequently received a median of five maintenance courses (range, 1–19) with a lower dose of decitabine (20 mg/m^2) infused over one hour on three consecutive days every 4–6 weeks. The complete and partial remission rate was 26%. Response rates did not differ between patients with or without adverse cytogenetics; patients with monosomal karyotypes also responded. The median overall survival from the start of decitabine treatment was 5.5 months; the one-year survival rate was 28%, and the two-year survival rate was 13%.

In an attempt to find the optimal therapy with decitabine in MDS, Kantarjian and co-workers compared three decitabine schedules administered in an outpatient setting at the Monroe Dunaway Anderson Cancer Center (MDACC): (1) 20 mg/m^2 intravenously over one hour daily for five days; (2) 20 mg/m^2 subcutaneously daily, divided into two doses, for five days; or (3) 10 mg/m^2 intravenously over 1 h daily for 10 days [15]. Courses of decitabine were repeated every four weeks. In the subgroup analysis the, five-day intravenous schedule, which had the highest dose intensity, yielded the highest CR rate (39%) in comparison to the five-day subcutaneous schedule (21%) and the 10-day intravenous (10 mg/m^2) schedule (24% CR). It should be noted that the 10-day intravenous schedule investigated a dose of 10 mg/m^2, which is half the dose that was used in the 10-day schedule by Blum *et al.* and Ritchie *et al.* (extensively discussed later) [16,17]. The results of the five-day 20-mg/m^2 schedule in MDS were confirmed in a larger multi-center study (ADOPT trial, *i.e.*, Alternative Dosing for OutPatient Treatment) [18].

Recently, the results have been reported of a multicenter, randomized, open label, phase 3 trial, which compared the efficacy and safety of decitabine in the five day schedule (20 mg/m^2, Days 1–5) (n = 242) with treatment choice (supportive care (n = 28) and low-dose cytarabine (at a dose of 20 mg/m^2 once daily for 10 days, every four weeks) (n = 215)) of older patients with newly-diagnosed AML and poor- or intermediate-risk cytogenetics [19]. Although the planned primary analysis of this trial after 396 deaths did not show a significant improvement of OS with decitabine *vs.* treatment choice (median OS 7.7 months *vs.* 5.0 months), an unplanned analysis after 446 deaths showed a significant benefit for decitabine. The CR rate in this study was 24%. The data from this study led to approval of decitabine for the treatment of AML in Europe, but not in the U.S. (*i.e.*, >30% blasts). The FDA has approved both azacitidine and decitabine for the treatment of all MDS subtypes (up to 30% blasts). The EMA (*i.e.*, European Medicines Agency) has approved azacitidine for high risk MDS, chronic myelomonocytic leukemia (with less than 10% myeloblasts, monoblasts, and promonocytes in bone marrow, *i.e.*, CMML-1) and AML (up to 30% blasts). In Table 1 a summary is provided of clinical outcome of phase 3 trials of azacitidine and decitabine in AML.

5. Azacitidine and Decitabine in 10-Day Schedules

Azanucleotides need cell cycling to become incorporated into the DNA during the S phase. Since cell cycling is essential to effect methylation reversal, it could be argued that prolonged administration (e.g., 10 days) of azanucleotides could be pharmacodynamically superior to standard schedule (five days for decitabine and seven days for azacitidine), Table 2 Clinical Outcome dependent on dosing in AML.

Table 1. Clinical outcome of phase 3 trials of azacitidine and decitabine in acute myeloid leukemia (AML).

Study	Competitors	CR (%)	Median OS	1/2-Year OS
Azacitidine (7 Days 75 mg/m^2 SC; Every 4 Weeks)				
Post hoc analysis CALGB 9221 (AML 20%–30% blasts) [11]	AZA (n = 27) *vs.* Observation (n = 12)	7% *vs.* 0%	19.3 months *vs.* NA; Combining CALGB 8421, 8921, 9221: 12.9 months (n = 25; p = NA)	NA
Post hoc analysis AZA001 study (AML 20%–30% blasts) [12]	Aza (n = 55) *vs.* CCR (n = 58) (BSC = 27/LDAC = 20/IC = 11)	18% *vs.* 16%	24.5 months *vs.* 16 months (p = 0.005)	50% *vs.* 16% (p = 0.001) (2-year OS)
AML001 study (AML >30% blasts) [13]	Aza (n = 241) *vs.* CCR (n = 247) (BSC = 45/LDAC = 158/IC = 44)	20% *vs.* 22%	10.4 months *vs.* 6.5 months (p = 0.08). Analysis censored for subsequent Tx: 12.1 months *vs.* 6.9 months (p = 0.01)	46.5% *vs.* 34.2% (p = NA) (1 year OS)
Decitabine (5 Days 20 mg/m^2 IV; Every 4 Weeks)				
DACO-016 (AML >20% blasts; only intermediate and poor risk) [19]	Decit (n = 242) *vs.* TC (n = 243) (BSC = 28/LDAC = 215)	15.7% *vs.* 7.4%	7.7 months *vs.* 5.0 months (p = 0.11). Analysis censored for subsequent Tx: 8.5 months *vs.* 5.3 months (p = 0.04). Unplanned analysis after 446 deaths: 7.7 months *vs.* 5.0 months (p = 0.04)	NA

CR: complete remission; OS: overall survival; CALGB: Cancer and Leukemia Group B; AZA: azacitidine; CCR: conventional care regimen; BSC: Best Supportive Care; LDAC: low dose Ara-C; Tx: treatment; DACO: Dacogen, decitabine; Decit: decitabine; TC: treatment choice.

Table 2. Clinical outcome dependent on dosing in AML.

Study	Dosing	CR (%)	Median OS
Azacitidine			
Post hoc analysis AML001 study (phase 3) (AML 20%–30% blasts) [12]	Aza (n = 55) 7 days 75 mg/m^2 SC; every 4 weeks	18%	24.5 months
AML001 study (phase 3) (AML >30% blasts) [13]	Aza (n = 241) 7 days 75 mg/m^2 SC; every 4 weeks	20%	10.4 months
United States Leukemia Intergroup Trial E1905 (phase 2) [20]	Aza (n = 74) 10 days 50 mg/m^2 SC; every 4 weeks	12%	18 months
Decitabine			
German phase 2 study [14]	Decit (n = 227) 3 days (135 mg/m^2 total)	13%	5.5 months
DACO-016 (phase 3) (AML >20% blasts; only intermediate and poor risk) [19]	Decit (n = 242) 5 days 20 mg/m^2	15.7%	7.7 months
Ohio State University experience (phase 2) [16]	Decit (n = 53) 10 days 20 mg/m^2	47%	12.7 months
Cornell University experience (report of retrospective analysis) [17]	Decit (n = 52) 10 days 20 mg/m^2	40% (after excluding 6 patients who received prior azanucleotide CR = 46%)	10.5 months

In a recent open label phase 2 randomized trial, azacitidine in a dose of 50 mg/m^2/day was given for 10 days ± entinostat 4 mg/m^2/day on Day 3 and Day 10 [20]. One hundred forty nine patients were analyzed, including 97 patients with MDS and 52 patients with AML. In the 10-day azacitidine group, 32% (95% CI, 22% to 44%) experienced hematological normalization (HN) (*i.e.*, complete remission + partial remission + tri-lineage hematological improvement). Although CR rates of the 10-day schedule were comparable with the reported CR rates with the seven-day schedule, this study suggest that prolonged administration of azacitidine seems to increase the HN rate compared with standard dosing (almost doubling of HN compared with the historical control Cancer and Leukemia Group B 9221 trial). Median overall survivals were 18 months for the 10-day azacitidine schedule and 13 months for the group with combined treatment of azacitidine and entinostat.

The experience with decitabine in a 10-day schedule of decitabine (of 20 mg/m^2) in AML patients has also been reported [16,17]. The data on the 10-day schedule are intriguing. The 10-day schedule was explored in a phase 2 clinical trial (n = 53) with single-agent decitabine in older patients (≥60 years) with previously untreated AML, who were not candidates or who refused intensive chemotherapy [16]. Subjects were treated with decitabine 20 mg/m^2 intravenously over 1 h on Days 1 to 10. Nineteen patients (36%) had antecedent hematologic disorder or therapy-related AML; 16 had complex karyotypes (≥3 abnormalities). The CR rate was 47% (n = 25), achieved after a median of three cycles of therapy. Nine additional subjects had no morphologic evidence of disease with incomplete count recovery, for an overall response rate of 64% (n = 34). CR was achieved in 52% of subjects presenting with normal karyotype (11 of 21) and in 50% (8 of 16) of those with complex karyotypes (defined as ≥3 abnormalities). Death occurred within eight weeks in 15% of subjects. The CR rate in subjects presenting WBC counts ≥15 × 10^9/L (range, 15 × 10^9/L–150 × 10^9/L) was 57% (eight of 14 subjects), including 50% (four of eight) for those subjects presenting WBC count ≥50 × 10^9/L. The disease-free survival duration was 46 weeks. The median OS was 55 weeks. Furthermore, this study showed that decitabine was well tolerated. Although patients were neutropenic for prolonged times, they did not experience mucositis and, therefore, could be managed largely in the outpatient setting. Patients who had less than 5% bone marrow blasts around Day + 28 of the 10-day decitabine cycle continued with a five-day schedule. Those patients with more than 5% bone marrow blasts received another 10-day decitabine cycle.

Recently, the efficacy and safety data of another study exploring the 10-day decitabine schedule have been reported [17]. In this study, 52 newly-diagnosed, older AML patients were treated with the 10-day decitabine schedule. All patients received at least one 10-day induction cycle with decitabine 20 mg/m^2 intravenously. After CR, most of the patients were treated with ongoing five-day cycles of decitabine 20 mg/m^2 until toxicity or progression of disease. The median number of treatment cycles was two (range 1–18). Patients required a median number of two cycles (range, 1–4) to achieve a response, with a median time to CR of 55.5 days (range 18–122 days). Among the 52 patients, 21 (40%) achieved a CR. None of the six patients who had previously been treated with azacitidine or decitabine for MDS achieved a CR. If these patients are excluded from the study population, the CR rate becomes 46%. Responses were durable over one year. The median OS was 318 days. The extra medullary toxicity was mild, but myelosuppression was noted in all patients. The median time to neutrophil recovery was 42.5 days (range, 20–120 days), and the median time to platelet count recovery was 48 days (range, 1–130 days). Twenty-nine patients (55%) had neutropenic fever with bacteremia requiring intravenous antibiotics. Patients were hospitalized for a median of 39 days (range, 0–169 days). However, it should be noted that the authors state in the manuscript that the reasons for prolonged hospitalization were frequently social or logistical, rather than medical.

These single-center experiences of the 10-day schedule of decitabine show promising remission and survival results. The 20 mg/m^2 daily decitabine for five-day or 10-day schedules are currently compared in a prospective randomized study in older unfit AML patients at the MD Anderson Cancer Center (NCT01786343, see ClinicalTrials.gov). The reported CR rates achieved with the 10-day decitabine schedule are comparable with those achieved after intensive chemotherapy (e.g., HOVON43 (a study of the Dutch HOVON foundation, *i.e.*, Hemato-oncologie voor Volwassenen Nederland) reported a CR rate of 54% after conventional intensive chemotherapy in AML patients ≥60 years) [21]. These CR rates should be considered with the perspective that hypomethylating agents impact survival without inducing CR, suggesting that almost similar CR rates between 10-day decitabine and conventional chemotherapy might translate to a survival benefit for the 10-day decitabine schedule. Therefore, the 10-day decitabine schedule might provide a framework upon which to build future combination studies to improve outcomes for older AML patients. The European Organisation for Research and Treatment of Cancer (EORTC) Leukemia Group, together with the Gruppo Italiano Malattie EMatologiche dell'Adulta (GIMEMA), the Central European Leukemia Group (CELG) and the German MDS Study Group, recently opened a prospective randomized trial to compare conventional intensive chemotherapy based on cytarabine combined with an anthracycline ("3 + 7") with the hypomethylating agent, decitabine, to determine the optimal backbone for the treatment of older AML patients (NCT02172872).

6. Hypomethylating Agents as Maintenance Therapy

Because of its low toxicity profile, maintenance treatment with hypomethylating agents is an attractive treatment option for older AML patients who are at high risk for relapse and who are not candidates for allogeneic hematopoietic cell transplantation. A prospective phase 2 study demonstrated that maintenance azacitidine treatment for five days at a dose of 60 mg/m^2 (after previous treatment with intensive chemotherapy) is safe and feasible [22]. Although no positive effect on the duration of CR was observed, this limited efficacy should be considered with the perspective of the low number of patients (*n* = 23, including 10 patients with MDS/AML) included. Currently, the HOVON is performing a prospective randomized trial comparing maintenance treatment with azacitidine (five days at a dose of 50 mg/m^2) with observation in older AML patients who are in CR after at least two cycles of intensive chemotherapy. The efficacy of oral azacitidine in the maintenance setting, which is logistically very attractive, is currently being tested in a prospective randomized study (Quazar AML-001; NCT01757535).

Limited data are available on the efficacy of decitabine in the maintenance setting. Lübbert *et al.* have reported three-day decitabine maintenance (20 mg/m^2/day) in 43 older AML patients who had received four cycles of decitabine treatment [14]. Further improvement of treatment response on maintenance or relapse after complete remission was not systematically recorded. Recently, the results of a small prospective phase 3 trial were reported. In this study, maintenance treatment with decitabine (*n* = 20) was compared with conventional care (*n* = 25; six observation, nine low-dose cytarabine and 10 intensive chemotherapy) [23]. Baseline characteristics were relatively balanced, with patients in the decitabine arm being older (55% >60 years *vs.* 28% in the conventional care arm and all with intensive chemotherapy being <60 years) and somewhat more frequently having poor karyotypes (25% *vs.* 20%). Decitabine was administered as 20 mg/m^2 IV daily on day 1–5 every 4–8 weeks for a total of up to 12 cycles. The primary endpoint was the relapse rate at one year. After a median follow-up of 44.9 months, fewer patients in the decitabine arm relapsed (50% *vs.* 60%), and the OS rate was 45% in the decitabine *vs.* 36% in the conventional care group (HR = 0.63; *p* = 0.32); these differences were not statistically significant. Treatment with standard-dose decitabine was well tolerated, with the most common adverse events being uncomplicated grade 3 neutropenia and/or thrombocytopenia.

7. DNA Hypomethylating Agent Therapy as a Bridging Strategy to AlloHCT

Various studies, as discussed above, have strongly suggested that the DNA hypomethylating agents, azacitidine and decitabine, have a favorable outcome in older AML patients. However, improvement is relatively small when compared to life expectancy in the absence of disease (in the Netherlands, a 76-year-old person has a life expectancy of 11 years), and treatment with hypomethylating agents cannot be considered curative. Treatment with hypomethylating agents could be curative when used in a sequential approach: debulking the disease with hypomethylating agents followed by reduced toxicity conditioning and allografting. In this strategy, hypomethylating agents are used as a bridging strategy before allografting; an effective, but non-toxic drug, like azacitidine or decitabine, is used to allow also more fragile patients to reach the potential curative treatment of allografting [24]. Azanucleotide treatment aims at debulking the disease while a donor (most often, an unrelated donor) is identified. Notably, because non-hematologic toxicities are usually mild and manageable (decitabine does not result in mucositis), the patient has the chance to stay fit and ambulatory, and the performance status may be improved with a good quality of life. This approach is by now well established in the literature (more than 120 patients have been reported up to now) as both feasible and capable of inducing longer-term remissions without negative effects with respect to graft-*versus*-host disease [25–30].

The impact of prior-to-transplantation azacitidine treatment on patient outcome after allogeneic hematopoietic cell transplantation (alloHCT) in MDS has been reported by a large French study [31]. In this study, 265 consecutive patients underwent alloHCT for MDS between October, 2005, and December, 2009; 163 had received cytoreductive treatment prior to transplantation, including induction chemotherapy (ICT) alone (ICT group; *n* = 98), azacitidine alone (AZA group; *n* = 48), or azacitidine preceded or followed by ICT (AZA-ICT group; *n* = 17). At diagnosis, 126 patients (77%) had an excess of marrow blasts and 95 patients (58%) had intermediate-2 or high-risk MDS according to the International Prognostic Scoring System (IPSS). Progression to more advanced disease before alloHCT was recorded in 67 patients. Donors were siblings (*n* = 75) or HLA (Human Leucocyte Antigen)-matched unrelated (10/10; *n* = 88). They received blood (*n* = 142) or marrow (*n* = 21) grafts following either myeloablative (*n* = 33) or reduced intensity (*n* = 130) conditioning. With a median follow-up of 38.7 months, three-year outcomes in the AZA, ICT and AZA-ICT groups were: 55%, 48% and 32% (*p* = 0.07) for OS; 42%, 44% and 29% (*p* = 0.14) for event-free survival (EFS); 40%, 37% and 36% (*p* = 0.86) for relapse; and 19%, 20% and 35% (*p* = 0.24) for non-relapse mortality (NRM), respectively. Multivariate analysis confirmed the absence of statistical differences between the AZA and the ICT groups in terms of OS, EFS, relapse and NRM.

The value of alloHCT after hypomethylating therapy was studied in a German study [32]. The multivariate analysis of this study, to minimize selection bias, was limited to patients aged 60–70 years with high-risk *de novo* MDS or secondary AML, who either received alloHCT (*n* = 105; with at least intermediate intensity conditioning in about half of the cases after induction chemotherapy) or who received azacitidine, but not alloHCT (*n* = 75), because of a lack of a donor or institutional guidelines. After accounting for performance status, cytogenetics, time from diagnosis and blast%, alloHCT was associated with superior OS compared to azacitidine without alloHCT, with the difference in OS becoming apparent one year after initiation of treatment (two-year OS 39 *vs.* 23%).

8. Use of Hypomethylating Agents after AlloHCT

Demethylating agents have been used after alloHCT in different settings: (1) to maintain CR (*i.e.*, to prevent relapse); (2) preemptive; and (3) to treat relapse. Limited data are available for whether maintenance therapy with HMAs after alloHCT improves RFS. In a dose finding study in high risk MDS/AML patients who were in CR at Day + 30 after transplantation, azacitidine was given subcutaneously for five subsequent days, starting on the sixth week after alloHCT at one of five dose levels (8, 16, 24, 32, 40 mg/m^2) [33]. The dose of 32 mg/m^2 was chosen. Azacitidine did not affect engraftment. At a median follow-up of 20.5 months, the one-year EFS and OS were 58% and 77%, respectively. Because most acute graft-versus-host disease (GVHD) started before starting azacitidine and patients with severe GVHD were excluded, no firm conclusions regarding acute GVHD could be made. The probability of developing chronic GVHD was, however, decreased significantly with longer azacitidine treatments. Currently, the maintenance question with HMAs after alloHCT is being evaluated in several clinical trials (NCT01168219, NCT01995578 and NCT01541280).

The value of azacitidine as a minimal residual disease-based preemptive therapy after alloHCT has been reported in a cohort of 59 patients who were prospectively monitored for impending relapse by decreasing CD34$^+$ cell chimerism [34]. In this trial (RELAZA, Azacitidine for treatment of imminent relapse in MDS or AML patients after alloHCT), at a median of 169 days after alloHCT, 20/59 prospectively screened patients experienced a decrease of CD34$^+$ donor chimerism to <80% and received four azacitidine cycles (75 mg/m^2/day for seven days) while in complete hematologic remission. A total of 16 patients (80%) responded with either increasing CD34$^+$ donor chimerism to $\geq$80% (n = 10; 50%) or stabilization (n = 6; 30%) in the absence of relapse. Hematologic relapse occurred ultimately in 13 patients.

HMAs have been used to treat recurrent disease after alloHCT, and the achievement of remission and complete donor chimerism has been reported [35,36]. Although response rates of around 50% and CR rates around 15% have been reported, the survival rate was still low and comparable with second alloHCT in this setting. The combination of azacitidine and donor lymphocyte infusions (DLI) as the first salvage therapy for relapse after alloHCT has also been studied in a cohort of 30 patients with AML/MDS within a prospective single-arm phase 2 trial [37]. The overall response rate was 30%, and 5/30 patients achieved long-term CR. Acute and chronic GVHD were seen in 37% and 17% of patients, respectively. This study suggests that azacitidine in combination with donor lymphocytes is an active treatment in high-risk patients who have relapsed after alloHCT.

9. Treatment of Older AML Patients

The optimal treatment of older AML patients in daily clinical practice remains challenging and is dependent on patient characteristics (age, co-morbidity), disease characteristics (cytogenetic and molecular abnormalities, WBC, *etc.*) and the wishes of the patient.

The OS of older AML patients has not been improved during the last few decades with intensive chemotherapy based on cytarabine combined with an anthracycline [38]. Although older AML patients generally have a limited benefit with currently available treatment, only a few prospective randomized studies in older AML patients, comparing different treatment strategies, have been done. A prospective clinical trial, though with a limited number of patients (n = 60), reported that standard intensive treatment improves early death rates and long-term survival compared to the best supportive care [39], a finding that was confirmed by an analysis of the Swedish Acute Leukemia Registry [40]. A prospective study in older patients with *de novo* AML (n = 87) has compared intensive chemotherapy with low-dose cytarabine (20 mg/m^2 for 21 days) and reported a similar overall survival (OS) in both arms, despite a higher number of complete remissions (CRs) in the intensive chemotherapy arm [41]. Moreover, a prospective randomized trial (n = 202) demonstrated that low-dose cytarabine (20 mg twice daily for 10 days) treatment was superior to the best supportive care and hydroxyurea [42]. In this study, patients with adverse cytogenetic profiles did not benefit from low-dose cytarabine. These studies suggest that older AML patients benefit from treatment, either by intensive chemotherapy or by low-dose cytarabine. From the perspective that the superiority of intensive chemotherapy (*i.e.*, "3 + 7") over less intensive therapy (e.g., low-dose Ara-C) has not been conclusive, the recently reported study, comparing decitabine, administered as a five-day regimen, with low-dose Ara-C, in older AML patients (*n* = 485), is particularly interesting [19]. Indeed, this study showed, though at an unplanned analysis with a one-year extended follow-up for survival, that the five-day decitabine treatment resulted in a superior overall survival compared with the low-dose Ara-C treatment.

No published data of prospective randomized trials that have compared the efficacy of intensive chemotherapy ("3 + 7") with hypomethylating agents are currently available. The MD Andersen Cancer Center reported the results of a cohort study of 671 patients, including 114 patients treated with hypomethylation-based (either azacitidine or decitabine) therapy and 557 patients treated with intensive chemotherapy [43]. Both groups were balanced according to cytogenetics and performance status and were older than 65 years. The CR rates with chemotherapy and hypomethylating agents were 42% and 28%, respectively (*p* = 0.001), and the eight-week mortality 18% and 11%, respectively (*p* = 0.075). Two-year relapse-free survival rates were 28% (chemo) *vs.* 39% (DNA methyltransferase inhibitor), *p* = 0.84. The median OS (6.7 *vs.* 6.5 months, *p* = 0.41) were similar in the two groups. Multivariate analysis confirmed that the type of AML therapy (intensive chemotherapy or hypomethylating agents) was not an independent prognostic factor for survival. Interestingly, in this study, multivariate analysis revealed that decitabine was associated with improved median OS compared with azacitidine (8.8 *vs.* 5.5 months, respectively, *p* = 0.03). This is in line with our own published experience in 200 consecutive older AML patients [44,45]. It should be noted that the observations of this retrospective analysis also suggest that the currently used response criteria (*i.e.*, CR) are not sufficient for evaluating some (less intensive) treatment strategies.

10. Conclusions

In conclusion, treatment recommendations for older adults with AML need to be individualized based on disease and patient characteristics [46]. However, at this moment, available clinical trial data do not satisfactorily determine which older patients are likely to benefit from specific treatments, given the complexity of tumor and patient characteristics underlying treatment responsiveness and treatment tolerance. The question to be answered is: what is considered a favorable treatment outcome that justifies a certain treatment-related mortality? From this perspective, it should be noted that a hematopoietic cell transplantation comorbidity index (HCT-CI) ≥3 has been reported to be associated with 29% mortality within 28 days from time of intensive chemotherapy in a cohort of patients, 177 AML patients over 60 years of age [47]. Should we treat these patients (with HCT-CI ≥3) with hypomethylating agents? Should the genotype of the AML blasts influence this decision? Without a doubt, azacitidine and decitabine are valuable treatment options for older AML patients, especially patients with co-morbidities and intermediate and poor risk disease. Whether azanucleotide treatment is superior (or comparable) with intensive chemotherapy, especially when used as a bridge to allogeneic transplantation, is an open question. To determine the optimal relation between certain treatments and disease (e.g., genotype) and patient-related factors (e.g., co-morbidity), future studies in older AML patients should include extensive biomarker analyses and geriatric assessments.

Cytarabine, azacitidine and decitabine are cytidine analogs. Cytarabine combines a cytosine base with an arabinose sugar. The carbon-5 of the cytidine backbone is substituted by nitrogen in the azanucleotides (azacitidine and decitabine). Azacitidine is intracellularly converted to 5-aza-2'-deoxycytidine (decitabine) by ribonucleotide reductase. Decitabine is incorporated in place of cytidine into DNA, where it acts as a direct and irreversible inhibitor of DNMTs. Because of the nitrogen atom at position 5, the enzyme DNMT remains covalently bound to DNA, and its DNA methyltransferase function is blocked and results in the degradation of trapped DNA methyltransferases. Consequently, cells then replicate in the absence of DNMTs, which results in progressive loss of methylation marks and reactivation of previously silenced genes. Little is known about the impact of azacitidine incorporated into RNA.

J. Clin. Med. **2015**, *4*, 1–17

Author Contributions: Marjan Cruijsen, Michael Lübbert, Pierre Wijermans and Gerwin Huls designed, wrote and approved the manuscript.

Conflicts of Interest: The authors declare no conflict of interest.

References

1. Gronbaek, K.; Hother, C.; Jones, P.A. Epigenetic changes in cancer. *APMIS* **2007**, *115*, 1039–1059. [CrossRef] [PubMed]
2. Jones, P.; Baylin, S.B. The epigenomics of cancer. *Cell* **2007**, *128*, 683–692. [CrossRef] [PubMed]
3. Figueroa, M.E.; Skrabanek, L.; Li, Y.; Jiemjit, A.; Fandy, T.E.; Paietta, E.; Fernandez, H.; Tallman, M.S.; Greally, J.M.; Carraway, H.; *et al.* MDS and secondary AML display unique patterns and abundance of aberrant DNA methylation. *Blood* **2009**, *114*, 3448–3458. [CrossRef] [PubMed]
4. Figueroa, M.E.; Lugthart, S.; Li, Y.; Erpelinck-Verschueren, C.; Deng, X.; Christos, P.J.; Schifano, E.; Booth, J.; van Putten, W.; Skrabanek, L.; *et al.* DNA methylation signatures identify biologically distinct subtypes in acute myeloid leukemia. *Cancer Cell* **2010**, *17*, 13–17. [CrossRef]
5. Cancer Genome Atlas Research Network. Genomic and epigenomic landscapes of adult *de novo* acute myeloid leukemia. *N. Engl. J. Med.* **2013**, *368*, 2059–2074.
6. Patel, J.P.; Gönen, M.; Figueroa, M.E.; Fernandez, H.; Sun, Z.; Racevskis, J.; van Vlierberghe, P.; Dolgalev, I.; Thomas, S.; Aminova, O.; *et al.* Prognostic relevance of integrated genetic profiling in acute myeloid leukemia. *N. Engl. J. Med.* **2012**, *366*, 1079–1089. [CrossRef]
7. Jüttermann, R.; Li, E.; Jaenisch, R. Toxicity of 5-aza-2′-deoxycytidine to mammalian cells is mediated primarily by covalent trapping of DNA methyltransferase rather than DNA demethylation. *Proc. Natl. Acad. Sci. USA* **1994**, *91*, 11797–11801. [CrossRef] [PubMed]
8. Goodyear, O.; Agathanggelou, A.; Novitzky-Basso, I.; Siddique, S.; McSkeane, T.; Ryan, G.; Vyas, P.; Cavenagh, J.; Stankovic, T.; Moss, P.; *et al.* Induction of a CD8+ T-cell response to the MAGE cancer testis antigen by combined treatment with azacitidine and sodium valproate in patients with acute myeloid leukemia and myelodysplasia. *Blood* **2010**, *116*, 1908–1918. [CrossRef] [PubMed]
9. Silverman, L.R.; Demakos, E.P.; Peterson, B.L.; Kornblith, A.B.; Holland, J.C.; Odchimar-Reissig, R.; Stone, R.M.; Nelson, D.; Powell, B.L.; DeCastro, C.M.; *et al.* Randomized controlled trial of azacitidine in patients with the myelodysplastic syndrome: A study of the cancer and leukemia group B. *J. Clin. Oncol.* **2002**, *20*, 2429–2440. [CrossRef]
10. Fenaux, P.; Mufti, G.J.; Hellström-Lindberg, E.; Santini, V.; Finelli, C.; Giagounidis, A.; Schoch, R.; Gattermann, N.; Sanz, G.; List, A. Efficacy of azacitidine compared with that of conventional care regimens in the treatment of higher-risk myelodysplastic syndromes: A randomised, open-label, phase III study. *Lancet Oncol.* **2009**, *10*, 223–232. [CrossRef]
11. Silverman, L.R.; McKenzie, D.R.; Peterson, B.L.; Holland, J.F.; Backstrom, J.T.; Beach, C.L.; Larson, R.A. Cancer and Leukemia group B Further analysis of trials with azacitidine in patients with myelodysplastic syndrome: Studies 8421, 8921, and 9221 by the Cancer and Leukemia Group B. *J. Clin. Oncol.* **2006**, *20*, 3895–3903. [CrossRef]
12. Fenaux, P.; Mufti, G.J.; Hellström-Lindberg, E.; Santini, V.; Gattermann, N.; Germing, U.; Sanz, G.; List, A.F.; Gore, S.; Seymour, J.F.; *et al.* Azacitidine prolongs overall survival compared with conventional care regimens in elderly patients with low bone marrow blast count acute myeloid leukaemia. *J. Clin. Oncol.* **2010**, *28*, 562–569. [CrossRef] [PubMed]
13. Dombret, H.; Seymour, J.F.; Butrym, A.; Wierzbowska, A.; Selleslag, D.; Jang, J.H.; Kumar, R.; Cavenagh, J.; Schuh, A.; Candoni, A.; *et al.* Results of a phase 3, multicenter, randomized, open-label study of azacitidine *vs.* conventional care regimens in older patients with newly diagnosed acute myeloid leukemia. In Proceedings of the 19th Congres of the European Hematology Association, Milan, Italy, 12–15 June 2014.
14. Lübbert, M.; Rüter, B.H.; Claus, R.; Schmoor, C.; Schmid, M.; Germing, U.; Kuendgen, A.; Rethwisch, V.; Ganser, A.; Platzbecker, U.; *et al.* A multicenter phase II trial of decitabine as first-line treatment for older patients with acute myeloid leukemia judged unfit for induction chemotherapy. *Haematologica* **2012**, *97*, 393–401. [CrossRef]

15. Kantarjian, H.; Oki, Y.; Garcia-Manero, G.; Huang, X.; O'Brien, S.; Cortes, J.; Faderl, S.; Bueso-Ramos, C.; Ravandi, F.; Estrov, Z. Results of a randomized study of 3 schedules of low-dose decitabine in higher-risk myelodysplastic syndrome and chronic myelomonocytic leukemia. *Blood* **2007**, *109*, 52–57. [CrossRef]

16. Blum, W.; Garzon, R.; Klisovic, R.B.; Schwind, S.; Walker, A.; Geyer, S.; Liu, S.; Havelange, V.; Becker, H.; Schaaf, L.; *et al.* Clinical response and miR-29b predictive significance in older AML patients treated with a 10-day schedule of decitabine. *Proc. Natl. Acad. Sci. USA* **2010**, *107*, 7473–7478. [CrossRef] [PubMed]

17. Ritchie, E.K.; Feldman, E.J.; Christos, P.J.; Rohan, S.D.; Lagassa, C.B.; Ippoliti, C.; Scandura, J.M.; Carlson, K.; Roboz, G.J. Decitabine in patients with newly diagnosed and relapsed acute myeloid leukemia. *Leuk. Lymphoma* **2013**, *54*, 2003–2007. [CrossRef] [PubMed]

18. Steensma, D.P.; Baer, M.R.; Slack, J.L.; Buckstein, R.; Godley, L.A.; Garcia-Manero, G.; Albitar, M.; Larsen, J.S.; Arora, S.; Cullen, M.T.; *et al.* Multicenter study of decitabine administered daily for 5 days every 4 weeks to adults with myelodysplastic syndromes: The alternative dosing for outpatient treatment (ADOPT) trial. *J. Clin. Oncol.* **2009**, *27*, 3842–3848. [CrossRef] [PubMed]

19. Kantarjian, H.M.; Thomas, X.G.; Dmoszynska, A.; Wierzbowska, A.; Mazur, G.; Mayer, J.; Gau, J.P.; Chou, W.C.; Buckstein, R.; Cermak, J.; *et al.* Multicenter, randomized, open-label, phase III trial of decitabine *vs.* patient choice, with physician advice, of either supportive care or low-dose cytarabine for the treatment of older patients with newly diagnosed acute myeloid leukemia. *J. Clin. Oncol.* **2012**, *30*, 2670–2677. [CrossRef] [PubMed]

20. Prebet, T.; Sun, Z.; Figueroa, M.E.; Ketterling, R.; Melnick, A.; Greenberg, P.L.; Herman, J.; Juckett, M.; Smith, M.R.; Malick, L.; *et al.* Prolonged administration of azacitidine with or without entinostat for myelodysplastic syndrome and acute myeloid leukemia with myelodysplasia-related changes: Results of the US Leukemia Intergroup trial E1905. *J. Clin. Oncol.* **2014**, *32*, 1242–1248. [CrossRef] [PubMed]

21. Löwenberg, B.; Ossenkoppele, G.J.; van Putten, W.; Schouten, H.C.; Graux, C.; Ferrant, A.; Sonneveld, P.; Maertens, J.; Jongen-Lavrencic, M.; von Lilienfeld-Toal, M.; *et al.* High-dose daunorubicin in older patients with acute myeloid leukemia. *N. Engl. J. Med.* **2009**, *361*, 1235–1248. [CrossRef] [PubMed]

22. Grövdal, M.; Karimi, M.; Khan, R.; Aggerholm, A.; Antunovic, P.; Astermark, J.; Bernell, P.; Engström, L.M.; Kjeldsen, L.; Linder, O.; *et al.* Maintenance treatment with azacytidine* for patients with high-risk myelodysplastic syndromes (MDS) or acute myeloid leukaemia following MDS in complete remission after induction chemotherapy. *Br. J. Haematol.* **2010**, *150*, 293–302. [CrossRef] [PubMed]

23. Boumber, Y.; Kantarjian, H.; Jorgensen, J.; Wen, S.; Faderl, S.; Castoro, R.; Autry, J.; Garcia-Manero, G.; Borthakur, G.; Jabbour, E.; *et al.* A randomized study of decitabine *vs.* conventional care for maintenance therapy in patients with acute myeloid leukemia in complete remission. *Leukemia* **2012**, *26*, 2428–2431. [CrossRef] [PubMed]

24. Lübbert, M.; Bertz, H.; Müller, M.J.; Finke, J. When azanucleoside treatment can be curative: Nonintensive bridging strategy before allografting in older patients with myelodysplastic syndrome/acute myeloid leukemia. *J. Clin. Oncol.* **2013**, *31*, 822–823. [CrossRef] [PubMed]

25. De Padua Silva, L.; de Lima, M.; Kantarjian, H.; Faderl, S.; Kebriaei, P.; Giralt, S.; Davisson, J.; Garcia-Manero, G.; Champlin, R.; Issa, J.P.; *et al.* Feasibility of allo-SCT after hypomethylating therapy with decitabine for myelodysplastic syndrome. *Bone Marrow Transpl.* **2009**, *43*, 839–843. [CrossRef]

26. Lübbert, M.; Bertz, H.; Rüter, B.; Marks, R.; Claus, R.; Wäsch, R.; Finke, J. Non-intensive treatment with low-dose 5-aza-2′-deoxycytidine (DAC) prior to allogeneic blood SCT of older MDS/AML patients. *Bone Marrow Transpl.* **2009**, *44*, 585–588. [CrossRef]

27. Cogle, C.R.; Imanirad, I.; Wiggins, L.E.; Hsu, J.; Brown, R.; Scornik, J.C.; Wingard, J.R. Hypomethylating agent induction therapy followed by hematopoietic cell transplantation is feasible in patients with myelodysplastic syndromes. *Clin. Adv. Hematol. Oncol.* **2010**, *8*, 40–46.

28. Field, T.; Perkins, J.; Huang, Y.; Kharfan-Dabaja, M.A.; Alsina, M.; Ayala, E.; Fernandez, H.F.; Janssen, W.; Lancet, J.; Perez, L.; *et al.* 5-Azacitidine for myelodysplasia before allogeneic hematopoietic cell transplantation. *Bone Marrow Transpl.* **2010**, *45*, 255–260. [CrossRef]

29. Kim, D.Y.; Lee, J.H.; Park, Y.H.; Lee, J.H.; Kim, S.D.; Choi, Y.; Lee, S.B.; Lee, K.H.; Ahn, S.Y.; Lee, Y.S.; *et al.* Feasibility of hypomethylating agents followed by allogeneic hematopoietic cell transplantation in patients with myelodysplastic syndrome. *Bone Marrow Transpl.* **2012**, *47*, 374–379. [CrossRef]

30. Gerds, A.T.; Gooley, T.A.; Estey, E.H.; Appelbaum, F.R.; Deeg, H.J.; Scott, B.L. Pretransplantation therapy with azacitidine *vs.* induction chemotherapy and posttransplantation outcome in patients with MDS. *Biol. Blood Marrow Transpl.* **2012**, *18*, 1211–1218. [CrossRef]

31. Damaj, G.; Duhamel, A.; Robin, M.; Beguin, Y.; Michallet, M.; Mohty, M.; Vigouroux, S.; Bories, P.; Garnier, A.; el Cheikh, J.; *et al.* Impact of azacitidine before allogeneic stem-cell transplantation for myelodysplastic syndromes: A study by the Société Française de Greffe de Moelle et de Thérapie-Cellulaire and the Groupe-Francophone des Myélodysplasies. *J. Clin. Oncol.* **2012**, *30*, 4533–4540. [CrossRef]

32. Platzbecker, U.; Schetelig, J.; Finke, J.; Trenschel, R.; Scott, B.; Kobbe, G.; Schaefer-Eckart, K.; Bornhäuser, M.; Itzykson, R.; Germing, U. Allogeneic hematopoietic cell transplantation in patients age 60–70 years with de novo high-risk myelodysplastic syndrome or secondary acute myelogenous leukemia: Comparison with patients lacking donors who received azacitidine. *Biol. Blood Marrow Transpl.* **2012**, *18*, 1415–1421. [CrossRef]

33. De lima, M.; Giralt, S.; Thall, P.; de Padua Silva, L.; Jones, R.; Komanduri, K.; Braun, T.; Nguyen, H.; Champlin, R.; Garcia-Manero, G. Maintenance therapy with low-dose azacitidine after allogeneic hematopoietic stem cell transplantation for recurrent acute myelogenous leukemia or myelodysplastic syndrome: A dose and schedule finding study. *Cancer* **2010**, *116*, 5420–5431. [PubMed]

34. Platzbecker, U.; Wermke, M.; Radke, J.; Oelschlaegel, U.; Seltman, F.; Kiani, A.; Klut, I.; Knoth, H.; Röllig, C.; Schetelig, J.; *et al.* Azacitidine for treatment of imminent relapse in MDS or AML patients after allogeneic HSCT: Results of the RELAZA trial. *Leukemia* **2012**, *26*, 381–389. [CrossRef] [PubMed]

35. Jabbour, E.; Giralt, S.; Kantarjian, H.; Garcia-Manero, G.; Jagasia, M.; Kebriaei, P.; de Padua, L.; Shpall, E.; Champlin, R.; de Lima, M. Low-dose azacitidine after allogeneic stem cell transplantation for acute leukemia. *Cancer* **2009**, *115*, 1899–1905. [CrossRef] [PubMed]

36. Lübbert, M.; Bertz, H.; Wäsch, R.; Marks, R.; Rüter, B.; Claus, R.; Finke, J. Efficacy of a 3-day, low-dose treatment with 5-azacytidine followed by donor lymphocyte infusions in older patients with acute myeloid leukemia or chronic myelomonocytic leukemia relapsed after allografting. *Bone Marrow Transpl.* **2010**, *45*, 627–632. [CrossRef]

37. Schroeder, T.; Czibere, A.; Platzbecker, U.; Bug, U.; Uharek, L.; Luft, T.; Giagounidis, A.; Zohren, F.; Bruns, I.; Wolschke, C.; *et al.* Azacitidine and donor lymphocyte infusions as first salvage therapy for relapse of AML or MDS after allogeneic stem cell transplantation. *Leukemia* **2013**, *27*, 1229–1235. [CrossRef] [PubMed]

38. Burnett, A.; Wetzler, M.; Löwenberg, B. Therapeutic advances in acute myeloid leukemia. *J. Clin. Oncol.* **2011**, *29*, 487–94. [CrossRef] [PubMed]

39. Löwenberg, B.; Zittoun, R.; Kerkhofs, H.; Jehn, U.; Abels, J.; Debusscher, L.; Cauchie, C.; Peetermans, M.; Solbu, G.; Suciu, S. On the value of intensive remission-induction chemotherapy in elderly patients of 65+ years with acute myeloid leukaemia: A randomized phase III study of the european organization for research and treatment of cancer leukaemia group. *J. Clin. Oncol.* **1989**, *7*, 1268–1274. [PubMed]

40. Juliusson, G.; Antunovic, P.; Derolf, A.; Lehmann, S.; Mollgard, L.; Stockelberg, D.; Tidefelt, U.; Wahlin, A.; Hoglund, M. Age and acute myeloid leukaemia: Real world data on decision to treat and outcomes from the swedish acute leukaemia registry. *Blood* **2009**, *113*, 4179–4187. [CrossRef] [PubMed]

41. Tilly, H.; Castaigne, S.; Bordessoule, D.; Casassus, P.; le Prise, P.Y.; Tertian, G.; Desablens, B.; Henry-Amar, M.; Degos, L. Low-dose cytarabine *vs.* intensive chemotherapy in the treatment of acute nonlymphocytic leukaemia in the elderly. *J. Clin. Oncol.* **1990**, *8*, 272–279. [PubMed]

42. Burnett, A.K.; Milligan, D.; Prentice, A.G.; Goldstone, A.H.; McMullin, M.F.; Hills, R.K.; Wheatley, K. A comparison of low-dose cytarabine and hydroxyurea with or without all-trans retinoic acid for acute myeloid leukaemia and high-risk myelodysplastic syndrome in patients not considered fit for intensive treatment. *Cancer* **2007**, *109*, 1114–1124. [CrossRef] [PubMed]

43. Quintas-Cardama, A.; Ravandi, F.; Liu-Dumlao, T.; Brandt, M.; Faderl, S.; Pierce, S.; Borthakur, G.; Garcia-Manero, G.; Cortes, J.; Kantarjian, H. Epigenetic therapy is associated with similar survival compared with intensive chemotherapy in older patients with newly diagnosed acute myeloid leukemia. *Blood* **2012**, *120*, 4850–4855. [CrossRef] [PubMed]

44. Van der Helm, L.H.; Scheepers, E.R.; Veeger, N.J.; Daenen, S.M.; Mulder, A.B.; van den Berg, E.; Vellenga, E.; Huls, G. Azacitidine might be beneficial in a subgroup of older AML patients compared to intensive chemotherapy: A single centre retrospective study of 227 consecutive patients. *J. Hematol. Oncol.* **2013**, *16*. [CrossRef]

45. Van der Helm, L.; Alhan, C.; Wijermans, P.W.; van Marwijk Kooy, M.; Schaafsma, R.; Biemond, B.J.; Beeker, A.; Hoogendoorn, M.; van Rees, B.; de Weerdt, O.; *et al.* Platelet doubling after the first azacitidine cycle is a promising predictor for response in MDS, CMML and AML patients in the Dutch azacitidine compassionate named patient program. *Br. J. Haematol.* **2011**, *155*, 599–606. [CrossRef] [PubMed]

46. Klepin, H.D.; Rao, A.V.; Pardee, T.S. Acute myeloid leukemia and myelodysplastic syndromes in older adults. *J. Clin. Oncol.* **2014**. [CrossRef]

47. Giles, F.J.; Borthakur, G.; Ravandi, F.; Faderl, S.; Verstovsek, S.; Thomas, D.; Wierda, W.; Ferrajoli, A.; Kornblau, S.; Pierce, S.; *et al.* The haematopoietic cell transplantation comorbidity index score is predictive of early death and survival in patients over 60 years of age receiving induction therapy for acute myeloid leukaemia. *Br. J. Haematol.* **2007**, *136*, 624–627. [CrossRef] [PubMed]

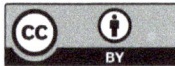

Journal of
Clinical Medicine

MDPI

Review

Rational Combinations of Targeted Agents in AML

Prithviraj Bose [1,†] **and Steven Grant** [2,*]

1   Department of Internal Medicine, Virginia Commonwealth University and VCU Massey Cancer Center
     Center, 1201 E Marshall St, MMEC 11-213, P.O. Box 980070, Richmond, VA 23298, USA;
     pbose@mcvh-vcu.edu
2   Departments of Internal Medicine, Microbiology and Immunology, Biochemistry and Molecular Biology,
     Human and Molecular Genetics and the Institute for Molecular Medicine, Virginia Commonwealth
     University and VCU Massey Cancer Center, 401 College St, P.O. Box 980035, Richmond, VA 23298, USA
*   Author to whom correspondence should be addressed; stgrant@vcu.edu;
     Tel.: +1-804-828-5211; Fax: +1-804-628-5920.
†   Current Affiliation: Department of Leukemia, University of Texas MD Anderson Cancer Center,
     1400 Holcombe Blvd, FC4.3062, Houston, TX 77030, USA; pbose@mdanderson.org.

Academic Editor: Celalettin Ustun
Received: 10 October 2014; Accepted: 6 January 2015; Published: 10 April 2015

Abstract: Despite modest improvements in survival over the last several decades, the treatment of
AML continues to present a formidable challenge. Most patients are elderly, and these individuals, as
well as those with secondary, therapy-related, or relapsed/refractory AML, are particularly difficult
to treat, owing to both aggressive disease biology and the high toxicity of current chemotherapeutic
regimens. It has become increasingly apparent in recent years that coordinated interruption of
cooperative survival signaling pathways in malignant cells is necessary for optimal therapeutic
results. The modest efficacy of monotherapy with both cytotoxic and targeted agents in AML testifies
to this. As the complex biology of AML continues to be elucidated, many "synthetic lethal" strategies
involving rational combinations of targeted agents have been developed. Unfortunately, relatively
few of these have been tested clinically, although there is growing interest in this area. In this
article, the preclinical and, where available, clinical data on some of the most promising rational
combinations of targeted agents in AML are summarized. While new molecules should continue
to be combined with conventional genotoxic drugs of proven efficacy, there is perhaps a need to
rethink traditional philosophies of clinical trial development and regulatory approval with a focus on
mechanism-based, synergistic strategies.

Keywords: AML; targeted therapies; rational combinations; HDAC inhibitors; CDK inhibitors;
proteasome inhibitors; checkpoint abrogators; apoptosis; BH3-mimetics; Mcl-1

---

1. Introduction

Despite significant progress in recent years in unraveling the genetic basis of AML [1], resulting in
improvements in our ability to prognosticate and predict outcomes with certain therapies [2], it remains
a devastating disease. Cure rates for young adults remain 40%–45% at best, and those for patients
older than 60 only around 10%–20% [3]. The anthracycline-cytarabine backbone, first introduced over
40 years ago [4], remains the cornerstone of initial therapy for most patients, and the only truly targeted
agent to receive regulatory approval, gemtuzumab ozogamycin, has been voluntarily withdrawn from
the market by the manufacturer [5,6]. Allogeneic hematopoietic stem cell transplantation (HSCT),
with all its attendant risks, remains the best post-remission therapy for AML till date [7]. In a recent
randomized, phase III trial [8], elacytarabine, a novel elaidic acid ester of cytarabine, failed to improve
outcomes over physicians' choice of one of seven different commonly used salvage regimens for
patients with relapsed or refractory disease, who have a dismal prognosis (5-year overall survival

from first relapse approximately 10%) [9]. Although initially greeted with considerable enthusiasm, no fms-like tyrosine kinase 3 (FLT3) inhibitor has been licensed for use [10], and resistance-conferring mutations in the FLT3 kinase have been described [11]. Recent approaches have involved exploring new therapeutic targets, e.g., isocitrate dehydrogenase (IDH) [12] or immune checkpoints, delivering conventional cytotoxic agents in fixed molar ratios [13,14], harnessing the power of T-cells against AML stem cell antigens (e.g., CD123) using dual affinity retargeting molecules (DARTs, *Blood* 2013; 122:360), *etc.*

Malignant cells are particularly vulnerable to the simultaneous disruption of multiple, cooperative survival signaling pathways [15,16]. In recent years, the concept of rationally combining targeted agents to defeat the redundancy of survival pathways in neoplastic cells has rapidly been gaining ground in a variety of tumor types [17]. Indeed, signaling pathways within cancer cells have been compared to other complex networks such as the internet or airplane flight patterns, characterized by both remarkable robustness and surprising vulnerability, such that very limited yet coordinated, specific targeting of the most critical "nodes" in the network can have dramatically outsized effects [18]. In this article, we review various "synthetic lethal" strategies using rational combinations of targeted drugs in AML.

2. Combinations Involving Epigenetic Therapies

2.1. DNMTIs + HDACIs

A particularly popular combination has been that of DNA methyltransferase inhibitors (DNMTIs) with histone deacetylase inhibitors (HDACIs). That epigenetic processes play a fundamental role in cancer causation and progression has been recognized for over a decade now [19]. Chromatin organization modulates gene transcription inasmuch as a more open, relaxed configuration of chromatin (e.g., induced by HDACIs through histone acetylation) or demethylation of CpG islands in the promoter regions of genes (e.g., induced by DNMTIs, also known as hypomethylating agents, HMAs) activates transcription of epigenetically silenced tumor suppressor genes, e.g., DNA repair genes [20]. The combination of DNMTIs and HDACIs synergistically triggers apoptosis and up-regulates microRNAs that, in turn, down-regulate oncogenes [21]. While the DNMTIs azacytidine and decitabine have clear single-agent activity in AML [22–25] and are widely used, response rates to HDACI monotherapy in AML and MDS have been more modest, of the order of 10%–20% [26] and none is approved for this indication, although the pan-HDACI pracinostat was recently granted "orphan drug" status by the FDA for AML [27]. As noted above, many trials of "dual epigenetic therapy" combining DNMTIs with HDACIs in AML have been conducted. In the recently published U.S. Leukemia Intergroup trial E1905 involving 97 patients with MDS and 52 with AML, addition of the class I-selective HDACI entinostat to azacytidine did not increase clinical response rates and was associated with pharmacodynamic antagonism [28]. Azacytidine was administered on days 1–10 of a 28-day cycle and entinostat on days 3 and 10 [28]. A randomized phase II study (NCT01305499) is currently underway to see if sequential, as opposed to concurrent, administration of entinostat will improve efficacy of this combination. In contrast, the combination of pracinostat with azacytidine yielded an 89% overall response rate (ORR) in a 9-patient pilot study in patients with higher risk categories of MDS and was very well tolerated [29].

2.2. Other DNMTI-Based Combinations

DNMTIs have also been combined with many other classes of targeted agents in AML. Based on the ability of the proteasome inhibitor bortezomib to up-regulate miR-29b, resulting in loss of transcriptional activation of several genes relevant to myeloid leukemogenesis, including DNA methyltransferases and receptor tyrosine kinases, a phase I trial of bortezomib and decitabine was conducted [30]. Seven of 19 patients overall achieved complete remission (CR) or complete remission with incomplete count recovery (CRi), although 5 of these were treatment-naïve [30]. The regimen was shown to down-regulate FLT3 [30]. These findings led to a phase II trial (NCT01420926) in the cooperative group setting in older patients with AML, but this trial was closed prematurely as it was deemed unlikely to meet its primary endpoint. In a phase II trial of sorafenib and azacytidine in 43 patients (37 evaluable) with *FLT3*-mutated AML and 0–7 (median 2) prior therapies, the ORR was 46%, including 27% CR/CRi [31]. FLT3 ligand levels did not rise to levels seen in prior studies of patients receiving cytotoxic chemotherapy [32]. Decitabine and midostaurin have been combined in a phase I study in patients with relapsed/refractory AML with or without *FLT3* mutations based on *in vitro* evidence of synergy against FLT3-internal tandem duplication (*FLT3-ITD*$^+$) cells [33]. Sequential administration was safe but concurrent administration was too toxic [33]. 57% of patients achieved stable disease (SD) or better; 25% had a complete hematologic response (CHR) [33]. Phase I trials combining decitabine with rapamycin [34] and with bexarotene [35] in patients with AML have been completed, with demonstration of safety but only modest outcomes. Both sequential [36] and concomitant [37] administration of azacytidine and lenalidomide have been studied in newly diagnosed elderly patients with AML in the phase I setting. Both combinations were well-tolerated, with ORRs of around 55% and CR/CRi rates ranging from 31% to 44% [36,37].

Given their efficacy and safety, and consequent widespread use as single agents for the treatment of patients with AML who are elderly and/or unfit for conventional chemotherapy, azacytidine and decitabine are increasingly being combined in clinical trials with a plethora of emerging, investigational targeted agents. Examples include volasertib (NCT02003573), a polo-like kinase 1 (PLK-1) inhibitor recently designated an "orphan drug" for AML [27], the first-in-class neddylation inhibitor MLN4924 (NCT01814826), the hedgehog inhibitor sonidegib (NCT02129101) and the Bcl-2-selective antagonist, ABT-199 (NCT02203773). *In vitro*, however, short interfering RNA (siRNA) silencing of the anti-apoptotic proteins Mcl-1 and Bcl-xL, but not Bcl-2, exhibited variable synergy with azacytidine [38].

2.3. BET Inhibitor-Based Combinations

A relatively recent development in the field of epigenetic targeting of chromatin networks in cancer has been the discovery of potent and specific small-molecule BET (bromodomain and extraterminal) inhibitors [39]. The bromodomain is a highly conserved motif of 110 amino acids found in proteins that interact with chromatin, such as transcription factors, histone acetylases and nucleosome remodelling complexes [40]. Bromodomain proteins function as chromatin "readers", some of which have key roles in the acetylation-dependent assembly of transcriptional regulator complexes [41]. Bromodomain proteins recruit chromatin-regulating enzymes, including "writers" and "erasers" of histone modification, to target promoters and to regulate gene expression [40]. Lysine acetylation, a key mechanism that regulates chromatin structure, creates docking sites for bromodomains, and BET proteins regulate the expression of key oncogenes and anti-apoptotic proteins [41]. It was recently demonstrated that the BET protein (BRD4) antagonist JQ1 synergistically induced apoptosis of AML cells in combination with the HDACI panobinostat and improved the survival of mouse xenografts [42]. Additionally, JQ1 also synergized with the FLT3 tyrosine kinase inhibitors (TKIs) ponatinib or quizartinib to induce apoptosis of *FLT3-ITD*$^+$ AML cells and overcame FLT3 TKI resistance-conferring mutations such as F691L and D835V [43]. Furthermore, the JQ1/panobinostat combination synergistically induced apoptosis of FLT3 TKI-resistant cells [43].

3. HDACI-Based Combinations Involving Non-Epigenetic Therapies (Table 1)

Distinct from their role as epigenetic modifiers, HDACIs exert a plethora of other actions (Figure 1) in neoplastic cells with a high degree of selectivity for the latter. These include down-regulation of anti-apoptotic and up-regulation of pro-apoptotic proteins (e.g., Bim), activation of the death receptor (extrinsic) pathway of apoptosis, induction of oxidative injury, interference with checkpoint and chaperone protein function (the latter through acetylation of Hsp90, leading to down-regulation of its "client" proteins), inhibition of DNA repair, interference with the function of co-repressors/co-factors, promotion of endoplasmic reticulum (ER) stress and disruption of aggresome function, JNK (C-Jun-N-terminal kinase) activation, STAT5 (signal transducer and activator of transcription 5) inhibition, proteasome inhibition, induction of autophagy and anti-angiogenic effects [26,44,45].

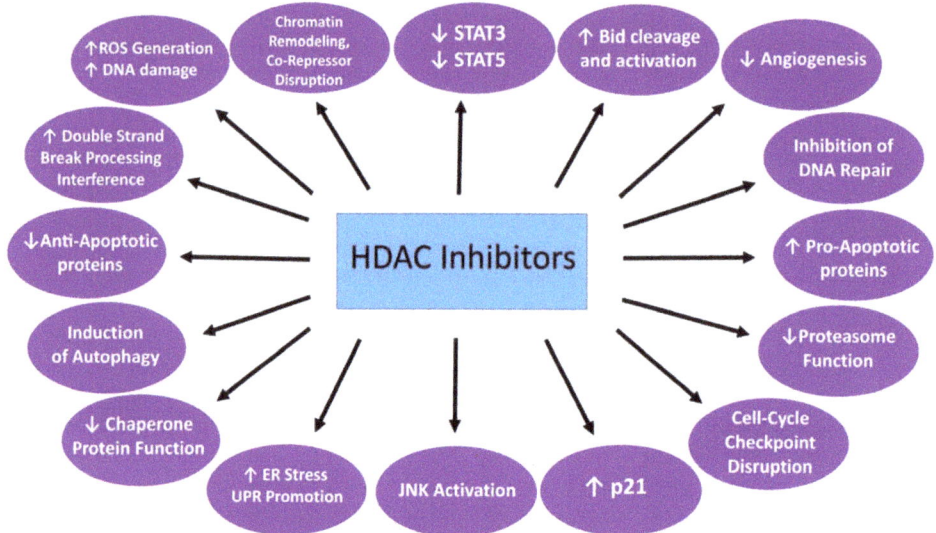

Figure 1. Mechanisms of HDACI lethality. Reproduced, with permission, from [45].

3.1. HDACIs + Proteasome Inhibitors

As noted above, the single-agent activity of HDACIs in AML is modest [26], and it has been appreciated for some time that the ultimate role of these agents may lie in combinatorial approaches [44,46]. An extensively studied rational combination has been that of HDACIs with proteasome inhibitors (PIs). While most advanced in multiple myeloma (MM) in terms of clinical development [47], this combination has been investigated in nearly every hematologic malignancy and may hold promise in AML [48,49]. Synergism between PIs and HDACIs stems from multiple mechanisms [50], including the inhibition by PIs of the pro-survival NF-κB pathway [51], which is activated by HDACIs and limits their lethality [52,53], disruption by HDACIs of aggresome formation [54], a physiologic response to proteasome inhibition [54], Hsp90 inhibition by HDACIs [55], both leading to marked accumulation of mis-folded proteins and accentuation of the proteotoxic stress induced by PIs, and multiple overlapping actions between these two classes of agents [26,44,45,56,57]. Additionally, there is evidence that the proteasome plays an important role in HDACI-induced apoptosis [58], and that HDACs are critical targets of bortezomib, at least in MM [59].

In pre-clinical studies, co-administration of sub-micromolar concentrations of the pan-HDACI belinostat with low nanomolar concentrations of bortezomib sharply increased apoptosis in AML and cell lines and primary blasts [48]. Synergistic interactions were associated with interruption of both canonical and non-canonical NF-κB signaling pathways, down-regulation of NF-κB-dependent pro-survival proteins (e.g., XIAP, Bcl-xL) and up-regulation of Bim [48]. These findings led to a phase I clinical trial of the combination in patients with relapsed/refractory or poor-prognosis previously untreated acute leukemias or higher risk MDS (NCT01075425) [49]. The maximum tolerated doses (MTDs) were determined to be 1.3 mg/m^2 IV of bortezomib on days 1, 4, 8 and 11 and 1000 mg/m^2 IV of belinostat on days 1–5 and 8–12 of a 3-week cycle. Of 35 response-evaluable subjects, one patient with mixed lineage leukemia (*MLL*)-rearranged biphenotypic acute leukemia refractory to "7 + 3" and FLAG-Ida (fludarabine, cytarabine, granulocyte colony stimulating factor, idarubicin) achieved a CR and went on to an allogeneic HSCT; 4 had a partial remission (PR), 14 achieved stable disease (SD), and 16 had disease progression. Four subjects discontinued study treatment due to adverse events (AEs). Overall, the regimen was very well-tolerated. One patient with Janus kinase 2 (*JAK2*)-mutated myelofibrosis transformed to AML remains on treatment beyond 31 cycles (manuscript in preparation). Efforts are currently underway to better characterize (at a genomic level) the leukemias of the two patients who did exceptionally well on this study.

3.2. HDACIs + CDK Inhibitors

Cyclin-dependent kinase inhibitors (CDKIs) represent an interesting class of agents capable of inducing cell cycle arrest and apoptosis in malignant cells, particularly hematologic tumor types, which may be more susceptible to inhibition of cell cycling and apoptosis induction [60]. Some of these agents, *i.e.*, those that inhibit cyclin T/CDK9, additionally inhibit global cellular transcription [61], thus down-regulating short-lived proteins critically dependent on transcription for their maintenance, e.g., the anti-apoptotic proteins XIAP and Mcl-1. Although no CDKI is currently approved, the FDA recently granted "orphan drug" designation to the pan-CDKI flavopiridol (alvocidib) for AML [27].

Multiple pre-clinical studies have demonstrated robust synergism in AML cells between pan-CDKIs such as flavopiridol or roscovitine and HDACIs, e.g., vorinostat, dacinostat, sodium butyrate [62–66]. Besides down-regulation of XIAP and Mcl-1, a major mechanism underlying these interactions was the blockade by CDKIs of HDACI-induced up-regulation of the endogenous CDKI, $p21^{WAF1/CIP1}$. These observations led to a phase I trial of the combination of alvocidib and vorinostat in patients with relapsed/refractory or poor prognosis newly diagnosed acute leukemia or higher risk MDS [67]. The alvocidib MTD was 20 mg/m^2 IV load over 30 min followed by 20 mg/m^2 infused over 4 h ("hybrid" schedule of administration [68]) on days 1 and 8, in combination with vorinostat, 200 mg orally, three times a day, for 14 days on a 21-day cycle [67]. No objective responses were achieved in 26 evaluable patients (of 28 treated), although 13 exhibited SD [67].

3.3. HDACIs + TKIs

As discussed above, HDACIs, especially those that inhibit HDAC6, acetylate and thereby interfere with the function of chaperone proteins, in particular Hsp90, consequently down-regulating several pro-growth and pro-survival Hsp90 "client" proteins of critical importance in myeloid leukemias, e.g., breakpoint cluster region-Abelson (Bcr-Abl), mutant FLT3, c-Raf and Akt [55]. In the context of FLT3, this phenomenon has also been reported with the class I-selective HDACI, entinostat [69]. Additionally, HDACIs disrupt mitotic spindle checkpoints in neoplastic cells [70] and induce "mitotic slippage" [71]. These findings have provided the rationale for multiple preclinical studies that have demonstrated the synergism between HDACIs and TKIs targeting Bcr-Abl [72–76], FLT3 [77], JAK [78,79] and aurora kinases [80–82], which play critical roles in mitosis [83,84]. Unfortunately, the dual Bcr-Abl/aurora kinase inhibitors MK-0457 (VX-680) [80,81] and KW-2449 [82] are no longer in development. To our knowledge, this concept has not been evaluated in clinical trials in AML. However, at least two ongoing clinical trials are testing the combination of the HDACI panobinostat and the JAK1/2 inhibitor ruxolitinib in patients with myelofibrosis (NCT01693601, NCT01433445). In chronic myeloid leukemia (CML), the HDACI+TKI strategy has been reported to target stem cells [85]. Synergistic anti-leukemic interactions between AT9283, a multi-targeted TKI that inhibits Bcr-Abl, FLT3, JAK and aurora kinases [86–88], and entinostat have been observed in Bcr-Abl+ cells, including those bearing the gatekeeper mutation T315I, as well as in AML cells, both *FLT3*-mutated and -wild type (Nguyen and Grant, unpublished observations). Considering that mutations that confer resistance to one of the most promising FLT3 TKIs, quizartinib, have been described [11], this strategy may yet prove valuable in AML.

3.4. HDACIs + G2/M Checkpoint Abrogators

Cell cycle checkpoints, part of the DNA damage response (DDR) network, are in-built safety mechanisms the activation of which helps preserve genomic integrity by halting cell division upon the occurrence of DNA damage and allowing time for DNA repair [89]. If repair fails, checkpoints trigger apoptosis [90]. The major cell cycle checkpoints are the G1/S, intra-S-phase and G2/M checkpoints. Checkpoint dysfunction is common in human cancers and is considered a pathologic hallmark of neoplastic transformation [91]. In particular, the G1/S-checkpoint is frequently dysfunctional because of p53 and/or Rb mutations, making malignant cells overtly reliant on the intra-S-phase and G2/M checkpoints [92]. Although p53 mutations are uncommon in de novo AML [93], overexpression of Mdm2, the negative regulator of p53, is common [94,95], as is disruption of regulated p53 expression [96], and p53 mutations are common in secondary AML [97–100]. p53 mutations are strongly associated with a complex aberrant karyotype in AML [101]. In these patients, p53 alterations are associated with older age, genomic complexity, specific DNA copy number alterations, monosomal karyotypes, and a dismal outcome [102]. When present, p53 mutations confer an extremely poor prognosis [93,103,104] that is not overcome even by allogeneic HSCT [105]. Finally, recent studies indicate that leukemic cells expressing FLT3-ITD display defective DNA repair mechanisms [106,107]. In the presence of a dysfunctional G1/S checkpoint, G2/M checkpoint abrogation (e.g., with small-molecule inhibitors of the Chk1 or Wee1 kinases) prevents cancer cells from repairing DNA damage, forcing them into a premature and lethal mitosis ("mitotic catastrophe") [92].

Given that HDACIs induce DNA damage [108] and inhibit DNA repair, both homologous [109] and non-homologous end-joining (NHEJ) [110], and the ability of these agents and Hsp90 inhibitors to down-regulate proteins that play major roles in the DDR network such as ATR (ATM and Rad3 related), Chk1 and Wee1 [111–114], the combination of HDACIs with G2/M checkpoint abrogators has considerable theoretical appeal [45]. Indeed, synergistic potentiation of vorinostat-mediated apoptosis by the Chk1 inhibitor MK-8776 has been demonstrated in various AML cell lines, both *p53*-wild type and -deficient, as well as in those bearing *FLT3-ITD* [115]. Furthermore, the regimen was active against primary AML blasts, particularly against the putative leukemia initiating cell (LIC, CD34$^+$CD38$^-$CD123$^+$) population [115]. However, clinical trials of Chk1 inhibitors have concentrated on combining them with conventional genotoxic agents, and no trials have explored simultaneous HDAC and Chk1 inhibition.

The Wee1 kinase has recently emerged as a novel therapeutic target in AML [116–118]. Although efforts at the preclinical level to develop AZD-1775, a potent, small-molecule inhibitor of Wee1 [119,120], in AML have focused largely on using it to circumvent resistance to cytarabine [121,122], a sound rationale exists for combining this agent with HDACIs in AML. Of note, AZD-1775 may be effective regardless of p53 functionality [120,122]. During interphase, Wee1 phosphorylates the cyclin B/CDK1 (also known as cdc2) complex at Tyr^{15} to inactivate it, and Wee1 inhibition causes forced activation of CDK1, premature mitotic entry and impairment of homologous recombination [123]. Activation of cyclin B/CDK1 (cdc2) requires dephosphorylation by the CDC25 phosphatases (A, B and C) [89]. Notably, inactivation of cdc2 (CDK1) involves phosphorylation at two inhibitory sites, *i.e.*, Tyr^{15} and Thr^{14}, and dephosphorylation of both sites is necessary for full cyclin B/CDK1 (cdc2) activation. Upon G2/M checkpoint activation, ATR/Chk1 phosphorylates (and thereby inhibits) CDC25A, -B and -C, thus preventing premature mitotic entry [89].

While Chk1 is a positive regulator of Wee1 (through stimulatory phosphorylation), Wee1 inhibition results in compensatory activation of Chk1, leading to phosphorylation of cyclin B/CDK1 (cdc2) at Thr^{14} [124], a therapeutically undesirable, putatively cytoprotective effect. Concomitant administration of an HDACI may circumvent this problem by down-regulating Chk1 [111]. While this could also be achieved by combined Chk1 and Wee1 inhibition [124–127], HDACIs carry the additional advantages of inducing DNA damage and inhibiting DNA repair. Preclinical studies in AML with the combination of vorinostat and AZD-1775 have shown striking synergism, irrespective of *p53* and *FLT3* mutational status, including in "LIC"s, primary AML blasts and in a xenograft mouse (flank) model [128].

Importantly, whereas AZD-1775 treatment of leukemia cells triggered cyclin B/CDK1 (cdc2) Tyr^{15} dephosphorylation, it also induced Chk1 activation and Thr^{14} phosphorylation [128]. However, HDACI co-administration abrogated these undesirable phenomena, resulting in pronounced Tyr^{15} and Thr^{14} dephosphorylation, and full cyclin B/CDK1 (cdc2) activation, accompanied by premature mitotic entry and DNA damage [128]. These data and similarly promising results obtained upon substituting the recently approved HDACI belinostat for vorinostat have sparked interest in a National Cancer Institute-sponsored phase I clinical trial of the AZD-1775/belinostat combination in patients with relapsed/refractory AML/MDS as well as treatment-naïve poor prognosis patients with AML.

3.5. Other HDACI-Based Rational Combinations in AML

Aside from the strategies discussed above, HDACIs may potentially be successfully combined with a number of other investigational agents in AML. The first-in-class polo-like kinase 1 (PLK1) inhibitor volasertib was recently granted first "breakthrough" [129], and then "orphan drug" designation [27] for AML. This agent is currently in clinical trials in combination with low dose cytarabine (NCT01721876), decitabine (NCT02003573) or intensive chemotherapy (NCT02198482). PLK1 is critical to mitotic progression [130,131], and plays an important role in the DDR network [132,133], interacting with multiple checkpoint proteins [134]. As Bcr-Abl signals downstream to PLK1 [135], the PLK1 inhibitor BI2536 was studied in combination with vorinostat in CML cell lines and primary cells [136]. Pronounced synergism was observed in both imatinib-sensitive and -resistant Bcr-Abl$^+$ cells, both *in vitro* and *in vivo* [136]. Enhanced Bcr-Abl pathway inhibition did not appear to be the predominant mechanism for lethality of the PLK1 inhibitor/HDACI combination; rather, it seemed to be potentiation of DNA damage and disabling of the DDR [136]. Given that pracinostat has also received "orphan drug" designation for AML [27], the combination of volasertib and pracinostat warrants attention in this disease.

The first-in-class inhibitor of protein "neddylation", MLN4924 [137], is another promising agent in AML [138,139] currently in clinical trials with azacytidine (NCT01814826). Targeting protein neddylation, a critical pathway of protein degradation located upstream of the proteasome [140], allows for more selective interference with protein turnover, potentially yielding a better therapeutic index for these drugs as compared to PIs [141,142]. At least in theory, combination of this agent with HDACIs is particularly appealing for several reasons [45]. MLN4924 inhibits NF-κB (activated by HDACIs [52,53]) and leads to ROS generation and DNA damage in AML cells [138]. Additionally, MLN4924 induces DNA re-replication, an irreversible cellular insult that leads to apoptosis, by interfering with the turnover of the cullin-RING ligase substrate CDT1, a critical DNA replication licensing factor, in S phase [143,144]. Finally, MLN4924 appears to trigger a cytoprotective autophagic response [145,146], that could be counteracted by HDACIs [147,148].

The phosphatidylinositol-3-kinase/Akt/mammalian target of rapamycin (PI3K/Akt/mTOR) pathway is a cellular growth, proliferation, motility and survival signaling axis [149] that represents one of the most frequently dysregulated pathways in cancer [150], including AML [151,152], where activation of the pathway has been shown to be required for cell survival [153,154]. In AML, Akt activation (phosphorylatyion at Thr^{308}/Ser^{473}) variably occurs in 50–80% of patients [155,156]; hence, there is considerable interest in targeting the PI3K/Akt/mTOR axis in AML [157]. Although mTOR inhibitors have been commercially available for some time for the treatment of various solid tumors, the first PI3K (delta isoform) inhibitor to receive regulatory approval, idelalisib [158,159], has only very recently arrived on the market, fueling intense interest in this class of agents. Synergistic interactions between PI3K or Akt inhibitors and HDACIs have been documented in AML cells [160,161]. Combined HDAC and PI3K inhibition led to a marked increase in apoptosis associated with Bcl-2 and Bid cleavage, XIAP and Mcl-1 down-regulation, mitogen activated protein kinase (MAPK) inactivation and blockade of HDACI-mediated induction of p21$^{CIP1/WAF1}$ [160]. Inactivation of extracellular signal-regulated kinase (ERK) was also seen with HDACI/perifosine (Akt inhibitor) co-treatment of AML cells, along with Akt inhibition, JNK activation, ROS and ceramide generation, leading to striking increases in mitochondrial injury and apoptosis [161].

4. Priming Apoptosis

The Bcl-2 family of proteins stands at the crossroads of cellular survival and death, and the pro- and anti-apoptotic members of this family regulate the intrinsic, or mitochondrial, pathway of apoptosis [162]. The seminal event in this pathway of programmed cell death, "mitochondrial outer membrane permeabilization (MOMP)", commits the cell to apoptosis and constitutes a "point of no return" triggered by the apoptosis "effectors" Bax and Bak [163]. Under normal conditions, the pro-survival anti-apoptotic proteins (mainly Bcl-2, Bcl-xL and Mcl-1) sequester the apoptosis effectors; thus, the latter need to be released from such binding in order to induce MOMP [163]. While some of the so-called "BH3-only" proteins (e.g., Bim, tBid and Puma) can directly activate Bax and Bak [163], most function as "sensitizers", *i.e.*, they displace the apoptosis effectors from their association with the anti-apoptotic proteins [164], a function mimicked by the "BH3-mimetic" class of drugs. The Bcl-2 family is of profound importance in the pathogenesis, prognosis, chemoresistance and treatment of AML [165].

The discovery of ABT-737, a specific "BH3-mimetic" antagonist of Bcl-2 and Bcl-xL, demonstrated for the first time that specific protein-protein interactions could be targeted by small molecules, and ushered in a new era in cell death research [166]. Subsequently, an oral analog with improved pharmacological properties, ABT-263 (navitoclax), was developed [167]. This agent demonstrated promising efficacy in patients with relapsed/refractory CLL in a phase I trial [168], but the occurrence of dose-dependent thrombocytopenia owing to on-target Bcl-xL inhibition [169] in early clinical trials [168,170–172] precluded continued development of this agent. There is also some evidence that Bcl-xL-inhibitory BH3-mimetics can undermine platelet function [173]. These observations led to the development, by reverse engineering of navitoclax, of ABT-199 (GDC-0199), a highly selective Bcl-2 antagonist that retains significant anti-tumor activity while sparing platelets [174]. This agent appears highly effective in CLL [175], and at least at the preclinical level, holds substantial promise in AML [176]. Of note, oblimersen, an anti-sense oligonucleotide against Bcl-2, failed in phase III clinical trials when added to chemotherapy in older patients in AML [177], despite improving 5-year survival when combined with fludarabine and cyclophosphamide in patients with relapsed/refractory CLL [178]. This agent was not, however, ever approved for use.

Neither ABT-199 (GDC-0199) nor navitoclax inhibits Mcl-1, which is fundamental to the pathogenesis and maintenance of AML [179] and the main determinant of resistance to ABT-737 [180,181]. The pan-BH3-mimetic obatoclax, which inhibited Mcl-1 in addition to Bcl-2/-xL [182], has been discontinued due to the occurrence of severe, infusional neurologic toxicity, e.g., ataxia, euphoria and somnolence. For these reasons, a number of combination strategies (Figure 2) have been explored preclinically to simultaneously target multiple arms of the apoptotic regulatory machinery, *i.e.*, Mcl-1 and Bcl-2/-xL [183,184]. Since Mcl-1 is a short-lived protein critically dependent on active transcription and translation for its maintenance, some of these strategies have used cyclin T/DCK9 inhibitors or sorafenib to repress cellular transcription [61] or translation [185], respectively. Thus, roscovitine dramatically increases ABT-737 lethality in AML cells by simultaneously and cooperatively inducing Bak activation and Bax translocation [186]. In the case of sorafenib, synergistic interactions with both ABT-737 [187] and obatoclax [188] have been reported, in the latter case with the induction of cytoprotective autophagy that could be inhibited pharmacologically, potentiating the lethality of the regimen [188]. In these studies, both Bim up-regulation and Mcl-1 down-regulation were noted, and synergism was demonstrated not only in AML cell lines, but also in patient-derived cells and in a xenograft mouse model [187,188]. HDACIs, which up-regulate Bim, have also been combined with both ABT-737 [189] and obatoclax [190]. HDACI-induced Bim is largely sequestered by Bcl-2 and Bcl-xL, which it is released by ABT-737, activating Bax and Bak and triggering MOMP [189]. Both mocetinostat and vorinostat display synergistic anti-leukemia activity with obatoclax, but in this setting, cell death is attributable to activation of both apoptosis and autophagy [190]. Finally, mitogen activated protein kinase kinase (MEK) inhibitors have been shown to synergize with ABT-737, both *in vitro* (including in "LICs") and *in vivo*, through the same mechanism, *i.e.*, down-regulation of Mcl-1, which is induced by ABT-737 via ERK activation [191].

Table 1. HDACI-based rational combinations with non-cytotoxic, non-epigenetic agents in AML.

Partner Agent Class	Mechanism(s) of Synergy	Clinical Trials, if any	Reference(s)
Proteasome inhibitors (PIs), e.g., bortezomib, carfilzomib, ixazomib, oprozomib, marizomib	NF-κB inhibition by PIs (activated by HDACIs); inhibition by HDACIs of aggresome formation and of Hsp90→increased proteotoxic stress, multiple other actions	NCT01075425; closed to accrual; phase I; enrolled primarily relapsed/refractory patients with AML; one CR, one prolonged SD (see text)	[48,49]
Cyclin-dependent kinase inhibitors (CDKIs), e.g., flavopiridol (alvocidib), roscovitine (seliciclib), dinaciclib, palbociclib	Down-regulation of XIAP and Mcl-1 by cyclin T/CDK9 inhibitors via transcriptional repression; blockade by CDKIs of HDACI-induced up-regulation of p21	NCT00278330; completed; phase I; enrolled primarily relapsed/refractory patients with AML; no objective responses; 50% achieved SD	[62–67]
Multi-kinase inhibitors (that inhibit aurora kinases and critical signaling molecules in AML, e.g., FLT3, JAK2), e.g., MK-0457, KW-2449, AT9283	Down-regulation of Hsp90 "client" proteins by HDACIs, e.g., FLT3, c-Raf, Akt, JAK2, disruption of mitotic spindle checkpoints and induction of mitotic "slippage"		[77,79,81]
Checkpoint abrogators, e.g., MK-8776 (Chk1 inhibitor), AZD-1775 (Wee1 inhibitor)	Induction of DNA damage and inhibition of DNA repair by HDACIs; down-regulation of ATR, Chk1 and Wee1 by HDACIs via Hsp90 inhibition	Phase I clinical trial of Wee1 inhibitor AZD-1775 and belinostat in patients with relapsed/refractory or poor-prognosis AML in development	[115,128]
Polo-like kinase inhibitors, e.g., BI2536, volasertib	Potentiation of DNA damage and disruption of the DNA damage response by HDACIs		[136]
Protein neddylation inhibitors (MLN4924)	Inhibition of NF-κB (activated by HDACIs) by MLN4924, ROS generation and induction of DNA damage by MLN4924 as well as by HDACIs, opposing effects on autophagy		Manuscript in preparation
BH3-mimetics, e.g., obatoclax, navitoclax, venetoclax	Up-regulation of Bim by HDACIs, which is released from Bcl-2 and Bcl-xL by ABT-737, activation of cytotoxic autophagy (obatoclax)		[189,190]
PI3K/Akt/mTOR pathway inhibitors, e.g., LY294002, buparlisib, idelalisib, duvelisib (PI3K inhibitors), perifosine (Akt inhibitor), BEZ235 (PI3K/mTOR inhibitor)	Bcl-2 and Bid cleavage, down-regulation of Mcl-1 and XIAP, MAPK/ERK inactivation, JNK activation, ROS generation, blockade of HDACI-mediated induction of p21		[160,161]

Abbreviations: HDACI, histone deacetylase inhibitor; NF-κB, nuclear factor kappa B; Hsp90, heat shock protein 90; AML, acute myeloid leukemia; CR, complete remission; SD, stable disease; DNA, deoxyribonucleic acid; ROS, reactive oxygen species; Bcl-2, B-cell lymphoma 2; XIAP, X-linked inhibitor of apoptosis; Mcl-1, myeloid cell leukemia 1; Bcl-xL, B-cell lymphoma extra long; MAPK, mitogen activated protein kinase; ERK, extracellular signal-regulated kinase; FLT3, fms-like tyrosine kinase 3; JAK2, Janus associated kinase 2; JNK, C-Jun N-terminal kinase; PI3K, phosphatidylinositol-3-kinase; mTOR, mammalian target of rapamycin; ATR, ATM (ataxia telangiectasia mutated) and Rad3-related; Chk1, checkpoint kinase 1.

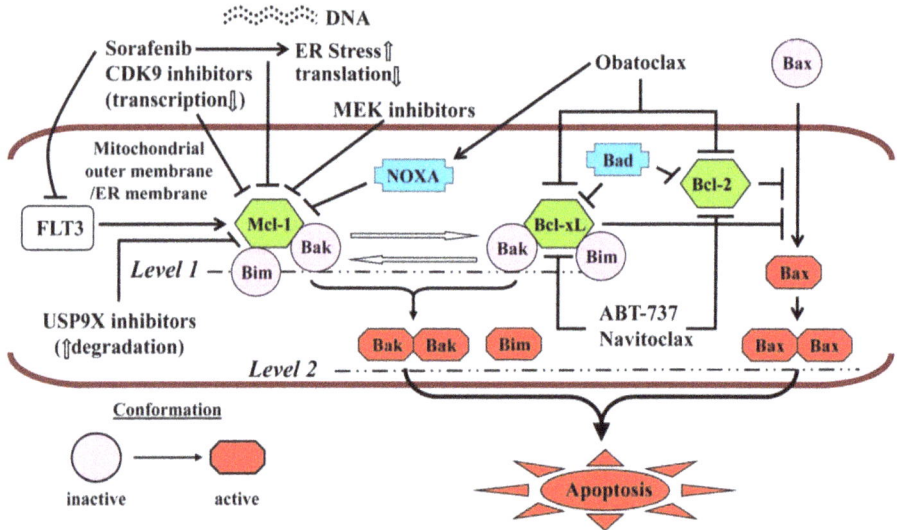

Figure 2. Should be: Mechanisms of potentiation of BH3-mimetic lethality by strategies targeting Mcl-1. Reproduced, with permission, from [184].

A particularly strong rationale exists [192] for combining BH3-mimetics, e.g., ABT-737, with dual inhibitors of PI3K and mTOR, e.g., NVP-BEZ235, PI-103 or GDC-0980 in AML (Figure 3). Akt regulates a wide range of target proteins that control cellular proliferation, survival, growth and other processes, including Bim, Bad and Bax, the forkhead box O (FOXO) transcription factors (which mediate apoptosis by activating the transcription of pro-apoptotic genes such as *FasL* and *Bim*), Mdm2, glycogen synthase kinase 3 (GSK3) isoforms (which down-regulate cyclin D1 and Myc), procaspase 9, IκB kinase (the negative regulator of NF-κB), the endogenous CDKI p27^{KIP1} and Chk1 [193,194]. Importantly, mTORC1, a major downstream effector of Akt, is often not only under the control of PI3K/Akt signaling [195], and conversely, mTOR inhibition can lead to feedback activation of PI3K/Akt and MEK/ERK, arguing for simultaneous inhibition of both PI3K/Akt and mTOR [196]. Some of these agents have shown clear preclinical evidence of activity in AML [197,198]. Finally, as noted above [160,161] and in sharp contrast to other tumor types [199], in AML cells, PI3K/Akt inhibitors may disrupt, rather than activate, the complementary Ras/Raf/MEK/ERK survival signaling pathway, activated in >80% of AML samples [200], through an unknown mechanism. For these reasons, while PI3K inhibitors (e.g., GDC-0941) [201] and mTOR inhibitors plus MEK inhibitors (e.g., AZD-8055 plus selumetinib) [202] demonstrate synergistic pro-apoptotic effects with ABT-737 in AML cell lines and patient-derived blasts, accompanied by Bim up-regulation, Mcl-1 down-regulation and Bax activation, dual PI3K/mTOR inhibitors may, in fact, be the superior partner for ABT-737 [192]. Indeed, these agents (e.g., NVP-BEZ235, PI-103) synergistically increased ABT-737-mediated cell death in multiple leukemia cell lines and primary AML specimens, as well as significantly diminished tumor growth and prolonged animal survival in a subcutaneous xenograft model [203]. PI3K/mTOR inhibitors markedly down-regulated Mcl-1, apparently through a GSK3-mediated mechanism, but increased Bim binding to Bcl-2/Bcl-xL; the latter effect was abrogated by ABT-737 [203]. Responding, but not non-responding, primary samples exhibited basal AKT phosphorylation, suggesting that basal Akt activation/addiction may predict for success of this therapeutic strategy [203]. Studies are underway to see if these findings can be extended to the combination of GDC-0980 and ABT-199 (GDC-0199).

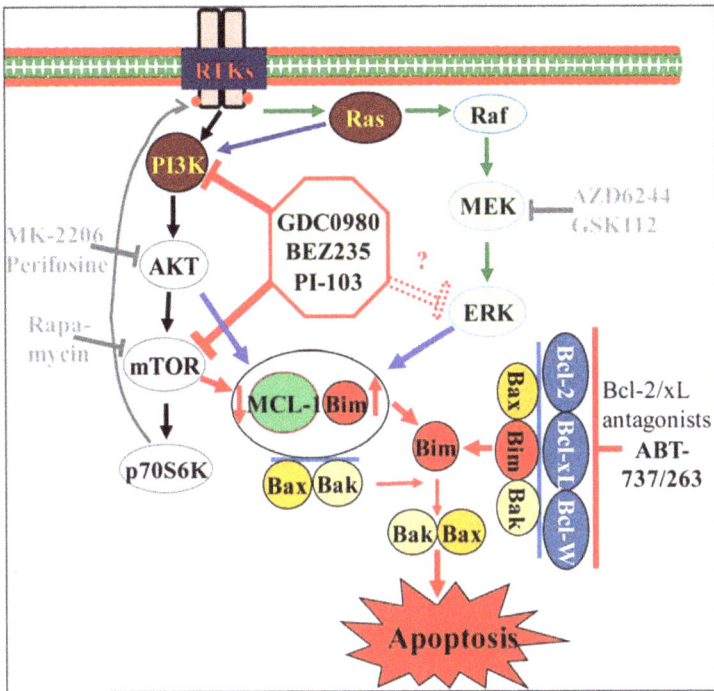

Figure 3. Hypothetical model of interactions between PI3K/AKT/mTOR pathway inhibitors and Bcl-2 antagonists. Reproduced, with permission, from [192].

5. Other Rational Combinations

The PI-CDKI combination of bortezomib and alvocidib is synergistic in myeloid leukemia cells [204,205] but, to our knowledge, this combination has been tested clinically only in patients with relapsed or refractory indolent B-cell neoplasms, including MM [206,207] In AML cells, synergistic induction of cell death was accompanied by down-regulation of Mcl-1 and XIAP, JNK activation, NF-κB inhibition, cdc2 activation and diminished expression of p21$^{WAF1/CIP1}$ [204]. In CML cells, similar findings were noted, in addition to Bcr-Abl down-regulation, STAT3/5 inhibition and diminished phosphorylation of Lyn, Hck, CrkL, and Akt [205]. The regimen effectively induced apoptosis in imatinib-resistant cells characterized by reduced expression of Bcr-Abl but a marked increase in expression/activation of Lyn and Hck [205].

Dramatic potentiation of CDKI-induced apoptosis by inhibitors of PI3K has been demonstrated in AML cell lines and primary patient-derived blasts, accompanied by diminished Bad phosphorylation, induction of Bcl-2 cleavage, and down-regulation of XIAP and Mcl-1 [208]. In contrast, synergistic enhancement of alvocidib-induced apoptosis was not observed with inhibitors of MEK/ERK or of mTOR [208]. Much more recently, PIK-75, a compound that transiently blocks CDK7/9, leading to transcriptional suppression of Mcl-1, and also targets the p110α isoform of PI3K has been shown to rapidly induce apoptosis of AML cells, significantly reduce leukemic burden and increase the survival of mouse xenografts without overt toxicity [209].

The observation that inhibition of Chk1 triggers marked ERK1/2 activation, which can be blocked by MEK inhibitors [210] or Ras-targeting agents such as statins [211] or farnesyltransferase inhibitors [212], leading to striking increases in apoptosis and dramatically enhanced lethality, both *in vitro* and *in vivo*, along with a requirement for ERK1/2 activation in progression across the G2/M

J. Clin. Med. **2015**, *4*, 634–664

boundary and through mitosis [213], as well as functional roles for MEK/ERK signaling in the DDR [214,215] provide the rationale for combined inhibition of Chk1 and the Ras/Raf/MEK/ERK pathway in AML [90]. Furthermore, these strategies act independently of *p53* mutational status [90]. However, these early studies [210–212] used UCN-01 (7-hydroxystaurosporine), which functions as a CDKI and as an inhibitor of protein kinase C (PKC), in addition to inhibiting Chk1. The recent withdrawals of several investigational Chk1 inhibitors has hampered translation of this concept. However, given the modest efficacy of selumetinib monotherapy in AML [216], combined Chk1 and MEK inhibition, most recently explored in MM [217], could also warrant attention in AML.

6. Conclusions

The number of rational combinations of targeted agents that are possible in AML and may be effective, at least in theory, is virtually limitless. The biggest challenge, therefore, is how to most judiciously choose the most promising combinations and bring them forward into clinical trials, which are costly and time-consuming. For these reasons, consideration should also be given to identifying the biologic subtypes of AML most likely to benefit from a given combination, as illustrated by the suggestion that basal Akt activation might predict for efficacy of a strategy simultaneously targeting Bcl-2/-xL nd PI3K/mTOR. Additionally, attention needs to be paid to better trial designs, e.g., adaptive designs, to get us answers to the biggest challenges confronting our patients in the most expeditious manner possible. Finally, the current paradigm for regulatory approval of new drugs in the United States discourages manufacturers from venturing into combinations of unapproved agents, and slows the pace of therapeutic progress. As a result, very few of the combinations discussed in this article have been tested in patients. While a complex problem, this is one that will require a concerted effort by lawmakers, researchers, industry and the concerned public to effect real change in the fight against cancer in general, and AML in particular.

Author Contributions: Prithviraj Bose wrote the manuscript. Steven Grant critically reviewed the manuscript for important intellectual content.

Conflicts of Interest: The authors declare no conflict of interest.

Acknowledgments: This work was supported in part by the following awards (SG): R01 CA167708 and P50 CA142509 from the National Institutes of Health, and an award from the Leukemia and Lymphoma Society (R1906-14).

References

1. Cancer Genome Atlas Research Network. Genomic and epigenomic landscapes of adult *de novo* acute myeloid leukemia. *N. Engl. J. Med.* **2013**, *368*, 2059–2074.
2. Patel, J.P.; Gonen, M.; Figueroa, M.E.; Fernandez, H.; Sun, Z.; Racevskis, J.; van Vlierberghe, P.; Dolgalev, I.; Thomas, S.; Aminova, O.; *et al.* Prognostic relevance of integrated genetic profiling in acute myeloid leukemia. *N. Engl. J. Med.* **2012**, *366*, 1079–1089. [CrossRef] [PubMed]
3. Burnett, A.K. Treatment of acute myeloid leukemia: Are we making progress? *Hematol. Am. Soc. Hematol. Educ. Program* **2012**, *2012*, 1–6.
4. Yates, J.W.; Wallace, H.J., Jr.; Ellison, R.R.; Holland, J.F. Cytosine arabinoside (NSC-63878) and daunorubicin (NSC-83142) therapy in acute nonlymphocytic leukemia. *Cancer Chemother. Rep.* **1973**, *57*, 485–488. [PubMed]
5. Ravandi, F.; Estey, E.H.; Appelbaum, F.R.; Lo-Coco, F.; Schiffer, C.A.; Larson, R.A.; Burnett, A.K.; Kantarjian, H.M. Gemtuzumab ozogamicin: Time to resurrect? *J. Clin. Oncol.* **2012**, *30*, 3921–3923. [CrossRef] [PubMed]
6. Rowe, J.M.; Lowenberg, B. Gemtuzumab ozogamicin in acute myeloid leukemia: A remarkable saga about an active drug. *Blood* **2013**, *121*, 4838–4841. [CrossRef] [PubMed]
7. Stelljes, M.; Krug, U.; Beelen, D.W.; Braess, J.; Sauerland, M.C.; Heinecke, A.; Ligges, S.; Sauer, T.; Tschanter, P.; Thoennissen, G.B.; *et al.* Allogeneic transplantation *versus* chemotherapy as postremission therapy for acute myeloid leukemia: A prospective matched pairs analysis. *J. Clin. Oncol.* **2014**, *32*, 288–296. [CrossRef] [PubMed]

8. Roboz, G.J.; Rosenblat, T.; Arellano, M.; Gobbi, M.; Altman, J.K.; Montesinos, P.; O'Connell, C.; Solomon, S.R.; Pigneux, A.; Vey, N.; *et al.* International randomized phase III study of elacytarabine *versus* investigator choice in patients with relapsed/refractory acute myeloid leukemia. *J. Clin. Oncol.* **2014**, *32*, 1919–1926. [CrossRef] [PubMed]

9. Forman, S.J.; Rowe, J.M. The myth of the second remission of acute leukemia in the adult. *Blood* **2013**, *121*, 1077–1082. [CrossRef] [PubMed]

10. Levis, M. FLT3 mutations in acute myeloid leukemia: What is the best approach in 2013? *Hematol. Am. Soc. Hematol. Educ. Program* **2013**, *2013*, 220–226. [CrossRef]

11. Smith, C.C.; Wang, Q.; Chin, C.S.; Salerno, S.; Damon, L.E.; Levis, M.J.; Perl, A.E.; Travers, K.J.; Wang, S.; Hunt, J.P.; *et al.* Validation of ITD mutations in FLT3 as a therapeutic target in human acute myeloid leukaemia. *Nature* **2012**, *485*, 260–263. [CrossRef] [PubMed]

12. Chaturvedi, A.; Araujo Cruz, M.M.; Jyotsana, N.; Sharma, A.; Yun, H.; Gorlich, K.; Wichmann, M.; Schwarzer, A.; Preller, M.; Thol, F.; *et al.* Mutant IDH1 promotes leukemogenesis *in vivo* and can be specifically targeted in human AML. *Blood* **2013**, *122*, 2877–2887. [CrossRef] [PubMed]

13. Lancet, J.E.; Cortes, J.E.; Hogge, D.E.; Tallman, M.S.; Kovacsovics, T.J.; Damon, L.E.; Komrokji, R.; Solomon, S.R.; Kolitz, J.E.; Cooper, M.; *et al.* Phase 2 trial of CPX-351, a fixed 5:1 molar ratio of cytarabine/daunorubicin, *vs.* cytarabine/daunorubicin in older adults with untreated AML. *Blood* **2014**, *123*, 3239–3246. [CrossRef] [PubMed]

14. Cortes, J.E.; Goldberg, S.L.; Feldman, E.J.; Rizzeri, D.A.; Hogge, D.E.; Larson, M.; Pigneux, A.; Recher, C.; Schiller, G.; Warzocha, K.; *et al.* Phase II, multicenter, randomized trial of CPX-351 (cytarabine:daunorubicin) liposome injection *versus* intensive salvage therapy in adults with first relapse AML. *Cancer* **2015**, *121*, 234–242.

15. Grant, S. Is the focus moving toward a combination of targeted drugs? *Best Pract. Res. Clin. Haematol* **2008**, *21*, 629–637. [CrossRef] [PubMed]

16. Bose, P.; Grant, S. Complementary combinations: What treatments will become key to the battle against acute myelogenous leukemia? *Expert Rev. Hematol.* **2012**, *5*, 475–478. [CrossRef] [PubMed]

17. Kaiser, J. Combining targeted drugs to stop resistant tumors. *Science* **2011**, *331*, 1542–1545. [CrossRef] [PubMed]

18. Westin, J.R. Busting robustness: Using cancer's greatest strength to our advantage. *Future Oncol.* **2015**, *11*, 73–77. [CrossRef] [PubMed]

19. Baylin, S.B.; Jones, P.A. A decade of exploring the cancer epigenome—Biological and translational implications. *Nat. Rev. Cancer* **2011**, *11*, 726–734. [CrossRef] [PubMed]

20. Jones, P.A.; Baylin, S.B. The fundamental role of epigenetic events in cancer. *Nat. Rev. Genet.* **2002**, *3*, 415–428. [CrossRef] [PubMed]

21. Jones, P.A.; Baylin, S.B. The epigenomics of cancer. *Cell* **2007**, *128*, 683–692. [CrossRef] [PubMed]

22. Fenaux, P.; Mufti, G.J.; Hellstrom-Lindberg, E.; Santini, V.; Gattermann, N.; Germing, U.; Sanz, G.; List, A.F.; Gore, S.; Seymour, J.F.; *et al.* Azacitidine prolongs overall survival compared with conventional care regimens in elderly patients with low bone marrow blast count acute myeloid leukemia. *J. Clin. Oncol.* **2010**, *28*, 562–569. [CrossRef] [PubMed]

23. Cashen, A.F.; Schiller, G.J.; O'Donnell, M.R.; DiPersio, J.F. Multicenter, phase II study of decitabine for the first-line treatment of older patients with acute myeloid leukemia. *J. Clin. Oncol.* **2010**, *28*, 556–561. [CrossRef] [PubMed]

24. Blum, W.; Garzon, R.; Klisovic, R.B.; Schwind, S.; Walker, A.; Geyer, S.; Liu, S.; Havelange, V.; Becker, H.; Schaaf, L.; *et al.* Clinical response and miR-29b predictive significance in older AML patients treated with a 10-day schedule of decitabine. *Proc. Natl. Acad. Sci. USA* **2010**, *107*, 7473–7478. [CrossRef] [PubMed]

25. Kantarjian, H.M.; Thomas, X.G.; Dmoszynska, A.; Wierzbowska, A.; Mazur, G.; Mayer, J.; Gau, J.P.; Chou, W.C.; Buckstein, R.; Cermak, J.; *et al.* Multicenter, randomized, open-label, phase III trial of decitabine *versus* patient choice, with physician advice, of either supportive care or low-dose cytarabine for the treatment of older patients with newly diagnosed acute myeloid leukemia. *J. Clin. Oncol.* **2012**, *30*, 2670–2677. [CrossRef] [PubMed]

26. Quintas-Cardama, A.; Santos, F.P.; Garcia-Manero, G. Histone deacetylase inhibitors for the treatment of myelodysplastic syndrome and acute myeloid leukemia. *Leukemia* **2011**, *25*, 226–235. [CrossRef] [PubMed]

27. Bose, P.; Grant, S. Orphan drug designation for pracinostat, volasertib and alvocidib in AML. *Leuk. Res.* **2014**, *38*, 862–865. [CrossRef] [PubMed]

28. Prebet, T.; Sun, Z.; Figueroa, M.E.; Ketterling, R.; Melnick, A.; Greenberg, P.L.; Herman, J.; Juckett, M.; Smith, M.R.; Malick, L.; *et al.* Prolonged administration of azacitidine with or without entinostat for myelodysplastic syndrome and acute myeloid leukemia with myelodysplasia-related changes: Results of the US Leukemia Intergroup trial E1905. *J. Clin. Oncol.* **2014**, *32*, 1242–1248. [CrossRef] [PubMed]

29. Quintas-Cardama, A.; Kantarjian, H.M.; Ravandi, F.; Foudray, C.; Pemmaraju, N.; Kadia, T.M.; Borthakur, G.; Daver, N.G.; Faderl, S.; Jabbour, E.; *et al.* Very High Rates of Clinical and Cytogenetic Response with the Combination of the Histone Deacetylase Inhibitor Pracinostat (SB939) and 5-Azacitidine in High-Risk Myelodysplastic Syndrome. *ASH Annu. Meet. Abstr.* **2012**, *120*, 3821.

30. Blum, W.; Schwind, S.; Tarighat, S.S.; Geyer, S.; Eisfeld, A.K.; Whitman, S.; Walker, A.; Klisovic, R.; Byrd, J.C.; Santhanam, R.; *et al.* Clinical and pharmacodynamic activity of bortezomib and decitabine in acute myeloid leukemia. *Blood* **2012**, *119*, 6025–6031. [CrossRef] [PubMed]

31. Ravandi, F.; Alattar, M.L.; Grunwald, M.R.; Rudek, M.A.; Rajkhowa, T.; Richie, M.A.; Pierce, S.; Daver, N.; Garcia-Manero, G.; Faderl, S.; *et al.* Phase 2 study of azacytidine plus sorafenib in patients with acute myeloid leukemia and FLT-3 internal tandem duplication mutation. *Blood* **2013**, *121*, 4655–4662. [CrossRef] [PubMed]

32. Levis, M. FLT3/ITD AML and the law of unintended consequences. *Blood* **2011**, *117*, 6987–6990. [CrossRef] [PubMed]

33. Williams, C.B.; Kambhampati, S.; Fiskus, W.; Wick, J.; Dutreix, C.; Ganguly, S.; Aljitawi, O.; Reyes, R.; Fleming, A.; Abhyankar, S.; *et al.* Preclinical and phase I results of decitabine in combination with midostaurin (PKC412) for newly diagnosed elderly or relapsed/refractory adult patients with acute myeloid leukemia. *Pharmacotherapy* **2013**, *33*, 1341–1352. [CrossRef] [PubMed]

34. Liesveld, J.L.; O'Dwyer, K.; Walker, A.; Becker, M.W.; Ifthikharuddin, J.J.; Mulford, D.; Chen, R.; Bechelli, J.; Rosell, K.; Minhajuddin, M.; *et al.* A phase I study of decitabine and rapamycin in relapsed/refractory AML. *Leuk. Res.* **2013**, *37*, 1622–1627. [CrossRef] [PubMed]

35. Welch, J.S.; Niu, H.; Uy, G.L.; Westervelt, P.; Abboud, C.N.; Vij, R.; Stockerl-Goldstein, K.E.; Jacoby, M.; Pusic, I.; Schroeder, M.A.; *et al.* A phase I dose escalation study of oral bexarotene in combination with intravenous decitabine in patients with AML. *Am. J. Hematol.* **2014**, *89*, E103–E108. [CrossRef] [PubMed]

36. Pollyea, D.A.; Kohrt, H.E.; Gallegos, L.; Figueroa, M.E.; Abdel-Wahab, O.; Zhang, B.; Bhattacharya, S.; Zehnder, J.; Liedtke, M.; Gotlib, J.R.; *et al.* Safety, efficacy and biological predictors of response to sequential azacitidine and lenalidomide for elderly patients with acute myeloid leukemia. *Leukemia* **2012**, *26*, 893–901. [CrossRef] [PubMed]

37. Ramsingh, G.; Westervelt, P.; Cashen, A.F.; Uy, G.L.; Stockerl-Goldstein, K.; Abboud, C.N.; Bernabe, N.; Monahan, R.; DiPersio, J.F.; Vij, R. A phase 1 study of concomitant high-dose lenalidomide and 5-azacitidine induction in the treatment of AML. *Leukemia* **2013**, *27*, 725–728. [CrossRef] [PubMed]

38. Bogenberger, J.M.; Kornblau, S.M.; Pierceall, W.E.; Lena, R.; Chow, D.; Shi, C.X.; Mantei, J.; Ahmann, G.; Gonzales, I.M.; Choudhary, A.; *et al.* BCL-2 family proteins as 5-Azacytidine-sensitizing targets and determinants of response in myeloid malignancies. *Leukemia* **2014**, *28*, 1657–1665. [CrossRef] [PubMed]

39. Dawson, M.A.; Kouzarides, T.; Huntly, B.J. Targeting epigenetic readers in cancer. *N. Engl. J. Med.* **2012**, *367*, 647–657. [CrossRef] [PubMed]

40. Belkina, A.C.; Denis, G.V. BET domain co-regulators in obesity, inflammation and cancer. *Nat. Rev. Cancer* **2012**, *12*, 465–477. [CrossRef] [PubMed]

41. Filippakopoulos, P.; Knapp, S. Targeting bromodomains: Epigenetic readers of lysine acetylation. *Nat. Rev. Drug Discov.* **2014**, *13*, 337–356. [CrossRef] [PubMed]

42. Fiskus, W.; Sharma, S.; Qi, J.; Valenta, J.A.; Schaub, L.J.; Shah, B.; Peth, K.; Portier, B.P.; Rodriguez, M.; Devaraj, S.G.; *et al.* Highly active combination of BRD4 antagonist and histone deacetylase inhibitor against human acute myelogenous leukemia cells. *Mol. Cancer Ther.* **2014**, *13*, 1142–1154. [CrossRef] [PubMed]

43. Fiskus, W.; Sharma, S.; Qi, J.; Shah, B.; Devaraj, S.G.; Leveque, C.; Portier, B.P.; Iyer, S.P.; Bradner, J.E.; Bhalla, K.N. BET protein antagonist JQ1 is synergistically lethal with FLT3 tyrosine kinase inhibitor (TKI) and overcomes resistance to FLT3-TKI in AML cells expressing FLT-ITD. *Mol. Cancer Ther.* **2014**, *13*, 2315–2327. [CrossRef] [PubMed]

44. Grant, S.; Dai, Y. Histone deacetylase inhibitors and rational combination therapies. *Adv. Cancer Res.* **2012**, *116*, 199–237. [PubMed]

45. Bose, P.; Dai, Y.; Grant, S. Histone deacetylase inhibitor (HDACI) mechanisms of action: Emerging insights. *Pharmacol. Ther.* **2014**, *143*, 323–336. [CrossRef] [PubMed]

46. Bots, M.; Johnstone, R.W. Rational combinations using HDAC inhibitors. *Clin. Cancer Res.* **2009**, *15*, 3970–3977. [CrossRef] [PubMed]

47. San-Miguel, J.F.; Hungria, V.T.; Yoon, S.S.; Beksac, M.; Dimopoulos, M.A.; Elghandour, A.; Jedrzejczak, W.W.; Gunther, A.; Nakorn, T.N.; Siritanaratkul, N.; *et al.* Panobinostat plus bortezomib and dexamethasone *versus* placebo plus bortezomib and dexamethasone in patients with relapsed or relapsed and refractory multiple myeloma: A multicentre, randomised, double-blind phase 3 trial. *Lancet Oncol.* **2014**, *15*, 1195–1206. [CrossRef] [PubMed]

48. Dai, Y.; Chen, S.; Wang, L.; Pei, X.Y.; Kramer, L.B.; Dent, P.; Grant, S. Bortezomib interacts synergistically with belinostat in human acute myeloid leukaemia and acute lymphoblastic leukaemia cells in association with perturbations in NF-kappaB and Bim. *Br. J. Haematol.* **2011**, *153*, 222–235. [CrossRef] [PubMed]

49. Holkova, B.; Bose, P.; Tombes, M.B.; Shrader, E.; Wan, W.; Weir-Wiggins, C.; Stoddert, E.; Sankala, H.; Kmieciak, M.; Roberts, J.D.; *et al.* Phase I Trial of Belinostat and Bortezomib in Patients with Relapsed or Refractory Acute Leukemia, Myelodysplastic Syndrome, or Chronic Myelogenous Leukemia in Blast Crisis—One Year Update. *ASH Annu. Meet. Abstr.* **2012**, *120*, 3588.

50. Batalo, M.S.; Bose, P.; Holkova, B.; Grant, S. Targeting mantle cell lymphoma with a strategy of combined proteasome and histone deacetylase inhibition. In *Resistance to Proteasome Inhibitors in Cancer*; Ping Dou, Q., Ed.; Springer-Verlag: New York, NY, USA, 2014; pp. 149–179.

51. Karin, M. Nuclear factor-kappaB in cancer development and progression. *Nature* **2006**, *441*, 431–436. [CrossRef] [PubMed]

52. Dai, Y.; Rahmani, M.; Dent, P.; Grant, S. Blockade of histone deacetylase inhibitor-induced RelA/p65 acetylation and NF-kappaB activation potentiates apoptosis in leukemia cells through a process mediated by oxidative damage, XIAP downregulation, and c-Jun N-terminal kinase 1 activation. *Mol. Cell. Biol.* **2005**, *25*, 5429–5444. [CrossRef] [PubMed]

53. Dai, Y.; Guzman, M.L.; Chen, S.; Wang, L.; Yeung, S.K.; Pei, X.Y.; Dent, P.; Jordan, C.T.; Grant, S. The NF (Nuclear factor)-kappaB inhibitor parthenolide interacts with histone deacetylase inhibitors to induce MKK7/JNK1-dependent apoptosis in human acute myeloid leukaemia cells. *Br. J. Haematol.* **2010**, *151*, 70–83. [CrossRef] [PubMed]

54. Hideshima, T.; Bradner, J.E.; Wong, J.; Chauhan, D.; Richardson, P.; Schreiber, S.L.; Anderson, K.C. Small-molecule inhibition of proteasome and aggresome function induces synergistic antitumor activity in multiple myeloma. *Proc. Natl. Acad. Sci. USA* **2005**, *102*, 8567–8572. [CrossRef] [PubMed]

55. Bali, P.; Pranpat, M.; Bradner, J.; Balasis, M.; Fiskus, W.; Guo, F.; Rocha, K.; Kumaraswamy, S.; Boyapalle, S.; Atadja, P.; *et al.* Inhibition of histone deacetylase 6 acetylates and disrupts the chaperone function of heat shock protein 90: A novel basis for antileukemia activity of histone deacetylase inhibitors. *J. Biol. Chem.* **2005**, *280*, 26729–26734. [CrossRef] [PubMed]

56. Adams, J. The development of proteasome inhibitors as anticancer drugs. *Cancer Cell* **2004**, *5*, 417–421. [CrossRef] [PubMed]

57. Adams, J. The proteasome: A suitable antineoplastic target. *Nat. Rev. Cancer* **2004**, *4*, 349–360. [CrossRef] [PubMed]

58. Fotheringham, S.; Epping, M.T.; Stimson, L.; Khan, O.; Wood, V.; Pezzella, F.; Bernards, R.; la Thangue, N.B. Genome-wide loss-of-function screen reveals an important role for the proteasome in HDAC inhibitor-induced apoptosis. *Cancer Cell* **2009**, *15*, 57–66. [CrossRef] [PubMed]

59. Kikuchi, J.; Wada, T.; Shimizu, R.; Izumi, T.; Akutsu, M.; Mitsunaga, K.; Noborio-Hatano, K.; Nobuyoshi, M.; Ozawa, K.; Kano, Y.; *et al.* Histone deacetylases are critical targets of bortezomib-induced cytotoxicity in multiple myeloma. *Blood* **2010**, *116*, 406–417. [CrossRef] [PubMed]

60. Bose, P.; Simmons, G.L.; Grant, S. Cyclin-dependent kinase inhibitor therapy for hematologic malignancies. *Expert Opin. Investig. Drugs* **2013**, *22*, 723–738. [CrossRef] [PubMed]

61. Chao, S.H.; Price, D.H. Flavopiridol inactivates P-TEFb and blocks most RNA polymerase II transcription *in vivo*. *J. Biol. Chem.* **2001**, *276*, 31793–31799. [CrossRef] [PubMed]

62. Almenara, J.; Rosato, R.; Grant, S. Synergistic induction of mitochondrial damage and apoptosis in human leukemia cells by flavopiridol and the histone deacetylase inhibitor suberoylanilide hydroxamic acid (SAHA). *Leukemia* **2002**, *16*, 1331–1343. [CrossRef] [PubMed]

63. Rosato, R.R.; Almenara, J.A.; Cartee, L.; Betts, V.; Chellappan, S.P.; Grant, S. The cyclin-dependent kinase inhibitor flavopiridol disrupts sodium butyrate-induced p21WAF1/CIP1 expression and maturation while reciprocally potentiating apoptosis in human leukemia cells. *Mol. Cancer Ther.* **2002**, *1*, 253–266. [PubMed]

64. Rosato, R.R.; Almenara, J.A.; Yu, C.; Grant, S. Evidence of a functional role for p21WAF1/CIP1 down-regulation in synergistic antileukemic interactions between the histone deacetylase inhibitor sodium butyrate and flavopiridol. *Mol. Pharmacol.* **2004**, *65*, 571–581. [CrossRef] [PubMed]

65. Rosato, R.R.; Almenara, J.A.; Maggio, S.C.; Atadja, P.; Craig, R.; Vrana, J.; Dent, P.; Grant, S. Potentiation of the lethality of the histone deacetylase inhibitor LAQ824 by the cyclin-dependent kinase inhibitor roscovitine in human leukemia cells. *Mol. Cancer Ther.* **2005**, *4*, 1772–1785. [CrossRef] [PubMed]

66. Rosato, R.R.; Almenara, J.A.; Kolla, S.S.; Maggio, S.C.; Coe, S.; Gimenez, M.S.; Dent, P.; Grant, S. Mechanism and functional role of XIAP and Mcl-1 down-regulation in flavopiridol/vorinostat antileukemic interactions. *Mol. Cancer Ther.* **2007**, *6*, 692–702. [CrossRef] [PubMed]

67. Holkova, B.; Supko, J.G.; Ames, M.M.; Reid, J.M.; Shapiro, G.I.; Perkins, E.B.; Ramakrishnan, V.; Tombes, M.B.; Honeycutt, C.; McGovern, R.M.; *et al.* A phase I trial of vorinostat and alvocidib in patients with relapsed, refractory, or poor prognosis acute leukemia, or refractory anemia with excess blasts-2. *Clin. Cancer Res.* **2013**, *19*, 1873–1883. [CrossRef] [PubMed]

68. Byrd, J.C.; Lin, T.S.; Dalton, J.T.; Wu, D.; Phelps, M.A.; Fischer, B.; Moran, M.; Blum, K.A.; Rovin, B.; Brooker-McEldowney, M.; *et al.* Flavopiridol administered using a pharmacologically derived schedule is associated with marked clinical efficacy in refractory, genetically high-risk chronic lymphocytic leukemia. *Blood* **2007**, *109*, 399–404. [CrossRef] [PubMed]

69. Nishioka, C.; Ikezoe, T.; Yang, J.; Takeuchi, S.; Koeffler, H.P.; Yokoyama, A. MS-275, a novel histone deacetylase inhibitor with selectivity against HDAC1, induces degradation of FLT3 via inhibition of chaperone function of heat shock protein 90 in AML cells. *Leuk. Res.* **2008**, *32*, 1382–1392. [CrossRef] [PubMed]

70. Qiu, L.; Burgess, A.; Fairlie, D.P.; Leonard, H.; Parsons, P.G.; Gabrielli, B.G. Histone deacetylase inhibitors trigger a G2 checkpoint in normal cells that is defective in tumor cells. *Mol. Biol. Cell* **2000**, *11*, 2069–2083. [CrossRef] [PubMed]

71. Stevens, F.E.; Beamish, H.; Warrener, R.; Gabrielli, B. Histone deacetylase inhibitors induce mitotic slippage. *Oncogene* **2008**, *27*, 1345–1354. [CrossRef] [PubMed]

72. Yu, C.; Rahmani, M.; Almenara, J.; Subler, M.; Krystal, G.; Conrad, D.; Varticovski, L.; Dent, P.; Grant, S. Histone deacetylase inhibitors promote STI571-mediated apoptosis in STI571-sensitive and -resistant Bcr/Abl+ human myeloid leukemia cells. *Cancer Res.* **2003**, *63*, 2118–2126. [PubMed]

73. Nimmanapalli, R.; Fuino, L.; Bali, P.; Gasparetto, M.; Glozak, M.; Tao, J.; Moscinski, L.; Smith, C.; Wu, J.; Jove, R.; *et al.* Histone deacetylase inhibitor LAQ824 both lowers expression and promotes proteasomal degradation of Bcr-Abl and induces apoptosis of imatinib mesylate-sensitive or -refractory chronic myelogenous leukemia-blast crisis cells. *Cancer Res.* **2003**, *63*, 5126–5135. [PubMed]

74. Nimmanapalli, R.; Fuino, L.; Stobaugh, C.; Richon, V.; Bhalla, K. Cotreatment with the histone deacetylase inhibitor suberoylanilide hydroxamic acid (SAHA) enhances imatinib-induced apoptosis of Bcr-Abl-positive human acute leukemia cells. *Blood* **2003**, *101*, 3236–3239. [CrossRef] [PubMed]

75. Fiskus, W.; Pranpat, M.; Balasis, M.; Bali, P.; Estrella, V.; Kumaraswamy, S.; Rao, R.; Rocha, K.; Herger, B.; Lee, F.; *et al.* Cotreatment with vorinostat (suberoylanilide hydroxamic acid) enhances activity of dasatinib (BMS-354825) against imatinib mesylate-sensitive or imatinib mesylate-resistant chronic myelogenous leukemia cells. *Clin. Cancer Res.* **2006**, *12*, 5869–5878. [CrossRef] [PubMed]

76. Fiskus, W.; Pranpat, M.; Bali, P.; Balasis, M.; Kumaraswamy, S.; Boyapalle, S.; Rocha, K.; Wu, J.; Giles, F.; Manley, P.W.; *et al.* Combined effects of novel tyrosine kinase inhibitor AMN107 and histone deacetylase inhibitor LBH589 against Bcr-Abl-expressing human leukemia cells. *Blood* **2006**, *108*, 645–652. [CrossRef] [PubMed]

77. Bali, P.; George, P.; Cohen, P.; Tao, J.; Guo, F.; Sigua, C.; Vishvanath, A.; Scuto, A.; Annavarapu, S.; Fiskus, W.; *et al.* Superior activity of the combination of histone deacetylase inhibitor LAQ824 and the FLT-3 kinase inhibitor PKC412 against human acute myelogenous leukemia cells with mutant FLT-3. *Clin. Cancer Res.* **2004**, *10*, 4991–4997. [CrossRef] [PubMed]

78. Wang, Y.; Fiskus, W.; Chong, D.G.; Buckley, K.M.; Natarajan, K.; Rao, R.; Joshi, A.; Balusu, R.; Koul, S.; Chen, J.; *et al.* Cotreatment with panobinostat and JAK2 inhibitor TG101209 attenuates JAK2V617F levels and signaling and exerts synergistic cytotoxic effects against human myeloproliferative neoplastic cells. *Blood* **2009**, *114*, 5024–5033. [CrossRef] [PubMed]

79. Novotny-Diermayr, V.; Hart, S.; Goh, K.C.; Cheong, A.; Ong, L.C.; Hentze, H.; Pasha, M.K.; Jayaraman, R.; Ethirajulu, K.; Wood, J.M. The oral HDAC inhibitor pracinostat (SB939) is efficacious and synergistic with the JAK2 inhibitor pacritinib (SB1518) in preclinical models of AML. *Blood Cancer J.* **2012**, *2*, e69. [CrossRef] [PubMed]

80. Dai, Y.; Chen, S.; Venditti, C.A.; Pei, X.Y.; Nguyen, T.K.; Dent, P.; Grant, S. Vorinostat synergistically potentiates MK-0457 lethality in chronic myelogenous leukemia cells sensitive and resistant to imatinib mesylate. *Blood* **2008**, *112*, 793–804. [CrossRef] [PubMed]

81. Fiskus, W.; Wang, Y.; Joshi, R.; Rao, R.; Yang, Y.; Chen, J.; Kolhe, R.; Balusu, R.; Eaton, K.; Lee, P.; *et al.* Cotreatment with vorinostat enhances activity of MK-0457 (VX-680) against acute and chronic myelogenous leukemia cells. *Clin. Cancer Res.* **2008**, *14*, 6106–6115. [CrossRef] [PubMed]

82. Nguyen, T.; Dai, Y.; Attkisson, E.; Kramer, L.; Jordan, N.; Nguyen, N.; Kolluri, N.; Muschen, M.; Grant, S. HDAC inhibitors potentiate the activity of the BCR/ABL kinase inhibitor KW-2449 in imatinib-sensitive or -resistant BCR/ABL+ leukemia cells *in vitro* and *in vivo*. *Clin. Cancer Res.* **2011**, *17*, 3219–3232. [CrossRef] [PubMed]

83. Lok, W.; Klein, R.Q.; Saif, M.W. Aurora kinase inhibitors as anti-cancer therapy. *Anticancer Drugs* **2010**, *21*, 339–350. [CrossRef] [PubMed]

84. Kelly, K.R.; Ecsedy, J.; Mahalingam, D.; Nawrocki, S.T.; Padmanabhan, S.; Giles, F.J.; Carew, J.S. Targeting aurora kinases in cancer treatment. *Curr. Drug Targets* **2011**, *12*, 2067–2078. [CrossRef] [PubMed]

85. Zhang, B.; Strauss, A.C.; Chu, S.; Li, M.; Ho, Y.; Shiang, K.D.; Snyder, D.S.; Huettner, C.S.; Shultz, L.; Holyoake, T.; *et al.* Effective targeting of quiescent chronic myelogenous leukemia stem cells by histone deacetylase inhibitors in combination with imatinib mesylate. *Cancer Cell* **2010**, *17*, 427–442. [CrossRef] [PubMed]

86. Dawson, M.A.; Curry, J.E.; Barber, K.; Beer, P.A.; Graham, B.; Lyons, J.F.; Richardson, C.J.; Scott, M.A.; Smyth, T.; Squires, M.S.; *et al.* AT9283, a potent inhibitor of the Aurora kinases and Jak2, has therapeutic potential in myeloproliferative disorders. *Br. J. Haematol.* **2010**, *150*, 46–57. [PubMed]

87. Tanaka, R.; Squires, M.S.; Kimura, S.; Yokota, A.; Nagao, R.; Yamauchi, T.; Takeuchi, M.; Yao, H.; Reule, M.; Smyth, T.; *et al.* Activity of the multitargeted kinase inhibitor, AT9283, in imatinib-resistant BCR-ABL-positive leukemic cells. *Blood* **2010**, *116*, 2089–2095. [CrossRef] [PubMed]

88. Podesta, J.E.; Sugar, R.; Squires, M.; Linardopoulos, S.; Pearson, A.D.; Moore, A.S. Adaptation of the plasma inhibitory activity assay to detect Aurora, ABL and FLT3 kinase inhibition by AT9283 in pediatric leukemia. *Leuk. Res.* **2011**, *35*, 1273–1275. [CrossRef] [PubMed]

89. Tse, A.N.; Carvajal, R.; Schwartz, G.K. Targeting checkpoint kinase 1 in cancer therapeutics. *Clin. Cancer Res.* **2007**, *13*, 1955–1960. [CrossRef] [PubMed]

90. Dai, Y.; Grant, S. New insights into checkpoint kinase 1 in the DNA damage response signaling network. *Clin. Cancer Res.* **2010**, *16*, 376–383. [CrossRef] [PubMed]

91. Kastan, M.B.; Bartek, J. Cell-cycle checkpoints and cancer. *Nature* **2004**, *432*, 316–323. [CrossRef] [PubMed]

92. Bucher, N.; Britten, C.D. G2 checkpoint abrogation and checkpoint kinase-1 targeting in the treatment of cancer. *Br. J. Cancer* **2008**, *98*, 523–528. [CrossRef] [PubMed]

93. Stirewalt, D.L.; Kopecky, K.J.; Meshinchi, S.; Appelbaum, F.R.; Slovak, M.L.; Willman, C.L.; Radich, J.P. FLT3, RAS, and TP53 mutations in elderly patients with acute myeloid leukemia. *Blood* **2001**, *97*, 3589–3595. [CrossRef] [PubMed]

94. Seliger, B.; Papadileris, S.; Vogel, D.; Hess, G.; Brendel, C.; Storkel, S.; Ortel, J.; Kolbe, K.; Huber, C.; Huhn, D.; *et al.* Analysis of the p53 and MDM-2 gene in acute myeloid leukemia. *Eur. J. Haematol.* **1996**, *57*, 230–240. [CrossRef] [PubMed]

95. Faderl, S.; Kantarjian, H.M.; Estey, E.; Manshouri, T.; Chan, C.Y.; Rahman Elsaied, A.; Kornblau, S.M.; Cortes, J.; Thomas, D.A.; Pierce, S.; *et al.* The prognostic significance of p16(INK4a)/p14(ARF) locus deletion and MDM-2 protein expression in adult acute myelogenous leukemia. *Cancer* **2000**, *89*, 1976–1982. [CrossRef] [PubMed]

96. Schottelius, A.; Brennscheidt, U.; Ludwig, W.D.; Mertelsmann, R.H.; Herrmann, F.; Lubbert, M. Mechanisms of p53 alteration in acute leukemias. *Leukemia* **1994**, *8*, 1673–1681. [PubMed]
97. Christiansen, D.H.; Andersen, M.K.; Pedersen-Bjergaard, J. Mutations with loss of heterozygosity of p53 are common in therapy-related myelodysplasia and acute myeloid leukemia after exposure to alkylating agents and significantly associated with deletion or loss of 5q, a complex karyotype, and a poor prognosis. *J. Clin. Oncol.* **2001**, *19*, 1405–1413. [PubMed]
98. Side, L.E.; Curtiss, N.P.; Teel, K.; Kratz, C.; Wang, P.W.; Larson, R.A.; le Beau, M.M.; Shannon, K.M. RAS, FLT3, and TP53 mutations in therapy-related myeloid malignancies with abnormalities of chromosomes 5 and 7. *Genes Chromosomes Cancer* **2004**, *39*, 217–223. [CrossRef] [PubMed]
99. Horiike, S.; Misawa, S.; Kaneko, H.; Sasai, Y.; Kobayashi, M.; Fujii, H.; Tanaka, S.; Yagita, M.; Abe, T.; Kashima, K.; *et al.* Distinct genetic involvement of the TP53 gene in therapy-related leukemia and myelodysplasia with chromosomal losses of Nos 5 and/or 7 and its possible relationship to replication error phenotype. *Leukemia* **1999**, *13*, 1235–1242. [CrossRef] [PubMed]
100. Misawa, S.; Horiike, S.; Kaneko, H.; Sasai, Y.; Ueda, Y.; Nakao, M.; Yokota, S.; Taniwaki, M.; Fujii, H.; Nakagawa, H.; *et al.* Significance of chromosomal alterations and mutations of the N-RAS and TP53 genes in relation to leukemogenesis of acute myeloid leukemia. *Leuk. Res.* **1998**, *22*, 631–637. [CrossRef] [PubMed]
101. Haferlach, C.; Dicker, F.; Herholz, H.; Schnittger, S.; Kern, W.; Haferlach, T. Mutations of the TP53 gene in acute myeloid leukemia are strongly associated with a complex aberrant karyotype. *Leukemia* **2008**, *22*, 1539–1541. [CrossRef] [PubMed]
102. Rucker, F.G.; Schlenk, R.F.; Bullinger, L.; Kayser, S.; Teleanu, V.; Kett, H.; Habdank, M.; Kugler, C.M.; Holzmann, K.; Gaidzik, V.I.; *et al.* TP53 alterations in acute myeloid leukemia with complex karyotype correlate with specific copy number alterations, monosomal karyotype, and dismal outcome. *Blood* **2012**, *119*, 2114–2121. [CrossRef] [PubMed]
103. Melo, M.B.; Ahmad, N.N.; Lima, C.S.; Pagnano, K.B.; Bordin, S.; Lorand-Metze, I.; SaAd, S.T.; Costa, F.F. Mutations in the p53 gene in acute myeloid leukemia patients correlate with poor prognosis. *Hematology* **2002**, *7*, 13–19. [CrossRef] [PubMed]
104. Wattel, E.; Preudhomme, C.; Hecquet, B.; Vanrumbeke, M.; Quesnel, B.; Dervite, I.; Morel, P.; Fenaux, P. P53 Mutations are Associated with Resistance to Chemotherapy and Short Survival in Hematologic Malignancies. *Blood* **1994**, *84*, 3148–3157. [PubMed]
105. Middeke, J.M.; Fang, M.; Cornelissen, J.J.; Mohr, B.; Appelbaum, F.R.; Stadler, M.; Sanz, J.; Baurmann, H.; Bug, G.; Schafer-Eckart, K.; *et al.* Outcome of patients with abnl(17p) acute myeloid leukemia after allogeneic hematopoietic stem cell transplantation. *Blood* **2014**, *123*, 2960–2967. [CrossRef] [PubMed]
106. Fan, J.; Li, L.; Small, D.; Rassool, F. Cells expressing FLT3/ITD mutations exhibit elevated repair errors generated through alternative NHEJ pathways: Implications for genomic instability and therapy. *Blood* **2010**, *116*, 5298–5305. [CrossRef] [PubMed]
107. Sallmyr, A.; Fan, J.; Datta, K.; Kim, K.T.; Grosu, D.; Shapiro, P.; Small, D.; Rassool, F. Internal tandem duplication of FLT3 (FLT3/ITD) induces increased ROS production, DNA damage, and misrepair: Implications for poor prognosis in AML. *Blood* **2008**, *111*, 3173–3182. [CrossRef] [PubMed]
108. Petruccelli, L.A.; Dupere-Richer, D.; Pettersson, F.; Retrouvey, H.; Skoulikas, S.; Miller, W.H., Jr. Vorinostat induces reactive oxygen species and DNA damage in acute myeloid leukemia cells. *PLoS ONE* **2011**, *6*, e20987. [CrossRef] [PubMed]
109. Kachhap, S.K.; Rosmus, N.; Collis, S.J.; Kortenhorst, M.S.; Wissing, M.D.; Hedayati, M.; Shabbeer, S.; Mendonca, J.; Deangelis, J.; Marchionni, L.; *et al.* Downregulation of homologous recombination DNA repair genes by HDAC inhibition in prostate cancer is mediated through the E2F1 transcription factor. *PLoS ONE* **2010**, *5*, e11208. [CrossRef] [PubMed]
110. Miller, K.M.; Tjeertes, J.V.; Coates, J.; Legube, G.; Polo, S.E.; Britton, S.; Jackson, S.P. Human HDAC1 and HDAC2 function in the DNA-damage response to promote DNA nonhomologous end-joining. *Nat. Struct. Mol. Biol.* **2010**, *17*, 1144–1151. [CrossRef] [PubMed]
111. Brazelle, W.; Kreahling, J.M.; Gemmer, J.; Ma, Y.; Cress, W.D.; Haura, E.; Altiok, S. Histone deacetylase inhibitors downregulate checkpoint kinase 1 expression to induce cell death in non-small cell lung cancer cells. *PLoS ONE* **2010**, *5*, e14335. [CrossRef] [PubMed]

J. Clin. Med. **2015**, *4*, 634–664

112. Ha, K.; Fiskus, W.; Rao, R.; Balusu, R.; Venkannagari, S.; Nalabothula, N.R.; Bhalla, K.N. Hsp90 inhibitor-mediated disruption of chaperone association of ATR with hsp90 sensitizes cancer cells to DNA damage. *Mol. Cancer Ther.* **2011**, *10*, 1194–1206. [CrossRef] [PubMed]

113. Sugimoto, K.; Sasaki, M.; Isobe, Y.; Tsutsui, M.; Suto, H.; Ando, J.; Tamayose, K.; Ando, M.; Oshimi, K. Hsp90-inhibitor geldanamycin abrogates G2 arrest in p53-negative leukemia cell lines through the depletion of Chk1. *Oncogene* **2008**, *27*, 3091–3101. [CrossRef] [PubMed]

114. Tse, A.N.; Sheikh, T.N.; Alan, H.; Chou, T.C.; Schwartz, G.K. 90-kDa heat shock protein inhibition abrogates the topoisomerase I poison-induced G2/M checkpoint in p53-null tumor cells by depleting Chk1 and Wee1. *Mol. Pharmacol.* **2009**, *75*, 124–133. [CrossRef] [PubMed]

115. Dai, Y.; Chen, S.; Kmieciak, M.; Zhou, L.; Lin, H.; Pei, X.Y.; Grant, S. The novel Chk1 inhibitor MK-8776 sensitizes human leukemia cells to HDAC inhibitors by targeting the intra-S checkpoint and DNA replication and repair. *Mol. Cancer Ther.* **2013**, *12*, 878–889. [CrossRef] [PubMed]

116. Caldwell, J.T.; Edwards, H.; Buck, S.A.; Ge, Y.; Taub, J.W. Targeting the wee1 kinase for treatment of pediatric Down syndrome acute myeloid leukemia. *Pediatr. Blood Cancer* **2014**, *61*, 1767–1773. [CrossRef] [PubMed]

117. Porter, C.C.; Kim, J.; Fosmire, S.; Gearheart, C.M.; van Linden, A.; Baturin, D.; Zaberezhnyy, V.; Patel, P.R.; Gao, D.; Tan, A.C.; *et al.* Integrated genomic analyses identify WEE1 as a critical mediator of cell fate and a novel therapeutic target in acute myeloid leukemia. *Leukemia* **2012**, *26*, 1266–1276. [CrossRef] [PubMed]

118. Weisberg, E.; Nonami, A.; Chen, Z.; Liu, F.; Zhang, J.; Sattler, M.; Nelson, E.; Cowens, K.; Christie, A.L.; Mitsiades, C.; *et al.* Identification of Wee1 as a novel therapeutic target for mutant RAS-driven acute leukemia and other malignancies. *Leukemia* **2015**, *29*, 27–37. [CrossRef] [PubMed]

119. Guertin, A.D.; Li, J.; Liu, Y.; Hurd, M.S.; Schuller, A.G.; Long, B.; Hirsch, H.A.; Feldman, I.; Benita, Y.; Toniatti, C.; *et al.* Preclinical Evaluation of the WEE1 Inhibitor MK-1775 as Single Agent Anticancer Therapy. *Mol. Cancer Ther.* **2013**, *12*, 1442–1452. [CrossRef] [PubMed]

120. Kreahling, J.M.; Gemmer, J.Y.; Reed, D.; Letson, D.; Bui, M.; Altiok, S. MK1775, a selective Wee1 inhibitor, shows single-agent antitumor activity against sarcoma cells. *Mol. Cancer Ther.* **2012**, *11*, 174–182. [CrossRef] [PubMed]

121. Tibes, R.; Bogenberger, J.M.; Chaudhuri, L.; Hagelstrom, R.T.; Chow, D.; Buechel, M.E.; Gonzales, I.M.; Demuth, T.; Slack, J.; Mesa, R.A.; *et al.* RNAi screening of the kinome with cytarabine in leukemias. *Blood* **2012**, *119*, 2863–2872. [CrossRef] [PubMed]

122. Van Linden, A.A.; Baturin, D.; Ford, J.B.; Fosmire, S.P.; Gardner, L.; Korch, C.; Reigan, P.; Porter, C.C. Inhibition of Wee1 sensitizes cancer cells to antimetabolite chemotherapeutics *in vitro* and *in vivo*, independent of p53 functionality. *Mol. Cancer Ther.* **2013**, *12*, 2675–2684. [CrossRef] [PubMed]

123. Krajewska, M.; Heijink, A.M.; Bisselink, Y.J.; Seinstra, R.I.; Sillje, H.H.; de Vries, E.G.; van Vugt, M.A. Forced activation of Cdk1 via wee1 inhibition impairs homologous recombination. *Oncogene* **2013**, *32*, 3001–3008. [CrossRef] [PubMed]

124. Qi, W.; Xie, C.; Li, C.; Caldwell, J.; Edwards, H.; Taub, J.W.; Wang, Y.; Lin, H.; Ge, Y. CHK1 plays a critical role in the anti-leukemic activity of the wee1 inhibitor MK-1775 in acute myeloid leukemia cells. *J. Hematol. Oncol.* **2014**, *7*, 53. [CrossRef] [PubMed]

125. Guertin, A.D.; Martin, M.M.; Roberts, B.; Hurd, M.; Qu, X.; Miselis, N.R.; Liu, Y.; Li, J.; Feldman, I.; Benita, Y.; *et al.* Unique functions of CHK1 and WEE1 underlie synergistic anti-tumor activity upon pharmacologic inhibition. *Cancer Cell Int.* **2012**, *12*, 45. [CrossRef] [PubMed]

126. Russell, M.; Levin, K.; Rader, J.; Belcastro, L.; Li, Y.; Martinez, D.; Pawel, B.R.; Shumway, S.D.; Maris, J.M.; Cole, K.A. Combination Therapy Targeting the Chk1 and Wee1 Kinases Demonstrates Therapeutic Efficacy in Neuroblastoma. *Cancer Res.* **2013**, *73*, 776–784. [CrossRef] [PubMed]

127. Carrassa, L.; Chila, R.; Lupi, M.; Ricci, F.; Celenza, C.; Mazzoletti, M.; Broggini, M.; Damia, G. Combined inhibition of Chk1 and Wee1: *In vitro* synergistic effect translates to tumor growth inhibition *in vivo*. *Cell Cycle* **2012**, *11*, 2507–2517. [CrossRef] [PubMed]

128. Zhou, L.; Zhang, Y.; Chen, S.; Kmieciak, M.; Leng, Y.; Lin, H.; Rizzo, K.A.; Dumur, C.I.; Ferreira-Gonzalez, A.; Dai, Y.; *et al.* A regimen combining the Wee1 inhibitor AZD1775 with HDAC inhibitors targets human acute myeloid leukemia cells harboring various genetic mutations. *Leukemia* **2014**. [CrossRef]

129. Three more drugs judged "breakthroughs". *Cancer Discov.* **2013**, *3*. [CrossRef]

130. Archambault, V.; Glover, D.M. Polo-like kinases: Conservation and divergence in their functions and regulation. *Nat. Rev. Mol. Cell Biol.* **2009**, *10*, 265–275. [CrossRef] [PubMed]

131. Lapenna, S.; Giordano, A. Cell cycle kinases as therapeutic targets for cancer. *Nat. Rev. Drug Discov.* **2009**, *8*, 547–566. [CrossRef] [PubMed]

132. Smits, V.A.; Klompmaker, R.; Arnaud, L.; Rijksen, G.; Nigg, E.A.; Medema, R.H. Polo-like kinase-1 is a target of the DNA damage checkpoint. *Nat. Cell Biol.* **2000**, *2*, 672–676. [CrossRef] [PubMed]

133. Takaki, T.; Trenz, K.; Costanzo, V.; Petronczki, M. Polo-like kinase 1 reaches beyond mitosis—Cytokinesis, DNA damage response, and development. *Curr. Opin. Cell Biol.* **2008**, *20*, 650–660. [CrossRef] [PubMed]

134. Liu, X.S.; Song, B.; Liu, X. The substrates of Plk1, beyond the functions in mitosis. *Protein Cell* **2010**, *1*, 999–1010. [CrossRef] [PubMed]

135. Gleixner, K.V.; Ferenc, V.; Peter, B.; Gruze, A.; Meyer, R.A.; Hadzijusufovic, E.; Cerny-Reiterer, S.; Mayerhofer, M.; Pickl, W.F.; Sillaber, C.; *et al.* Polo-like Kinase 1 (Plk1) as a Novel Drug Target in Chronic Myeloid Leukemia: Overriding Imatinib Resistance with the Plk1 Inhibitor BI 2536. *Cancer Res.* **2010**, *70*, 1513–1523. [CrossRef] [PubMed]

136. Dasmahapatra, G.; Patel, H.; Nguyen, T.; Attkisson, E.; Grant, S. PLK1 inhibitors synergistically potentiate HDAC inhibitor lethality in imatinib mesylate-sensitive or -resistant BCR/ABL+ leukemia cells *in vitro* and *in vivo*. *Clin. Cancer Res.* **2013**, *19*, 404–414. [CrossRef] [PubMed]

137. Soucy, T.A.; Smith, P.G.; Milhollen, M.A.; Berger, A.J.; Gavin, J.M.; Adhikari, S.; Brownell, J.E.; Burke, K.E.; Cardin, D.P.; Critchley, S.; *et al.* An inhibitor of NEDD8-activating enzyme as a new approach to treat cancer. *Nature* **2009**, *458*, 732–736. [CrossRef] [PubMed]

138. Swords, R.T.; Kelly, K.R.; Smith, P.G.; Garnsey, J.J.; Mahalingam, D.; Medina, E.; Oberheu, K.; Padmanabhan, S.; O'Dwyer, M.; Nawrocki, S.T.; *et al.* Inhibition of NEDD8-activating enzyme: A novel approach for the treatment of acute myeloid leukemia. *Blood* **2010**, *115*, 3796–3800. [CrossRef] [PubMed]

139. Swords, R.T.; Erba, H.P.; DeAngelo, D.J.; Smith, P.G.; Pickard, M.D.; Dezube, B.J.; Giles, F.J.; Medeiros, B.C. The Novel, Investigational NEDD8-Activating Enzyme Inhibitor MLN4924 in Adult Patients with Acute Myeloid Leukemia (AML) or High-Grade Myelodysplastic Syndromes (MDS): A Phase 1 Study. *ASH Annu. Meet. Abstr.* **2010**, *116*, 658.

140. Rabut, G.; Peter, M. Function and regulation of protein neddylation. "Protein modifications: Beyond the usual suspects" review series. *EMBO Rep.* **2008**, *9*, 969–976. [CrossRef] [PubMed]

141. Nawrocki, S.T.; Griffin, P.; Kelly, K.R.; Carew, J.S. MLN4924: A novel first-in-class inhibitor of NEDD8-activating enzyme for cancer therapy. *Expert Opin. Investig. Drugs* **2012**, *21*, 1563–1573. [CrossRef] [PubMed]

142. Wang, M.; Medeiros, B.C.; Erba, H.P.; DeAngelo, D.J.; Giles, F.J.; Swords, R.T. Targeting protein neddylation: A novel therapeutic strategy for the treatment of cancer. *Expert Opin. Ther. Targets* **2011**, *15*, 253–264. [CrossRef] [PubMed]

143. Lin, J.J.; Milhollen, M.A.; Smith, P.G.; Narayanan, U.; Dutta, A. NEDD8-targeting drug MLN4924 elicits DNA rereplication by stabilizing Cdt1 in S phase, triggering checkpoint activation, apoptosis, and senescence in cancer cells. *Cancer Res.* **2010**, *70*, 10310–10320. [CrossRef] [PubMed]

144. Milhollen, M.A.; Narayanan, U.; Soucy, T.A.; Veiby, P.O.; Smith, P.G.; Amidon, B. Inhibition of NEDD8-activating enzyme induces rereplication and apoptosis in human tumor cells consistent with deregulating CDT1 turnover. *Cancer Res.* **2011**, *71*, 3042–3051. [PubMed]

145. Luo, Z.; Pan, Y.; Jeong, L.S.; Liu, J.; Jia, L. Inactivation of the Cullin (CUL)-RING E3 ligase by the NEDD8-activating enzyme inhibitor MLN4924 triggers protective autophagy in cancer cells. *Autophagy* **2012**, *8*, 1677–1679. [CrossRef] [PubMed]

146. Luo, Z.; Yu, G.; Lee, H.W.; Li, L.; Wang, L.; Yang, D.; Pan, Y.; Ding, C.; Qian, J.; Wu, L.; *et al.* The Nedd8-activating enzyme inhibitor MLN4924 induces autophagy and apoptosis to suppress liver cancer cell growth. *Cancer Res.* **2012**, *72*, 3360–3371. [CrossRef] [PubMed]

147. Robert, T.; Vanoli, F.; Chiolo, I.; Shubassi, G.; Bernstein, K.A.; Rothstein, R.; Botrugno, O.A.; Parazzoli, D.; Oldani, A.; Minucci, S.; *et al.* HDACs link the DNA damage response, processing of double-strand breaks and autophagy. *Nature* **2011**, *471*, 74–79. [CrossRef] [PubMed]

148. Shubassi, G.; Robert, T.; Vanoli, F.; Minucci, S.; Foiani, M. Acetylation: A novel link between double-strand break repair and autophagy. *Cancer Res.* **2012**, *72*, 1332–1335. [CrossRef] [PubMed]

149. Cantley, L.C. The phosphoinositide 3-kinase pathway. *Science* **2002**, *296*, 1655–1657. [CrossRef] [PubMed]

150. Courtney, K.D.; Corcoran, R.B.; Engelman, J.A. The PI3K pathway as drug target in human cancer. *J. Clin. Oncol.* **2010**, *28*, 1075–1083. [PubMed]

151. Martelli, A.M.; Nyakern, M.; Tabellini, G.; Bortul, R.; Tazzari, P.L.; Evangelisti, C.; Cocco, L. Phosphoinositide 3-kinase/Akt signaling pathway and its therapeutical implications for human acute myeloid leukemia. *Leukemia* **2006**, *20*, 911–928. [CrossRef] [PubMed]

152. Martelli, A.M.; Evangelisti, C.; Chiarini, F.; Grimaldi, C.; Manzoli, L.; McCubrey, J.A. Targeting the PI3K/AKT/mTOR signaling network in acute myelogenous leukemia. *Expert Opin. Investig. Drugs* **2009**, *18*, 1333–1349. [CrossRef] [PubMed]

153. Xu, Q.; Simpson, S.E.; Scialla, T.J.; Bagg, A.; Carroll, M. Survival of acute myeloid leukemia cells requires PI3 kinase activation. *Blood* **2003**, *102*, 972–980. [CrossRef] [PubMed]

154. Xu, Q.; Thompson, J.E.; Carroll, M. mTOR regulates cell survival after etoposide treatment in primary AML cells. *Blood* **2005**, *106*, 4261–4268. [CrossRef] [PubMed]

155. Min, Y.H.; Eom, J.I.; Cheong, J.W.; Maeng, H.O.; Kim, J.Y.; Jeung, H.K.; Lee, S.T.; Lee, M.H.; Hahn, J.S.; Ko, Y.W. Constitutive phosphorylation of Akt/PKB protein in acute myeloid leukemia: Its significance as a prognostic variable. *Leukemia* **2003**, *17*, 995–997. [CrossRef] [PubMed]

156. Steelman, L.S.; Abrams, S.L.; Whelan, J.; Bertrand, F.E.; Ludwig, D.E.; Basecke, J.; Libra, M.; Stivala, F.; Milella, M.; Tafuri, A.; *et al.* Contributions of the Raf/MEK/ERK, PI3K/PTEN/Akt/mTOR and Jak/STAT pathways to leukemia. *Leukemia* **2008**, *22*, 686–707. [CrossRef] [PubMed]

157. Martelli, A.M.; Evangelisti, C.; Chiarini, F.; McCubrey, J.A. The phosphatidylinositol 3-kinase/Akt/mTOR signaling network as a therapeutic target in acute myelogenous leukemia patients. *Oncotarget* **2010**, *1*, 89–103. [PubMed]

158. Furman, R.R.; Sharman, J.P.; Coutre, S.E.; Cheson, B.D.; Pagel, J.M.; Hillmen, P.; Barrientos, J.C.; Zelenetz, A.D.; Kipps, T.J.; Flinn, I.; *et al.* Idelalisib and rituximab in relapsed chronic lymphocytic leukemia. *N. Engl. J. Med.* **2014**, *370*, 997–1007. [CrossRef] [PubMed]

159. Gopal, A.K.; Kahl, B.S.; de Vos, S.; Wagner-Johnston, N.D.; Schuster, S.J.; Jurczak, W.J.; Flinn, I.W.; Flowers, C.R.; Martin, P.; Viardot, A.; *et al.* PI3Kdelta inhibition by idelalisib in patients with relapsed indolent lymphoma. *N. Engl. J. Med.* **2014**, *370*, 1008–1018. [CrossRef] [PubMed]

160. Rahmani, M.; Yu, C.; Reese, E.; Ahmed, W.; Hirsch, K.; Dent, P.; Grant, S. Inhibition of PI-3 kinase sensitizes human leukemic cells to histone deacetylase inhibitor-mediated apoptosis through p44/42 MAP kinase inactivation and abrogation of p21(CIP1/WAF1) induction rather than AKT inhibition. *Oncogene* **2003**, *22*, 6231–6242. [CrossRef] [PubMed]

161. Rahmani, M.; Reese, E.; Dai, Y.; Bauer, C.; Payne, S.G.; Dent, P.; Spiegel, S.; Grant, S. Coadministration of histone deacetylase inhibitors and perifosine synergistically induces apoptosis in human leukemia cells through Akt and ERK1/2 inactivation and the generation of ceramide and reactive oxygen species. *Cancer Res.* **2005**, *65*, 2422–2432. [CrossRef] [PubMed]

162. Reed, J.C. Bcl-2-family proteins and hematologic malignancies: History and future prospects. *Blood* **2008**, *111*, 3322–3330. [CrossRef] [PubMed]

163. Davids, M.S.; Letai, A. Targeting the B-cell lymphoma/leukemia 2 family in cancer. *J. Clin. Oncol.* **2012**, *30*, 3127–3135. [CrossRef] [PubMed]

164. Willis, S.N.; Chen, L.; Dewson, G.; Wei, A.; Naik, E.; Fletcher, J.I.; Adams, J.M.; Huang, D.C. Proapoptotic Bak is sequestered by Mcl-1 and Bcl-xL, but not Bcl-2, until displaced by BH3-only proteins. *Genes Dev.* **2005**, *19*, 1294–1305. [CrossRef] [PubMed]

165. Bose, P.; Grant, S. Bcl-2 family: Translational aspects. In *Targeted Therapy of Acute Myeloid Leukemia*; Andreeff, M., Ed.; Springer-Verlag: New York, NY, USA, 2015; pp. 67–94.

166. Oltersdorf, T.; Elmore, S.W.; Shoemaker, A.R.; Armstrong, R.C.; Augeri, D.J.; Belli, B.A.; Bruncko, M.; Deckwerth, T.L.; Dinges, J.; Hajduk, P.J.; *et al.* J An inhibitor of Bcl-2 family proteins induces regression of solid tumours. *Nature* **2005**, *435*, 677–681. [CrossRef] [PubMed]

167. Tse, C.; Shoemaker, A.R.; Adickes, J.; Anderson, M.G.; Chen, J.; Jin, S.; Johnson, E.F.; Marsh, K.C.; Mitten, M.J.; Nimmer, P.; *et al.* ABT-263: A potent and orally bioavailable Bcl-2 family inhibitor. *Cancer Res.* **2008**, *68*, 3421–3428. [CrossRef] [PubMed]

168. Roberts, A.W.; Seymour, J.F.; Brown, J.R.; Wierda, W.G.; Kipps, T.J.; Khaw, S.L.; Carney, D.A.; He, S.Z.; Huang, D.C.; Xiong, H.; *et al.* Substantial susceptibility of chronic lymphocytic leukemia to BCL2 inhibition: Results of a phase I study of navitoclax in patients with relapsed or refractory disease. *J. Clin. Oncol.* **2012**, *30*, 488–496. [CrossRef] [PubMed]

169. Mason, K.D.; Carpinelli, M.R.; Fletcher, J.I.; Collinge, J.E.; Hilton, A.A.; Ellis, S.; Kelly, P.N.; Ekert, P.G.; Metcalf, D.; Roberts, A.W.; *et al.* Programmed anuclear cell death delimits platelet life span. *Cell* **2007**, *128*, 1173–1186. [CrossRef] [PubMed]

170. Wilson, W.H.; O'Connor, O.A.; Czuczman, M.S.; LaCasce, A.S.; Gerecitano, J.F.; Leonard, J.P.; Tulpule, A.; Dunleavy, K.; Xiong, H.; Chiu, Y.L.; *et al.* Navitoclax, a targeted high-affinity inhibitor of BCL-2, in lymphoid malignancies: A phase 1 dose-escalation study of safety, pharmacokinetics, pharmacodynamics, and antitumour activity. *Lancet Oncol.* **2010**, *11*, 1149–1159. [CrossRef] [PubMed]

171. Gandhi, L.; Camidge, D.R.; Ribeiro de Oliveira, M.; Bonomi, P.; Gandara, D.; Khaira, D.; Hann, C.L.; McKeegan, E.M.; Litvinovich, E.; Hemken, P.M.; *et al.* Phase I study of Navitoclax (ABT-263), a novel Bcl-2 family inhibitor, in patients with small-cell lung cancer and other solid tumors. *J. Clin. Oncol.* **2011**, *29*, 909–916. [CrossRef] [PubMed]

172. Rudin, C.M.; Hann, C.L.; Garon, E.B.; Ribeiro de Oliveira, M.; Bonomi, P.D.; Camidge, D.R.; Chu, Q.; Giaccone, G.; Khaira, D.; Ramalingam, S.S.; *et al.* Phase II study of single-agent navitoclax (ABT-263) and biomarker correlates in patients with relapsed small cell lung cancer. *Clin. Cancer Res.* **2012**, *18*, 3163–3169. [CrossRef] [PubMed]

173. Schoenwaelder, S.M.; Jarman, K.E.; Gardiner, E.E.; Hua, M.; Qiao, J.; White, M.J.; Josefsson, E.C.; Alwis, I.; Ono, A.; Willcox, A.; Andrews, R.K.; *et al.* Bcl-xL-inhibitory BH3 mimetics can induce a transient thrombocytopathy that undermines the hemostatic function of platelets. *Blood* **2011**, *118*, 1663–1674. [CrossRef] [PubMed]

174. Souers, A.J.; Leverson, J.D.; Boghaert, E.R.; Ackler, S.L.; Catron, N.D.; Chen, J.; Dayton, B.D.; Ding, H.; Enschede, S.H.; Fairbrother, W.J.; *et al.* ABT-199, a potent and selective BCL-2 inhibitor, achieves antitumor activity while sparing platelets. *Nat. Med.* **2013**, *19*, 202–208. [CrossRef] [PubMed]

175. BCL-2 Inhibitor Yields High Response in CLL and SLL. *Cancer Discov.* **2014**, *4*. [CrossRef]

176. Pan, R.; Hogdal, L.J.; Benito, J.M.; Bucci, D.; Han, L.; Borthakur, G.; Cortes, J.; Deangelo, D.J.; Debose, L.; Mu, H.; *et al.* Selective BCL-2 Inhibition by ABT-199 Causes On-Target Cell Death in Acute Myeloid Leukemia. *Cancer Discov.* **2014**, *4*, 362–375. [CrossRef] [PubMed]

177. Marcucci, G.; Moser, B.; Blum, W.; Stock, W.; Wetzler, M.; Kolitz, J.E.; Thakuri, M.; Carter, T.; Stuart, R.K.; Larson, R.A. A phase III randomized trial of intensive induction and consolidation chemotherapy {+/-} oblimersen, a pro-apoptotic Bcl-2 antisense oligonucleotide in untreated acute myeloid leukemia patients >60 years old. *ASCO Meet. Abstr.* **2007**, *25* (Suppl. 18), 7012.

178. O'Brien, S.; Moore, J.O.; Boyd, T.E.; Larratt, L.M.; Skotnicki, A.B.; Koziner, B.; Chanan-Khan, A.A.; Seymour, J.F.; Gribben, J.; Itri, L.M.; *et al.* 5-year survival in patients with relapsed or refractory chronic lymphocytic leukemia in a randomized, phase III trial of fludarabine plus cyclophosphamide with or without oblimersen. *J. Clin. Oncol.* **2009**, *27*, 5208–5212. [CrossRef] [PubMed]

179. Glaser, S.P.; Lee, E.F.; Trounson, E.; Bouillet, P.; Wei, A.; Fairlie, W.D.; Izon, D.J.; Zuber, J.; Rappaport, A.R.; Herold, M.J.; *et al.* Anti-apoptotic Mcl-1 is essential for the development and sustained growth of acute myeloid leukemia. *Genes Dev.* **2012**, *26*, 120–125. [CrossRef] [PubMed]

180. Konopleva, M.; Contractor, R.; Tsao, T.; Samudio, I.; Ruvolo, P.P.; Kitada, S.; Deng, X.; Zhai, D.; Shi, Y.X.; Sneed, T.; *et al.* Mechanisms of apoptosis sensitivity and resistance to the BH3 mimetic ABT-737 in acute myeloid leukemia. *Cancer Cell* **2006**, *10*, 375–388. [CrossRef] [PubMed]

181. Van Delft, M.F.; Wei, A.H.; Mason, K.D.; Vandenberg, C.J.; Chen, L.; Czabotar, P.E.; Willis, S.N.; Scott, C.L.; Day, C.L.; Cory, S.; *et al.* The BH3 mimetic ABT-737 targets selective Bcl-2 proteins and efficiently induces apoptosis via Bak/Bax if Mcl-1 is neutralized. *Cancer Cell* **2006**, *10*, 389–399. [CrossRef] [PubMed]

182. Konopleva, M.; Watt, J.; Contractor, R.; Tsao, T.; Harris, D.; Estrov, Z.; Bornmann, W.; Kantarjian, H.; Viallet, J.; Samudio, I.; *et al.* Mechanisms of antileukemic activity of the novel Bcl-2 homology domain-3 mimetic GX15-070 (obatoclax). *Cancer Res.* **2008**, *68*, 3413–3420. [CrossRef] [PubMed]

183. Dai, Y.; Grant, S. Targeting multiple arms of the apoptotic regulatory machinery. *Cancer Res.* **2007**, *67*, 2908–2911. [CrossRef] [PubMed]

184. Bose, P.; Grant, S. Mcl-1 as a Therapeutic Target in Acute Myelogenous Leukemia (AML). *Leuk. Res. Rep.* **2013**, *2*, 12–14. [PubMed]

185. Rahmani, M.; Davis, E.M.; Bauer, C.; Dent, P.; Grant, S. Apoptosis induced by the kinase inhibitor BAY 43-9006 in human leukemia cells involves down-regulation of Mcl-1 through inhibition of translation. *J. Biol. Chem.* **2005**, *280*, 35217–35227. [CrossRef] [PubMed]

186. Chen, S.; Dai, Y.; Harada, H.; Dent, P.; Grant, S. Mcl-1 down-regulation potentiates ABT-737 lethality by cooperatively inducing Bak activation and Bax translocation. *Cancer Res.* **2007**, *67*, 782–791. [CrossRef] [PubMed]

187. Zhang, W.; Konopleva, M.; Ruvolo, V.R.; McQueen, T.; Evans, R.L.; Bornmann, W.G.; McCubrey, J.; Cortes, J.; Andreeff, M. Sorafenib induces apoptosis of AML cells via Bim-mediated activation of the intrinsic apoptotic pathway. *Leukemia* **2008**, *22*, 808–818. [CrossRef] [PubMed]

188. Rahmani, M.; Aust, M.M.; Attkisson, E.; Williams, D.C., Jr.; Ferreira-Gonzalez, A.; Grant, S. Inhibition of Bcl-2 antiapoptotic members by obatoclax potently enhances sorafenib-induced apoptosis in human myeloid leukemia cells through a Bim-dependent process. *Blood* **2012**, *119*, 6089–6098. [CrossRef] [PubMed]

189. Chen, S.; Dai, Y.; Pei, X.Y.; Grant, S. Bim upregulation by histone deacetylase inhibitors mediates interactions with the Bcl-2 antagonist ABT-737: Evidence for distinct roles for Bcl-2, Bcl-xL, and Mcl-1. *Mol. Cell. Biol.* **2009**, *29*, 6149–6169. [CrossRef] [PubMed]

190. Wei, Y.; Kadia, T.; Tong, W.; Zhang, M.; Jia, Y.; Yang, H.; Hu, Y.; Tambaro, F.P.; Viallet, J.; O'Brien, S.; *et al.* The combination of a histone deacetylase inhibitor with the Bcl-2 homology domain-3 mimetic GX15–070 has synergistic antileukemia activity by activating both apoptosis and autophagy. *Clin. Cancer Res.* **2010**, *16*, 3923–3932. [CrossRef] [PubMed]

191. Konopleva, M.; Milella, M.; Ruvolo, P.; Watts, J.C.; Ricciardi, M.R.; Korchin, B.; McQueen, T.; Bornmann, W.; Tsao, T.; Bergamo, P.; *et al.* MEK inhibition enhances ABT-737-induced leukemia cell apoptosis via prevention of ERK-activated MCL-1 induction and modulation of MCL-1/BIM complex. *Leukemia* **2012**, *26*, 778–787. [CrossRef] [PubMed]

192. Vachhani, P.; Bose, P.; Rahmani, M.; Grant, S. Rational combination of dual PI3K/mTOR blockade and Bcl-2/-xL inhibition in AML. *Physiol. Genomics* **2014**, *46*, 448–456. [PubMed]

193. Luo, J.; Manning, B.D.; Cantley, L.C. Targeting the PI3K-Akt pathway in human cancer: Rationale and promise. *Cancer Cell* **2003**, *4*, 257–262. [CrossRef]

194. Manning, B.D.; Cantley, L.C. AKT/PKB signaling: Navigating downstream. *Cell* **2007**, *129*, 1261–1274. [CrossRef] [PubMed]

195. Engelman, J.A. Targeting PI3K signalling in cancer: Opportunities, challenges and limitations. *Nat. Rev. Cancer* **2009**, *9*, 550–562. [CrossRef] [PubMed]

196. Tamburini, J.; Chapuis, N.; Bardet, V.; Park, S.; Sujobert, P.; Willems, L.; Ifrah, N.; Dreyfus, F.; Mayeux, P.; Lacombe, C.; *et al.* Mammalian target of rapamycin (mTOR) inhibition activates phosphatidylinositol 3-kinase/Akt by up-regulating insulin-like growth factor-1 receptor signaling in acute myeloid leukemia: Rationale for therapeutic inhibition of both pathways. *Blood* **2008**, *111*, 379–382. [CrossRef] [PubMed]

197. Park, S.; Chapuis, N.; Bardet, V.; Tamburini, J.; Gallay, N.; Willems, L.; Knight, Z.A.; Shokat, K.M.; Azar, N.; Viguie, F.; *et al.* PI-103, a dual inhibitor of Class IA phosphatidylinositide 3-kinase and mTOR, has antileukemic activity in AML. *Leukemia* **2008**, *22*, 1698–1706. [CrossRef] [PubMed]

198. Chapuis, N.; Tamburini, J.; Green, A.S.; Vignon, C.; Bardet, V.; Neyret, A.; Pannetier, M.; Willems, L.; Park, S.; Macone, A.; *et al.* Dual inhibition of PI3K and mTORC1/2 signaling by NVP-BEZ235 as a new therapeutic strategy for acute myeloid leukemia. *Clin. Cancer Res.* **2010**, *16*, 5424–5435. [CrossRef] [PubMed]

199. Grant, S. Cotargeting survival signaling pathways in cancer. *J. Clin. Investig.* **2008**, *118*, 3003–3006. [CrossRef] [PubMed]

200. Ricciardi, M.R.; McQueen, T.; Chism, D.; Milella, M.; Estey, E.; Kaldjian, E.; Sebolt-Leopold, J.; Konopleva, M.; Andreeff, M. Quantitative single cell determination of ERK phosphorylation and regulation in relapsed and refractory primary acute myeloid leukemia. *Leukemia* **2005**, *19*, 1543–1549. [CrossRef] [PubMed]

201. Jin, L.; Tabe, Y.; Kojima, K.; Shikami, M.; Benito, J.; Ruvolo, V.; Wang, R.Y.; McQueen, T.; Ciurea, S.O.; Miida, T.; *et al.* PI3K inhibitor GDC-0941 enhances apoptotic effects of BH-3 mimetic ABT-737 in AML cells in the hypoxic bone marrow microenvironment. *J. Mol. Med. (Berl.)* **2013**, *91*, 1383–1397. [CrossRef]

202. Zhang, W.; Ruvolo, V.R.; Gao, C.; Zhou, L.; Bornmann, W.; Tsao, T.; Schober, W.D.; Smith, P.; Guichard, S.; Konopleva, M.; *et al.* Evaluation of apoptosis induction by concomitant inhibition of MEK, mTOR, and Bcl-2 in human acute myelogenous leukemia cells. *Mol. Cancer Ther.* **2014**, *13*, 1848–1859. [CrossRef] [PubMed]

203. Rahmani, M.; Aust, M.M.; Attkisson, E.; Williams, D.C., Jr.; Ferreira-Gonzalez, A.; Grant, S. Dual inhibition of Bcl-2 and Bcl-xL strikingly enhances PI3K inhibition-induced apoptosis in human myeloid leukemia cells through a GSK3- and Bim-dependent mechanism. *Cancer Res.* **2013**, *73*, 1340–1351. [CrossRef] [PubMed]

204. Dai, Y.; Rahmani, M.; Grant, S. Proteasome inhibitors potentiate leukemic cell apoptosis induced by the cyclin-dependent kinase inhibitor flavopiridol through a SAPK/JNK- and NF-kappaB-dependent process. *Oncogene* **2003**, *22*, 7108–7122. [CrossRef] [PubMed]

205. Dai, Y.; Rahmani, M.; Pei, X.; Dent, P.; Grant, S. Bortezomib and flavopiridol interact synergistically to induce apoptosis in chronic myeloid leukemia cells resistant to imatinib mesylate through both Bcr/Abl-dependent and -independent mechanisms. *Blood* **2004**, *104*, 509–518. [CrossRef] [PubMed]

206. Holkova, B.; Perkins, E.B.; Ramakrishnan, V.; Tombes, M.B.; Shrader, E.; Talreja, N.; Wellons, M.D.; Hogan, K.T.; Roodman, G.D.; Coppola, D.; *et al.* Phase I trial of bortezomib (PS-341; NSC 681239) and alvocidib (flavopiridol; NSC 649890) in patients with recurrent or refractory B-cell neoplasms. *Clin. Cancer Res.* **2011**, *17*, 3388–3397. [CrossRef] [PubMed]

207. Holkova, B.; Kmieciak, M.; Perkins, E.B.; Bose, P.; Baz, R.; Roodman, G.D.; Stuart, R.K.; Ramakrishnan, V.; Wan, W.; Peer, C.J.; *et al.* Phase I Trial of Bortezomib and "Non-Hybrid" (Bolus) Infusion Schedule of Alvocidib (Flavopiridol) in Patients with Recurrent or Refractory Indolent B-cell Neoplasms. *Clin. Cancer Res.* **2014**, *20*, 5652–5662. [CrossRef] [PubMed]

208. Yu, C.; Rahmani, M.; Dai, Y.; Conrad, D.; Krystal, G.; Dent, P.; Grant, S. The lethal effects of pharmacological cyclin-dependent kinase inhibitors in human leukemia cells proceed through a phosphatidylinositol 3-kinase/Akt-dependent process. *Cancer Res.* **2003**, *63*, 1822–1833. [PubMed]

209. Thomas, D.; Powell, J.A.; Vergez, F.; Segal, D.H.; Nguyen, N.Y.; Baker, A.; Teh, T.C.; Barry, E.F.; Sarry, J.E.; Lee, E.M.; *et al.* Targeting acute myeloid leukemia by dual inhibition of PI3K signaling and Cdk9-mediated Mcl-1 transcription. *Blood* **2013**, *122*, 738–748. [CrossRef] [PubMed]

210. Dai, Y.; Yu, C.; Singh, V.; Tang, L.; Wang, Z.; McInistry, R.; Dent, P.; Grant, S. Pharmacological inhibitors of the mitogen-activated protein kinase (MAPK) kinase/MAPK cascade interact synergistically with UCN-01 to induce mitochondrial dysfunction and apoptosis in human leukemia cells. *Cancer Res.* **2001**, *61*, 5106–5115. [PubMed]

211. Dai, Y.; Khanna, P.; Chen, S.; Pei, X.Y.; Dent, P.; Grant, S. Statins synergistically potentiate 7-hydroxystaurosporine (UCN-01) lethality in human leukemia and myeloma cells by disrupting Ras farnesylation and activation. *Blood* **2007**, *109*, 4415–4423. [CrossRef] [PubMed]

212. Dai, Y.; Rahmani, M.; Pei, X.Y.; Khanna, P.; Han, S.I.; Mitchell, C.; Dent, P.; Grant, S. Farnesyltransferase inhibitors interact synergistically with the Chk1 inhibitor UCN-01 to induce apoptosis in human leukemia cells through interruption of both Akt and MEK/ERK pathways and activation of SEK1/JNK. *Blood* **2005**, *105*, 1706–1716. [CrossRef] [PubMed]

213. Roberts, E.C.; Shapiro, P.S.; Nahreini, T.S.; Pages, G.; Pouyssegur, J.; Ahn, N.G. Distinct cell cycle timing requirements for extracellular signal-regulated kinase and phosphoinositide 3-kinase signaling pathways in somatic cell mitosis. *Mol. Cell. Biol.* **2002**, *22*, 7226–7241. [CrossRef] [PubMed]

214. Wu, D.; Chen, B.; Parihar, K.; He, L.; Fan, C.; Zhang, J.; Liu, L.; Gillis, A.; Bruce, A.; Kapoor, A.; Tang, D. ERK activity facilitates activation of the S-phase DNA damage checkpoint by modulating ATR function. *Oncogene* **2006**, *25*, 1153–1164. [CrossRef] [PubMed]

215. Golding, S.E.; Rosenberg, E.; Neill, S.; Dent, P.; Povirk, L.F.; Valerie, K. Extracellular signal-related kinase positively regulates ataxia telangiectasia mutated, homologous recombination repair, and the DNA damage response. *Cancer Res.* **2007**, *67*, 1046–1053. [CrossRef] [PubMed]

216. Jain, N.; Curran, E.; Iyengar, N.M.; Diaz-Flores, E.; Kunnavakkam, R.; Popplewell, L.; Kirschbaum, M.H.; Karrison, T.; Erba, H.P.; Green, M.; *et al.* Phase II study of the oral MEK inhibitor selumetinib in advanced acute myelogenous leukemia: A University of Chicago phase II consortium trial. *Clin. Cancer Res.* **2014**, *20*, 490–498. [PubMed]

217. Pei, X.Y.; Dai, Y.; Felthousen, J.; Chen, S.; Takabatake, Y.; Zhou, L.; Youssefian, L.E.; Sanderson, M.W.; Bodie, W.W.; Kramer, L.B.; *et al.* Circumvention of Mcl-1-dependent drug resistance by simultaneous Chk1 and MEK1/2 inhibition in human multiple myeloma cells. *PLoS ONE* **2014**, *9*, e89064. [CrossRef] [PubMed]

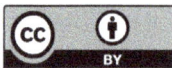

Journal of
Clinical Medicine

MDPI

Review

Treatment of Acute Myeloid Leukemia in Adolescent and Young Adult Patients

Guldane Cengiz Seval and Muhit Ozcan *

Department of Hematology, Ankara University School of Medicine, Ankara 06100, Turkey;
guldanecengiz@gmail.com
* Author to whom correspondence should be addressed; muhit.ozcan@medicine.ankara.edu.tr;
  Tel.: +90-312-595-7380.

Academic Editor: Celalettin Ustun
Received: 5 September 2014; Accepted: 3 February 2015; Published: 11 March 2015

Abstract: The objectives of this review were to discuss standard and investigational treatment strategies for adolescent and young adult with acute myeloid leukemia, excluding acute promyelocytic leukemia. Acute myeloid leukemia (AML) in adolescent and young adult patients (AYAs) may need a different type of therapy than those currently used in children and older patients. As soon as AML is diagnosed, AYA patient should be offered to participate in well-designed clinical trials. The standard treatment approach for AYAs with AML is remission induction chemotherapy with an anthracycline/cytarabine combination, followed by either consolidation chemotherapy or stem cell transplantation, depending on the ability of the patient to tolerate intensive treatment and cytogenetic features. Presently, continuing progress of novel drugs targeting specific pathways in acute leukemia may bring AML treatment into a new era.

Keywords: acute myeloid leukemia; adolescent and young adults; treatment

---

1. Introduction

The adolescent and young adult (AYA) population is defined by an age group range approximately between 15 and 35 years of age [1]. About 70,000 adolescents and young adults (ages 15–39) are diagnosed with cancer each year in the United States.

Acute myeloid leukemia (AML) represents about 33% of adolescent and 50% adult leukemia [2]. In United States, using 1975–2011 US Surveillance Epidemiology and End Results (SEER) data, annual rates for new diagnosis of AML in AYAs are 4.4/100,000, but survival data for the specific age groups of AYA are scarce. Although population-based data from England and Wales 1993–1998 years showed a five-year survival of 46%, while US SEER 1975–2000 years registry data showed a 20-year survival of 20%–27% for 15–29-year-old AYA with AML [2].

The improvement of prognosis in childhood and adolescent AML has been seen over the past two decades; CR with intensive induction therapy 80%–90% and 60%–65% are cured after post remission therapy. Recently, Children Oncology Group (COG) reported the outcomes of 238 AYA patients (16 through 20 years) from four serial childhood COG trials (CCG-2891, CCG-2941, CCG-2961 and AAML03P1) between 1989 and 2006 [3]. In the evaluation of this report, AYA patients were more likely to have poor-risk disease and are less likely to have standard-risk disease. Nevertheless, the outcome of AYA was similar to children patients with newly diagnosed AML. Notably, there are exact differences in treatment-related mortality as higher rates of infection-related deaths were seen in AYAs with AML.

Large prospective studies that include both pediatric and adult patients with AML could not clarify a distinct biology of AYAs [4]. Garrido *et al.* [3] reported that CD34 positive AML stem cells from younger patients express high levels of bcl-2. In contrast to our knowledge, this overexpression reduced the rates of apoptosis, drug resistance and poor clinical outcomes. Cytogenetic is the most important prognosis factor of AML, but only a few studies analyzed the frequencies of genetic abnormalities specifically in AYAs [5,6]. One of the large prospective studies for children and up to age of 55 years old adults, MRC AML 10 trial, established equal cytogenetic group distributions among AYAs aged 14–35 and younger children. The most interesting result of the study was rapid decline of the three-year survival rate from 42% in children to 19% in AYAs [5]. In 2008, Rowley's review of the cytogenetic of AML mentioned the age-dependent pattern of AML translocations [6]. It was disclosed that t(15,17), the characteristic of APL, peaks in incidence between 20 and 39 years of age, and that t(11q23), a particularly difficult-to-treat type of AML, has its lowest frequency in this age group [6]. The European Leukemia Net brought out a standardized prognostic scoring system including the conventional cytogenetic and the commonly used molecular testing markers (FLT3-ITD, CEBPA and NPM1) [7]. It is important to note that, no specific genetic or phenotypic aberrations were found in AYAs with AML.

It is clear that in these age groups, patients deserve special attention differences in underlying cancer biology with special medical, physical, psychological and social needs. Unavoidable psychosocial care is the most difficult in the management of adolescents. The need of autonomy and independence, social development, sexual maturation, education and employment generated the conventional problems. In view of these specific adolescents' needs, it is recommended to treat these patients in special units whenever possible [8].

2. Management

Principles of Treatment

AML treatment in AYA should be based on cytogenetic and molecular factors to avoid overtreatment in patients with favorable prognosis and to improve outcome in those with unfavorable prognosis. Notably, the therapy should be to cure the patient by exterminating the leukemic clone while avoiding side effects and late effects as much as possible. In acute lymphoblastic leukemia, it has been shown that poorer prognosis of AYAs can be overcome with intensive pediatric protocols; whether a similar approach should be applied to AYAs with AML is not evidently provided [2]. Despite several strategies to increase the intensity of therapy, the long-term overall survival rate has not exceeded a plateau of 50%, suggesting that treatment-related toxicity does not balance against antileukemic efficacy [9]. Also, it appears that further intensification of therapy or "one-size-fits-all" treatment strategy will not improve the current AML survival rates.

As soon as AML is diagnosed, AYA patient should be offered to participate into well-designed clinical trials to ensure highest quality and safety of diagnostics and management. Although the majority of children with AML are treated in clinical trials, the number of AYAs enrolled in clinical trials is much lower. Reasons for the poor clinical trial participation in adolescents are undefined differences in biology, poor compliance or intolerance of therapy, receiving care at centers without AYA experience and psychosocial needs [4,8].

In contrast to children and adults, there is no data clarifying the kind of therapy appropriate for AYA. There are also limited prospective and retrospective studies looking into the outcomes for AYAs treated on pediatric *versus* adult protocols. Besides, treatment protocol of AYA depends especially on the individual fitness of the patient and the choice of treating physician or center. As usual, AML treatment consists of induction and consolidation to maintain remission arms. Differing from adults, additional CNS therapy is routine in most of the pediatric protocols [9]. Furthermore, the efficacy of maintenance therapy in AYA has not been proved as with adults and children.

When chemotherapy was introduced into the care of AYA with leukemia, the goal was focused on achieving remission. Long-term complications include effects on reproductive capacity should be separately evaluated. In patients determined to be at risk for future infertility, assisted reproductive technologies such as cryopreservation of gonadal tissue or gametes can be used [10].

3. Remission Induction Therapy

The combination of three days of an anthracycline (daunorubicin 60–90 mg/m^2/day idarubicin 10–12 mg/m^2/day or mitoxantrone 10–12 mg/m^2/day) and seven days of cytarabine (100–200 mg/m^2/day), named as "3 + 7" continues to be the backbone of AML induction therapy over the past four decades [11]. AYA AML patients usually received one or two cycles of induction therapy. On the basis of available evidence in children and adolescents with AML, complete remission (CR) achieved >80% with these regimens.

From 1986 to 2008, Cancer and Leukemia Group B (CALGB) had conducted sequential trials for newly diagnosed AML, named as CALGB 8525, CALGB 9022, CALGB 9222, CALGB 9621 and CALGB 19808. Daunorubicin and cytarabine-based induction treatment were used in all CALGB trials and the CR rate after receiving up to two courses was 76% for the AYA cohort, including 149 patients aged 16–21 years [12]. The summaries of protocols are shown in Table 1.

Table 1. Summary of the protocols.

Protocol/Courses (References)	Induction Drugs	Postremission Drugs	BMT
CALGB 9022 [12]	AraC and DNM	HiDAC, VP-16/Cyclophosphamide, and AZQ/mitoxantrone	None
CALGB 9621 [12]	AraC, DNM, VP-16, (±Valspodar)	HiDAC	Autologous (except CBF + AML)
AML BFM-93 [13]	AraC, VP-16, and DNM/Ida	HAM-Consolidation therapy (6-thioguanine; prednisolone; vincristine; adriamycin; Ara-C; intrathecal Ara-C; cyclophosphamide) Intensification (HiDAC and VP-16 and cranial irradiation)-Maintenance therapy (thioguanine and Ara-C)	Allogeneic
MRC AML12 [14]	AraC, VP-16 and DNM/Mitoxantrone (±GCSF)	Amsacrine, AraC, VP-16-AraC, Mitoxantrone/AraC, Ida, VP-16/BMT	Allogeneic Autolog
AML-BFM 2004 [14]	AraC, VP-16 and L-DNM/Ida HAM	AraC/, Ida (±2-chloro-2-deoxyadenosine) HAM-Intensification (HiDAC, VP-16 and cranial irradiation) Maintenance therapy (intrathecal AraC)	Allogeneic
AML 10 [15]	AraC, DNM/Ida/Mitoxantrone	Intermediate-dose AraC	Allogeneic Autolog
MRC AML15 [16]	AraC, DNM, VP-16, Fludarabine, Ida, GCSF (±Mylotarg)	Amsacrine, AraC, VP-16 (±Mylotarg) HiDAC (±Mylotarg)	Allogeneic
PALG [17]	AraC, DNM (±2-chloro-2-deoxyadenosine) CLAG	HAM-HiDAC (±2-chloro-2-deoxyadenosine) Maintenance therapy (AraC, DNM, 6-thioguanine)	Allogeneic Autolog
SWOG S0106 [18]	AraC, DNM, and GO	HiDAC (±GO)	Allogeneic
CALGB 8525 [19]	AraC and DNM	AraC	None
CCG-2891 [20]	Dexamethasone, AraC, 6-Thioguanine, VP-16, DNM, intrathecal AraC	AraC and L-asparaginase-AraC, 6-thioguanine, vincristine, L-asparaginase, cyclophosphamide and 5-azacytidine AraC, DNM, VP-16, 6-thioguanine and dexamethasone	Allogeneic Autolog

Abbreviations: AraC, Cytarabine; BMT, bone marrow transplantation; DNM, daunomycin; AZQ, 5 Azacytidine; HiDAC, high dose cytarabine; VP-16, etoposide; Ida, Idarubicin; GO, gemtuzumab + ozogamycin; CBF, Core Binding Factor; HAM, high dose cytarabine and mitoxantrone; G-CSF, granulocyte colony-stimulating factor; CLAG, 2-chloro-2-deoxyadenosin, cytarabine and granulocyte colony-stimulating factor.

Various trials have sought that intensifying induction therapy may improve the initial response rate and the long-term outcome among AML patients. Sequential studies by the Eastern Cooperative Oncology Group (ECOG) first postulated that increasing the dose of daunorubicin 45 to 60 mg/m^2/day for three days resulted in a median complete remission rate of 62% [21]. Furthermore, same group demonstrated the improvements in rates of complete remission and the overall survival with the administration of 90 mg/m^2/day for three days of daunorubicin among young adults [22]. Also, another anthracyclin, idarubicin, has been used in AML treatment since 1980s. The AML-BFM 93 trial evaluated the efficacy of idarubicin (12 mg/m^2/day × 3 days) compared with daunorubicin (60 mg/m^2/day × 3 days) in AML induction therapy in children and adolescent. Individuals in idarubicin arm improved blast cell clearance (<5% blasts on day 15); higher CR rates were found in younger patients without an overall survival benefit [13]. The similar results were also obtained in subsequent studies. The anthraquinone derivative mitoxantrone has also been commonly used as part of effective induction regimens for a long time. In the United Kingdom, Medical Research Council

Acute Myeloid Leukemia 12 (MRC AML12) trial comprising 1243 AML patients (between 15 to 59 years old) received cytarabine (100 mg/m^2/day × 10 days), etoposide (100 mg/m^2/day × 5 days) and either daunorubicin (50 mg/m^2/day × 3 days) or mitoxantrone (12 mg/m^2/day × 3 days) for induction; the results showed no survival benefit with comparable acute toxicity [14]. After these results, the children subgroup analysis of the overall study published revealed significant reduction in relapse with mitoxantrone, but due to higher rates of treatment related mortality, this did not turn out to be a significant improvement in overall survival [23]. It is noteworthy that in the EORTC and GIMEMA Groups Study AML-10 trial, one of the largest study in AML aged 15–60 years, where patients were randomly assigned to daunorubicin 50 mg/m^2/day, mitoxantrone 12 mg/m^2/day or idarubicin 10 mg/m^2/day (each given with cytrabine and etoposide) on days one, three, five and after one or two courses of induction therapy, similar outcomes were observed between the treatment arms [15]. There is enough evidence to indicate that intensification of daunorubicin may have a beneficial effect without increasing toxicity and that the choice of anthracycline varies depending on the current conditions [24].

It is important to note that the most feared adverse effect of anthracyclines is acute and late cardiotoxicity. Several reports have already reported that children and adolescents are more comfortable with anthracycline cardiotoxicity depending on continuous heart muscle growth. After liposomal encapsulation of daunorubicin was discovered as they consume higher doses without increasing cardiotoxicity. Interestingly, AML-BFM 2004 trial reported that liposomal daunorubicin (80 mg/m^2/day × 3 days) and standard induction with idarubicin (2 mg/m^2/day × 3 days) had similar response rates after induction with comparable early and late cardiotoxicity among <18 years old pediatric and adolescent population [24]. Nevertheless, in patients with cardiac disease, liposomal daunorubicin should be used.

Also, different leukemia groups studied cytarabine dose escalation. The randomized comparison between high dose (200 mg/m^2/day; days 1–10 every 12 h) and standard dose (100 mg/m^2/day; days 1–10 every 12 h) cytarabine displayed similar outcomes (overall response was 84% *vs.* 85%; eight-year survival was 31% *vs.* 32%) in the MRC AML12 trial [14]. In subgroup analysis of 708 children (2–15 years old) and 541 AYA (16–24 years old) patients, 10 year OS and relapse rates were found to be 47% *vs.* 59% and 47% *vs.* 42% ($p > 0.05$), respectively [4]. Evaluation of high-dose cytarabine (HiDAC) combined with daunorubicin in induction has been reported by different studies; the Southwest Oncology Group (SWOG; 2 g/m^2 bid × 6 days), the Australian Leukemia Study Group (ALSG; 3 g/m^2 bid on days one, three, five, and seven) and the Eastern Cooperative Oncology Group (ECOG; 3 g/m^2 on days one, three, and five) [6]. Neither of these trials revealed a higher CR rate with HiDAC nor observed increased toxicity in all. It is important to note that the administration of HiDAC in induction regimens has failed to improve the outcome and thus cannot be recommended outside clinical trials.

A third drug (e.g., etoposide or 6-thioguanine (6-TG)) is usually added in induction of pediatric protocols even if conducted studies failed to demonstrate any therapeutic benefit from addition of 6-TG or etoposide to "3 + 7". Between 2002 and 2009, 385 patients aged 15–29 years were enrolled on the MRC AML15 trial; the addition of etoposide to "3 + 7" showed no benefit in rate or durability of response (ORR of all cohort: 86% *vs.* 84%) [16]. Moreover, CALGB 7921 trial suggested that instead of adding 6-TG, cytarabine and daunorubicin dose or cycle intervals could be edited [25].

Other drugs added to standard induction treatment of AYAs include: A purine analog such as fludarabine or cladribine and a calicheamicin conjugated to a CD33 antibody as gemtuzumab ozogamicin (GO). Polish Adult Leukemia Group (PALG) have evaluated cladribine or fludaribine added to daunorubicin and cytarabine. They found 12% increase in three-year-OS and 10 months extension of the median survival in cladribine arm compared with the standard induction arm. Furthermore, treatment related toxicity was comparable in both arms [17]. In addition, same study group reported similar survival outcomes between fludarabine and the standard induction arms [26]. As a result of these studies, cladribine added regimen as remission induction should be considered as a new treatment option, but fludarabine addition seemed not to have any advantage. In 2010, the results of the SWOG S0106 trial has been shown that GO decreased CR rates with higher mortality among children and adolescent and hence, withdrawn [18]. Consequently, the recently published AAML0531 trial sought the efficacy of GO added induction therapy and showed improvement in EFS but not OS among children and adolescent through reduced relapse rate. Although treatment related mortality was increased in GO added arm, in spite of similar overall toxicity incidence between both arms [27]. Future investigation is required to optimize the administration of GO.

Interestingly, several reports have already suggested that after the first administration of cytotoxic agents in AML, leukemia cells can be recruited into the cell cycle and then become more sensitive to cell cycle-specific agent 6 to 10 days after the initial chemotherapy exposure. The Children Cancer Group (CCG) conducted four trials; each used an "intensive-timing" induction regimen. In the CCG-2891 trial, pediatric and adolescent AML patients received a four-day cycle of five-drug induction therapy (dexamethasone, cytrabine, 6-thioguanine, etoposide and daunorubicin (DCTER)); cycles are repeated either every 10 days (intensive-timing) regardless of low blood counts and side effects of the treatment or every 14 days (standard-timing) depending on bone marrow recovery [20]. Although AYAs treated on this CCG protocol had higher incidence of remission (74% in all population), 10 year OS was 45% ± 6% because of the higher rate of treatment related mortality (26% ± 6%) [20]. Altogether, these results and the aforementioned study indicate that pediatric protocols would be better for AYAs if the treatment related mortality with these regimens could be reduced.

Recently, Woods *et al.* reported the comparison results between pediatric and adult protocols in 517 AYAs with AML using data from three large cooperative groups (COG, CALGB, and SWOG) and demonstrated that aggressive pediatric protocols provide more anti-leukemia efficacy with halve of relapse rates but higher treatment related-mortality. Ten year OS was higher for the COG AYA cohort than for the other two adult cohorts (45% *vs.* 34%, *p* = 0.026) [12]. To our knowledge, there has been no approach beyond 1–2 course in 7–10 days cytarabine and three days of an anthracycline combination for induction treatment in AYAs with AML.

4. Postremission Therapy

Pretreatment karyotype and bone marrow assessment on the 7th or 10th day after completion of induction treatment determine the type of post-remission therapy. Many studies, herein mentioned used HiDAC or allogeneic hematopoietic stem cell transplantation (HSCT) as post-induction treatment.

Intensification of consolidation is as important as intensive induction therapy; since 1980s, the CALGB study group has conducted various trials to find the best intensive post-remission therapy for younger AML patients. In 1994, the results of CALGB 8525 trial was published and four courses of HiDAC (3 g/m^2 per every 12 hours on days one, three, and five) was found to be superior to lower/intermediate-dose cytarabine (either 100 or 400 mg/m^2/day on days 1–5) in young adults [19]. In addition, subsequent studies has shown that HiDAC improved survival rates in patients with Core Binding Factor (CBF)-AML more than Cytogenetically Normal (CN)-AML (five years OS; 64% *vs.* 35%) [28]. Also in 2008, the German-Austrian AML Study Group (AMLSG) reported the efficacy of HiDAC in AML with mutated NPM1 without FLT3-ITD and with mutated CEBPA [29].

NOPHO AML 93, MRC AML 10, AML-BFM 2004 and AML99 trials has been shown to decrease the relapse rates with intensive induction protocols that include HiDAC in pediatric population [30]. Unlike adult studies, non-cross-resistant drugs used in induction are mostly administered a total of 2–5 courses as consolidation and maintenance treatment in children and adolescent with AML. However MRC AML-12 trial has revealed that more than four courses of post-remission treatment did not improve the outcomes [14].

In MRC AML15 trial, young adults alive after two courses of induction therapy were randomly allocated either MRC consolidation (amsacrine, cytarabine, etoposide, and then mitoxantrone and cytarabine (MACE-MidAC)) or the international standard consolidation (HiDAC). The results of the study showed similar outcomes with increased treatment related to hematologic toxicity in MACE-MidAC arm. According to the evaluation of cytogenetic risk group, OS for poor-risk patients determined was significantly higher in MRC consolidation arm; the group concluded that one course of MACE-MidAC is a superior consolidation option for high-risk AML patients who are not eligible for HSCT [16].

The German Acute Myeloid Leukemia Cooperative Group (AMLCG) investigated the effectiveness of maintenance treatment in younger AML since 1985. In 2003, they postulated the comparison of maintenance treatment (monthly courses of cytarabine 100 mg/m^2 every 12 h for five days, different second drug every course, daunorubicin, 45 mg/m^2/day on days three and four (course 1), 6-thioguanine 100 mg/m^2 every 12 h on days one to five (course 2), cyclophosphamide 1 g/m^2/day on day three (course 3), 6-thioguanine again (course 4)) between intensive consolidation treatment (cytarabine 1 g/m^2 every 12 h on days one, two, eight, and nine) [31]. The aforementioned trial has revealed equal CR rates between both arms even though relapse free survival was higher in poor-risk AML patients who received maintenance treatment. A group from MD Anderson Cancer Center used azacitidine (32 mg/m^2/day for five days in each of four 30-day) after HSCT as a new remission consolidation/maintenance protocol in high risk AML [32]. They established that azacitidine might improve EFS and OS with acceptable toxicities. Recently, azacitidine combined with lenalidomid (azacitidine 50–75 mg/m^2/day for five days, lenalidomide 5–10 mg/day on days 5 to 25) was administered to 10 patients with AML in remission after induction as maintenance treatment and provided the immunological benefits of this regimen [33]. It is important to note that maintenance treatment is not a standard part of AML treatment and still need further investigations.

Developments in transplantation since 1980s have led to increasing improvements in survival and reduction of treatment-related mortality (TRM) among HSCT recipients. Therefore, HSCT as frontline post induction therapy is recommended for all aged patients with intermediate-unfavorable risk AML even if HSCT in low-risk group during first remission is unknown in children and young adults. Surprisingly, the results from MRC AML10 and AML12 trials showed no survival benefit with allo-HSCT in first CR for any risk group in AYAs [14,34]. They concluded that favorable-risk patients should not undergo transplantation in first CR, but children and adolescent with intermediate-high risk should be weighed on case-by-case basis. It has already been known that SCT from HLA-matched (8/8 or 10/10 allele matched) related donor is more beneficial than continued chemotherapy; the important advantage in preventing relapse may be offset by high rates of transplant-related deaths because of the wrong optimal timing.

In 2012, the CIBMTR published the outcomes of AYAs with AML treated with HLA-identical sibling (MSD) or unrelated (URD) HSCT between 1980 and 2005. They reported improvement of five years OS and reduction of transplant-related mortality (TRM) from 1998 to 2005, compared with 1980 to 1988 (Due to MSD data OS at five years: 43% *vs.* 37%, $p > 0.05$; TRM: 39% *vs.* 20%, $p = 0.01$) [35]. This can be explained with continued improvements in AML prognostic factors, HSCT conditioning regimens, HLA typing and HSCT supportive care.

Pediatric cooperative groups conducted various trials that compared allo-SCT with intensive consolidation chemotherapy in children and adolescents with newly diagnosed AML. In 2008, COG published a meta-analysis of four cooperative group studies (Pediatric Oncology Group (POG) 8821, Children's Cancer Group (CCG) 2891, CCG 2961, and Medical Research Council (MRC) 10), which used HLA matched related allo-HSCT in first remission for children and adolescent patients. The results of these analyses showed the improvement of outcomes in favorable-risk AML patients, but the point to be considered is that only 2/3 of the patients have their risk stratification and cytogenetic results [36]. The MRC 10 and 12 trials revealed better outcomes in children than in AYAs; therefore, the survival benefit could not be shown in both groups who underwent allo-HSCT [14,34]. Despite these results, the beneficial effect of allo-HSCT has been proven in severally randomized young adults trials compared to other approaches.

Although there is no consensus on optimal conditioning regimens for AYAs, most centers use non-TBI-containing myeloablative protocols (MAC) first or subsequent remission. Busulfan and cyclophosphamide are the most administered drugs [37]. Also, treosulphan and fludarabine containing reduced intensity conditioning regimens (RIC) have recently begun to be used with minimal TRM, but still need more prospective trials for recommendation [38]. There is a recently terminated prospective randomized Bone Marrow Transplantation-Clinical Trials Network's BMT-CTN 0901 clinical trial (NCT01339910) comparing RIC regimens with MAC in AML/MDS; the results explain the optimized conditioning intensity. TBI is no longer preferred because of its late effects and increased risk of seconder malignancies [30]. Notably, TBI did not improve EFS during first remission in some of the pediatric and young adult AML trials [39,40]; however, better EFS with higher doses of TBI was found among AYAs in a review of the literature [41]. Recently, different cooperative groups are seeking the effectiveness of adding fractionated TBI to conditioning regimens in selected advanced patients with AML [42].

Since AYAs with high-risk AML who lack a matched sibling donor (approximately 70%–75% of patients with AML) may benefit from alternative approaches including matched unrelated (including cord blood products) or mismatched family donor, decision should be made based on the urgency of the HSCT [43].

Recently, Kelly *et al.* compared the clinical outcomes after MRD or MUD HSCT during first remission in a total of 159 children (74 of them were AYAs) with high-risk AML using data from COG trials (CCG 2891, POG 9421, CCG 2961, and AAML03P1) and CIBMTR reports. Their results demonstrated similar OS and TRM between both arms with lower relapse risk after only MUD HSCT in a competing risks regression model (HR 0.43, $p < 0.01$) when compared to post-remission chemotherapy [44]. Various studies have also revealed no superiority between MRD and MUD HSCT outcomes (relapse, GVHD and survival) of young adults with CN-AML. However, the most limiting factor is the time taken (median four months in most countries) for the identification of a suitably matched unrelated donor and unfortunately, patients may relapse during this waiting period.

Ebihara *et al.* reported the clinical results of 16 AYA patients who underwent unrelated cord blood transplantation (CBT) during 1999 to 2009. All patients received myeloablative-conditioning regimen and the OS and the DFS at three years were determined to be 67.5% and 48.6%, respectively, a comparable published result of adults and children with AML [45]. During 1996 to 2010, 67 adolescent (38 treated with UCB and 29 treated with Haploidentical sibling SCT) diagnosed with acute leukemia were enrolled in a retrospective study from Spain. The overall outcome including leukemia free survival was better in haplo-SCT arm; TRM was higher in UCB-SCT arm and unexpectedly, the cumulative incidence of relapse was similar in both arms [46]. To our knowledge, the most important factor that restricts the widespread use of CBT is the amount of CD34+ stem cells from the individual graft; though double cord transplant was done to overcome this limitation. The ongoing BMT-CTN 1101 trial (NCT01745913) clarifies the optimal alternative donor source by comparing double UCB with haploidentical transplant.

Haploidentical SCT recently became an effective treatment option in the AYAs with AML candidate for HSCT with lacking an HLA-identical donor or with urgent need to perform SCT. Since every individual has, at least, one mutual HLA haplotype with each biological parent or child, then a suitable donor can be identified within days. In 1998, the Perugia group found leukemia free survival rates of 45%–50% and DFS rates of 30%–45% for young adults with AML receiving transplantation of bone marrow from related one HLA haplotype identical donor. TBI with myeloablative conditioning regimen was admitted and the product consist of large numbers of T-cell-depleted hematopoietic stem cells [47]. Consequently, slowed immune reconstruction, higher rates of TRM and stimulation of graft-*versus*-leukemia effector mechanism could be seen in this kind of transplant. Data from the EBMT registry showed that leukemia free survival at two years was 48% for patients in first remission; however, for patients in non-remission, this rate dropped to 1% [48]. Based on these results, it may be considered that haplo-SCT has more anti-leukemia effect in the early phase of high-risk AML treatment with increase risk of GVHD and graft rejection. Luznik *et al.* developed a new approach to reduce haplo-HSCT related toxicity; post-transplant cyclophosphamide was added to a marrow graft after reduced intensity conditioning regimen [49]. The approach decreased the cumulative incidence of severe GVHD and TRM. Further investigations are required to recommend haplo-HSCT for AYAs with AML in first remission.

Autologous HSCT during the first remission has been commonly used for the past two decades as post remission treatment in all aged patients with high risk AML who are not eligible for MRD HSCT. However, the results of studies comparing auto-HSCT with the other post remission approaches are conflicting. MRC AML10 trial showed the improvement in DFS with similar OS; although CCG 2891 trial has reported that auto-HSCT in CR1 did not have better impact on outcomes compared to post induction chemotherapy [34,50]. It has to be mentioned that these different trials have not used the same intensive induction treatments before auto-HSCT. When we looked into analyses of MRC AML10 trial comparing autologous *versus* allogeneic HSCT, we found that allo-HSCT has improved the survival rates and reduced the relapse rates [34]. Also, the EORTC-LG/GIMEMA AML-10 trial has been determined that younger or high/very high-risk AML patients had better outcome with allo-HSCT compared with auto-HSCT [51]. Altogether, these results showed that auto-HSCT has failed to improve the outcome among young adults population and cannot be recommended for AYAs with AML in first CR outside clinical trials [52].

5. Primary Refractory and Relapsed Acute Myeloid Leukemia

For acute myeloid leukemia (AML) patients in complete remission, maintaining remission is a necessity. To our knowledge, the prognosis of relapse depends on the molecular profile of leukemia, the duration of first CR, the age of patient and the type of post-remission therapy administered. Moreover, with the current intensive protocols, up to 20%–30% of young and 40%–50% of older AML patients experienced primary induction failure [53]. More than 50% of the patients in complete remission relapsed within one year (except for AYAs with favorable risk of cytogenetics); relapsed/refractory AML patients have a very poor outcome with 10% of survival incidence. Despite the knowledge of leukemia pathophysiology, the prognosis following relapse is still uniformly poor. MRC AML10 trial reported the median relapse time to be 10 months and the OS after relapse to be <40% in children and AYAs [34].

For younger patients with relapsed/refractory AML, the enrollment in a clinical trial should be the first approach. If there is a late relapse patient, retreatment with the previously used induction regimen should be employed. Notably, if the relapse is detected at the early phase of tumor burden, HSCT should be considered after salvage chemotherapy. Since there are few prospective controlled studies assessing different treatments, thus no standard salvage chemotherapy can be recommended.

In relapsed/refractory AML, the aim was to achieve second remission using various protocols; such as induction therapy antimetabolite (cytarabine, fludarabine) and anthracycline-based. HiDAC is widely used for induction treatment of relapsed/refractory AML. In 2012, Larson *et al.* published the outcomes of HiDAC/mitoxantrone in younger adults with relapsed or refractory high-risk AML and reported an overall response rate of 55% with the induction death rate of 9% [54]. The Japanese Childhood AML Cooperative Study Group AML99 trial determined the results of children and adolescent with relapsed AML patients who received treatment protocols including; cytarabine, etoposide and idarubicin/mitoxantrone [55]. The study showed that the second remission with cytarabine based reinduction regimens was 50% and that the five-year OS was 37%.

To evaluate the CR rates of refractory/relapsed AML in younger adults, the Japanese Adult Leukemia Study Group (JALSG) conducted a phase II study of FLAGM (fludarabine 15 mg/m^2 every 12 h on days 1–4, Ara-C 2 g/m^2 on days 1–4), G-CSF 300 µg/m^2 on days 1–4, and mitoxantrone 10 mg/m^2 on days 3–5 protocol [56]. Seventy percent response rate was provided by FLAGM in relapsed or refractory AML patients; furthermore, randomized studies are still warranted to confirm this option.

In the study of Relapsed AML01/2001, 394 children (younger than 21 years) were randomized equally for FLAG (Fludarabine 30 mg/m^2/day, on days 1–5, Ara-C 2 g/m^2/day, on days 1–5, and G-CSF 200 µg/m^2 on days 0–5) *versus* liposomal daunorubicine (60 mg/m^2/day, on days 1, 3 and 5) +

FLAG. Liposomal daunorubicine (DNX) added FLAG significantly improved the early response from 70% to 80% and CR rate from 70% to 80%. However, the OS was similar between two groups [57].

Malfuson *et al.* published a small retrospective analysis of the outcomes for 14 young adults with first relapsed AML; those who received 3 + 7 + GO induction regimen [58]. The overall response rate was reported to be 79% with a tolerable toxicity profile. GO + FLAG (Fludarabine 30 mg/m^2/day, on days 1–5, Ara-C 2 g/m^2/day, on days 1–5, GO 3 mg/m^2/day on day 1, and G-CSF 3 mg/kg/day) also studied in relapsed/refractory AML reported excellent clinical and molecular response in 29 of the 34 young adults with CBF-AML [59]. The major restriction of GO studies is the number of patients (small population); large, randomized and prospective trials would be required to recommend first relapsed.

In first relapse, all type of HSCT is widely preferred approach after achieving a second remission. For patients who are not eligible for allo-HSCT in second remission, auto-HSCT can be considered. Auto-HSCT data from the British Society of Blood and Marrow Transplantation (BSBMT) registry has shown five-year OS of 32% and disease-free probabilities of 30%–35% [60]. Notably, most relapses were detected within the first 24 months of auto-HSCT.

Allogeneic HSCT from HLA-matched or mismatched donor is the most effective consolidation therapy once a new remission has been obtained. However, most of the studies in relapsed pediatric AML have demonstrated poor outcome except those patients with late relapse and favorable AML. Recently, the International BFM-Study Group has shown 38% overall survival for allo-HSCT in children and adolescent with second remission [57]. RIC was commonly offered before allo-HSCT in relapsed patients depending on the age of the patient, the poor performance status, the co-morbidities and the prior treatments with lesser TRM and more GVL effect.

6. New Therapy Approaches

To the best of our knowledge, the treatment of AML was based on 1–2 course remission induction chemotherapy, followed by either consolidation therapy or HSCT depending on the prognostic features of the patients. However, enormous progress in the understanding of AML pathogenesis and improvements in molecular genomic technologies are leading to novel target agents and the development of personalized and risk-adapted treatment.

Clofarabine (2-chloro-2'-fluoro-deoxy-9-b-D-arabinofura-nosyladenine) is a second-generation nucleoside analog, which inhibits both ribonucleotide reductase and DNA polymerase. Investigators from the MD Anderson Cancer Center (MDACC) conducted various trials with single agent clofarabine or combined with cytarabine and/or idarubicin; a favorable outcome was derived even in adults with primary refractory or relapsed AML [61]. In 2009, Hijiya *et al.* published the result of clofarabine, cyclophosphamide and etoposide combined regimen in five pediatric (between age 5–21 years) patients with AML and 100% OR (1 CR and 4 CR in the absence of total platelet recovery (CRp)) [62]; this highly promising response reported in this small population warrants further study. To our knowledge there is no published trials and only one ongoing COG trial (clinicaltrials-gov #NCT00372619) to clarify the benefit of clofarabine and cytarabine combination in 1–30 years old patients with refractory or relapsed acute myeloid leukemia.

The hypomethylating agents; azacitidine and decitabine have shown single agent benefit in AML. There are various ongoing trials for azacitidine either as single or combined agent (clinicaltrials-gov #NCT01839240, #NCT01249430, #NCT01861002, #NCT00422890). In the French ATU retrospective trial, 11% response rate was found among patients with refractory or relapsed AML treated with azacytidine [56]. It seems that single agent azacytidine has only limited efficacy in relapsed or refractory AML. In a phase I study, 23 patients with relapsed or refractory AML were treated with the combination of 5-azacytidine and bortezomib; the results of the trial showed 26% response rate. Recently, Phillips *et al.* showed the efficacy of low dose decitabine (20 mg/m^2/day 10 days) in eight children and young adults with heavily pretreated relapsed/refractory AML and reported only 38% of the patients achieved CR with very favorable toxicity profile [63].

J. Clin. Med. **2015**, *4*, 441–459

Internal tandem duplication mutation of FMS-like tyrosine kinase 3 (FLT3-ITD mutations) was found in 20% adult and 15% pediatric AML patients associated with poor prognosis [64]. The patients are candidates for targeted therapy; although several FLT3-inhibitors (sorafenib, crelonatinib, quizartinib, midoustaurin) have been studied on various trials, herein mentioned some milestone trials in young adults.

Several groups have shown that Sorafenib, a multikinase (FLT3, c-KIT, NRAS, and Raf kinas) inhibitor, has impressive response and a tolerable safety profile in adults with AML as a single agent or in sorafenib-containing induction protocol. In SORAML trial, 264 younger patients were randomized to achieve sorafenib (800 mg/day during induction, consolidation and 12 months maintenance period) or plasebo adding 3 + 7 (cytarabine 100 mg/m^2/day 7 days, daunorubicin 60 mg/m^2/day 3 days) and following HiDAC as consolidation. The results of the study CR rates and 2 year OS were higher in sorafenib arm (sorafenib *vs.* placebo; CR: 60% *vs.* 56%, $p = 0.62$; OS: 66% *vs.* 72%, $p = 0.37$) with increased incidence of treatment related toxicity [65]. In a phase I study, 11 children (aged between 6–17 years) with acute myeloid leukemia were treated with sorafenib (200 mg/m^2 and 150 mg/m^2 twice daily, with maximum doses of 400 mg and 300 mg; alone on days one to seven and 13 to 28), clofarabine (40 mg/m^2 on days 8 to 12), and cytarabine (1 g/m^2 on days 8 to 12). Leukemia response was evaluated on day eight and seven patients (63%) revealed more than 50% reduction of baseline bone marrow blasts regardless of FLT3 status [66]. In summary, the benefit of sorafenib was proven in different, prospective, randomized trials for treatment of newly diagnosed or relapsed/refractory AML. Futher prospective studies on sorafenib would be required to confirm all the stated results.

Lestaurtinib is a potent inhibitor of FLT3 and triggers apoptosis in FLT3-ITD leukemic blasts. The Cephalon 204 trial patients (aged between 18 years and older) with AML were randomized either with chemotherapy (MEC/HiDAC) or lestaurtinib (80 mg/day every 12 h, beginning two days after the completion of chemotherapy (day seven)). Lestaurtinib failed to improve the outcomes; however, only 58% of the patients in lestaurtinib arm reached LT3 inhibition; as estimated from the PIA assay, on day 15 and those improved response rate and OS [67].

Midostaurin (PKC412) is an inhibitor of FLT3 tyrosine kinase, VEGFR, PDGFR, and c-KIT. In a phase I trial of midostaurin, 35% and 25% of the patients show reduction in the amount of peripheral and bone marrow blasts [68]. The ongoing CALGB study clarifies the addition of midostaurin to induction, consolidation therapy and followed single agent midostaurin as maintenance treatment as frontline therapy of younger adult patients with AML (ClinicalTrials.gov: NCT00651261).

In conclusion, with the continued progress of novel drugs targeting specific pathways in acute leukemia, AML treatment may be brought into a new era. It is important to note that more clinical trials should be conducted in order to understand the benefit of targeted agents in AYA population.

7. Conclusions

Age is an independent prognostic factor in AML; the prognosis of AYAs diagnosed with AML is better than those in young adult patients. However, there were no genetic or phenotypic abnormalities reported on AML in AYAs. Treating AYA patients with AML is still challenging since there is no data clarifying the kind of relevant therapy for AYA. Based on limited prospective and retrospective AYA studies, a prospect for cure of about 50% was achieved whether treated on an adult or pediatric protocol. We therefore suggest that encouraging AYAs to participate in clinical trials is the only way to improve response rate.

Author Contributions: All authors wrote the paper and revised the final manuscript.

Conflicts of Interest: The authors declare no conflict of interest.

References

1. Gramatges, M.M.; Rabin, K.R. The adolescent and young adult with cancer: State of the art—Acute leukemias. *Curr. Oncol. Rep.* **2013**, *15*, 317–324. [CrossRef] [PubMed]

2. Creutzig, U.; Büchner, T.; Sauerland, M.C.; Zimmermann, M.; Reinhardt, D.; Döhner, H.; Schlenk, R.F. Significance of age in acute myeloid leukemia patients younger than 30 years: A common analysis of the pediatric trials AML-BFM 93/98 and the adult trials AMLCG 92/99 and AMLSG HD93/98A. *Cancer* **2008**, *112*, 562–571. [CrossRef] [PubMed]
3. Garrido, S.M.; Cooper, J.J.; Appelbaum, F.R.; Willman, C.L.; Kopecky, K.; Banker, D.E. Blasts from elderly acute myeloid leukemia patients are characterized by low levels of culture- and drug-induced apoptosis. *Leuk. Res.* **2001**, *25*, 23–32. [CrossRef] [PubMed]
4. Ofran, Y.; Rowe, J.M. Acute myeloid leukemia in adolescents and young adults: Challenging aspects. *Acta Haematol.* **2014**, *132*, 292–297. [CrossRef] [PubMed]
5. Grimwade, D.; Howe, K.; Langrbeer, S.; Davis, L.; Oliver, F.; Walker, H.; Swirsky, D.; Wheatley, K.; Goldstone, A.; Burnett, A.; *et al.* Establishing the presence of the *t*(15;17) in suspected acute promyelocytic leukaemia: Cytogenetic, molecular and PML immunofluorescence assessment of patients entered into the M.R.C. ATRA trial. *Br. J. Haematol.* **1996**, *94*, 557–573. [PubMed]
6. Rowley, J.D. Chromosomal translocations: Revisited yet again. *Blood* **2008**, *112*, 2183–2189. [CrossRef] [PubMed]
7. Döhner, H.; Estey, E.H.; Amadori, S.; Appelbaum, F.R.; Büchner, T.; Burnett, A.K.; Dombret, H.; Fenaux, P.; Grimwade, D.; Larson, R.A.; *et al.* Diagnosis and management of acute myeloid leukemia in adults: Recommendations from an international expert panel, on behalf of the European LeukemiaNet. *Blood* **2010**, *115*, 453–474. [CrossRef] [PubMed]
8. Bleyer, A.; Budd, T.; Montello, M. Older adolescentsand young adults with cancer, and clinical trials: Lack of participation and progress in North America. In *Cancer in Adolescents and Young Adults*; Springer: Berlin, Germany, 2007; pp. 71–81.
9. Pui, C.-H.H.; Schrappe, M.; Ribeiro, R.C.; Niemeyer, C.M. Childhood and adolescent lymphoid and myeloid leukemia. In *Hematology/the Education Program of the American Society of Hematology*; American Society of Hematology: Washington, DC, USA, 2004; pp. 118–145.
10. Shapira, M.; Raanani, H.; Cohen, Y.; Meirow, D. Fertility preservation in young females with hematological malignancies. *Acta Haematol.* **2014**, *132*, 400–413. [CrossRef] [PubMed]
11. Dillman, R.O.; Davis, R.B.; Green, M.R.; Weiss, R.B.; Gottlieb, A.J.; Caplan, S.; Kopel, S.; Preisler, H.; McIntyre, O.R.; Schiffer, C. A comparative study of two different doses of cytarabine for acute myeloid leukemia: A phase III trial of Cancer and Leukemia Group B. *Blood* **1991**, *78*, 2520–2526. [PubMed]
12. Woods, W.G.; Franklin, A.R.; Alonzo, T.A.; Gerbing, R.B.; Donohue, K.A.; Othus, M.; Horan, J.; Appelbaum, F.R.; Estey, E.H.; Bloomfield, C.D.; *et al.* Outcome of adolescents and young adults with acute myeloid leukemia treated on COG trials compared to CALGB and SWOG trials. *Cancer* **2013**, *119*, 4170–4179. [CrossRef] [PubMed]
13. Creutzig, U.; Ritter, J.; Zimmermann, M.; Hermann, J.; Gadner, H.; Sawatzki, D.B.; Niemeyer, C.M.; Schwabe, D.; Selle, B.; Boos, J.; *et al.* Idarubicin improves blast cell clearance during induction therapy in children with AML: Results of study AML-BFM 93. AML-BFM study group. *Leukemia* **2001**, *15*, 348–354. [CrossRef] [PubMed]
14. Burnett, A.K.; Hills, R.K.; Milligan, D.W.; Goldstone, A.H.; Prentice, A.G.; McMullin, M.-F.F.; Duncombe, A.; Gibson, B.; Wheatley, K. Attempts to optimize induction and consolidation treatment in acute myeloid leukemia: Results of the MRC AML12 trial. *J. Clin. Oncol.* **2010**, *28*, 586–595. [CrossRef] [PubMed]
15. Mandelli, F.; Vignetti, M.; Suciu, S.; Stasi, R.; Petti, M.-C.C.; Meloni, G.; Muus, P.; Marmont, F.; Marie, J.-P.P.; Labar, B.; *et al.* Daunorubicin versus mitoxantrone versus idarubicin as induction and consolidation chemotherapy for adults with acute myeloid leukemia: The EORTC and GIMEMA Groups Study AML-10. *J. Clin. Oncol.* **2009**, *27*, 5397–5403. [CrossRef] [PubMed]
16. Burnett, A.K.; Russell, N.H.; Hills, R.K.; Hunter, A.E.; Kjeldsen, L.; Yin, J.; Gibson, B.E.; Wheatley, K.; Milligan, D. Optimization of chemotherapy for younger patients with acute myeloid leukemia: Results of the medical research council AML15 trial. *J. Clin. Oncol.* **2013**, *31*, 3360–3368. [CrossRef]
17. Holowiecki, J.; Grosicki, S.; Robak, T.; Kyrcz-Krzemien, S.; Giebel, S.; Hellmann, A.; Skotnicki, A.; Jedrzejczak, W.W.; Konopka, L.; Kuliczkowski, K.; *et al.* Addition of cladribine to daunorubicin and cytarabine increases complete remission rate after a single course of induction treatment in acute myeloid leukemia. Multicenter, phase III study. *Leukemia* **2004**, *18*, 989–997. [CrossRef] [PubMed]

18. Petersdorf, S.H.; Kopecky, K.J.; Slovak, M.; Willman, C.; Nevill, T.; Brandwein, J.; Larson, R.A.; Erba, H.P.; Stiff, P.J.; Stuart, R.K.; *et al.* A phase 3 study of gemtuzumab ozogamicin during induction and postconsolidation therapy in younger patients with acute myeloid leukemia. *Blood* **2013**, *121*, 4854–4860. [CrossRef] [PubMed]

19. Mayer, R.; Davis, R.; Schiffer, C.; Berg, D.; Powell, B.; Schulman, P.; Omura, G.; Moore, J.; McIntyre, O.; Frei, E. Intensive postremission chemotherapy in adults with acute myeloid leukemia. *N. Engl. J. Med.* **1994**, *331*, 896–903. [CrossRef] [PubMed]

20. Woods, W.G.; Kobrinsky, N.; Buckley, J.D.; Lee, J.W.; Sanders, J.; Neudorf, S.; Gold, S.; Barnard, D.R.; DeSwarte, J.; Dusenbery, K.; *et al.* Timed-sequential induction therapy improves postremission outcome in acute myeloid leukemia: A report from the Children's Cancer Group. *Blood* **1996**, *87*, 4979–4989. [PubMed]

21. Bennett, J.M.; Young, M.L.; Andersen, J.W.; Cassileth, P.A.; Tallman, M.S.; Paietta, E.; Wiernik, P.H.; Rowe, J.M. Long-term survival in acute myeloid leukemia: The eastern cooperative oncology group experience. *Cancer* **1997**, *80*, 2205–2209. [CrossRef] [PubMed]

22. Fernandez, H.; Sun, Z.; Yao, X.; Litzow, M.; Luger, S.; Paietta, E.; Racevskis, J.; Dewald, G.; Ketterling, R.; Bennett, J.; *et al.* Anthracycline dose intensification in acute myeloid leukemia. *N. Engl. J. Med.* **2009**, *361*, 1249–1259. [CrossRef] [PubMed]

23. Gibson, B.E.; Webb, D.K.; Howman, A.J.; de Graaf, S.S.; Harrison, C.J.; Wheatley, K. Results of a randomized trial in children with Acute Myeloid Leukaemia: Medical research council AML12 trial. *Br. J. Haematol.* **2011**, *155*, 366–376. [CrossRef] [PubMed]

24. Creutzig, U.; Zimmermann, M.; Bourquin, J.-P.P.; Dworzak, M.N.; Fleischhack, G.; Graf, N.; Klingebiel, T.; Kremens, B.; Lehrnbecher, T.; von Neuhoff, C.; *et al.* Randomized trial comparing liposomal daunorubicin with idarubicin as induction for pediatric acute myeloid leukemia: Results from Study AML-BFM 2004. *Blood* **2013**, *122*, 37–43. [CrossRef] [PubMed]

25. Preisler, H.; Davis, R.B.; Kirshner, J.; Dupre, E.; Richards, F.; Hoagland, H.C.; Kopel, S.; Levy, R.N.; Carey, R.; Schulman, P. Comparison of three remission induction regimens and two postinduction strategies for the treatment of acute nonlymphocytic leukemia: A cancer and leukemia group B study. *Blood* **1987**, *69*, 1441–1449. [PubMed]

26. Holowiecki, J.; Grosicki, S.; Giebel, S.; Robak, T.; Kyrcz-Krzemien, S.; Kuliczkowski, K.; Skotnicki, A.B.; Hellmann, A.; Sulek, K.; Dmoszynska, A.; *et al.* Cladribine, but not fludarabine, added to daunorubicin and cytarabine during induction prolongs survival of patients with acute myeloid leukemia: A multicenter, randomized phase III study. *J. Clin. Oncol.* **2012**, *30*, 2441–2448. [CrossRef] [PubMed]

27. Gamis, A.S.; Alonzo, T.A.; Meshinchi, S.; Sung, L.; Gerbing, R.B.; Raimondi, S.C.; Hirsch, B.A.; Kahwash, S.B.; Heerema-McKenney, A.; Winter, L.; *et al.* Gemtuzumab ozogamicin in children and adolescents with *de novo* acute myeloid leukemia improves event-free survival by reducing relapse risk: Results from the randomized phase iii Children's Oncology Group trial AAML0531. *J. Clin. Oncol.* **2014**, *32*, 3021–3032. [CrossRef] [PubMed]

28. Bloomfield, C.D.; Lawrence, D.; Byrd, J.C.; Carroll, A.; Pettenati, M.J.; Tantravahi, R.; Patil, S.R.; Davey, F.R.; Berg, D.T.; Schiffer, C.A.; *et al.* Frequency of prolonged remission duration after high-dose cytarabine intensification in acute myeloid leukemia varies by cytogenetic subtype. *Cancer Res.* **1998**, *58*, 4173–4179. [PubMed]

29. Schlenk, R.F.; Döhner, K.; Krauter, J.; Fröhling, S.; Corbacioglu, A.; Bullinger, L.; Habdank, M.; Späth, D.; Morgan, M.; Benner, A.; *et al.* Mutations and treatment outcome in cytogenetically normal acute myeloid leukemia. *N. Engl. J. Med.* **2008**, *358*, 1909–1918. [CrossRef] [PubMed]

30. Creutzig, U.; van den Heuvel-Eibrink, M.M.; Gibson, B.; Dworzak, M.N.; Adachi, S.; de Bont, E.; Harbott, J.; Hasle, H.; Johnston, D.; Kinoshita, A.; *et al.* Diagnosis and management of acute myeloid leukemia in children and adolescents: Recommendations from an international expert panel. *Blood* **2012**, *120*, 3187–3205. [CrossRef] [PubMed]

31. Büchner, T.; Hiddemann, W.; Berdel, W.E.; Wörmann, B.; Schoch, C.; Fonatsch, C.; Löffler, H.; Haferlach, T.; Ludwig, W.-D.D.; Maschmeyer, G.; *et al.* 6-Thioguanine, cytarabine, and daunorubicin (TAD) and high-dose cytarabine and mitoxantrone (HAM) for induction, TAD for consolidation, and either prolonged maintenance by reduced monthly TAD or TAD-HAM-TAD and one course of intensive consolidation by sequential HAM in adult patients at all ages with *de novo* acute myeloid leukemia (AML): A randomized trial of the German AML Cooperative Group. *J. Clin. Oncol.* **2003**, *21*, 4496–4504. [CrossRef] [PubMed]

32. De Lima, M.; Giralt, S.; Thall, P.F.; de Padua Silva, L.; Jones, R.B.; Komanduri, K.; Braun, T.M.; Nguyen, H.Q.; Champlin, R.; Garcia-Manero, G. Maintenance therapy with low-dose azacitidine after allogeneic hematopoietic stem cell transplantation for recurrent acute myelogenous leukemia or myelodysplastic syndrome: A dose and schedule finding study. *Cancer* **2010**, *116*, 5420–5431. [CrossRef] [PubMed]

33. Govindaraj, C.; Madondo, M.; Kong, Y.Y.; Tan, P.; Wei, A.; Plebanski, M. Lenalidomide-based maintenance therapy reduces TNF receptor 2 on CD4 T cells and enhances immune effector function in acute myeloid leukemia patients. *Am. J. Hematol.* **2014**, *89*, 795–802. [CrossRef] [PubMed]

34. Hann, I.M.; Stevens, R.F.; Goldstone, A.H.; Rees, J.K.; Wheatley, K.; Gray, R.G.; Burnett, A.K. Randomized comparison of DAT versus ADE as induction chemotherapy in children and younger adults with acute myeloid leukemia. Results of the Medical Research Council's 10th AML trial (MRC AML10). Adult and Childhood Leukaemia Working Parties of the Medical Research Council. *Blood* **1997**, *89*, 2311–2318. [PubMed]

35. Majhail, N.S.; Brazauskas, R.; Hassebroek, A.; Bredeson, C.N.; Hahn, T.; Hale, G.A.; Horowitz, M.M.; Lazarus, H.M.; Maziarz, R.T.; Wood, W.A.; *et al.* Outcomes of allogeneic hematopoietic cell transplantation for adolescent and young adults compared with children and older adults with acute myeloid leukemia. *Biol. Blood Marrow Transplant.* **2012**, *18*, 861–873. [CrossRef] [PubMed]

36. Horan, J.T.; Alonzo, T.A.; Lyman, G.H.; Gerbing, R.B.; Lange, B.J.; Ravindranath, Y.; Becton, D.; Smith, F.O.; Woods, W.G. Impact of disease risk on efficacy of matched related bone marrow transplantation for pediatric acute myeloid leukemia: The Children's Oncology Group. *J. Clin. Oncol.* **2008**, *26*, 5797–5801. [CrossRef] [PubMed]

37. Vettenranta, K. Current European practice in pediatric myeloablative conditioning. *Bone Marrow Transplant.* **2008**, *41* (Suppl. S2), 14–17. [CrossRef]

38. Nemecek, E.R.; Guthrie, K.A.; Sorror, M.L.; Wood, B.L.; Doney, K.C.; Hilger, R.A.; Scott, B.L.; Kovacsovics, T.J.; Maziarz, R.T.; Woolfrey, A.E.; *et al.* Conditioning with treosulfan and fludarabine followed by allogeneic hematopoietic cell transplantation for high-risk hematologic malignancies. *Biol. Blood Marrow Transplant.* **2011**, *17*, 341–350. [CrossRef] [PubMed]

39. Tewari, P.; Franklin, A.R.; Tarek, N.; Askins, M.A.; Mofield, S.; Kebriaei, P. Hematopoietic stem cell transplantation in adolescents and young adults. *Acta Haematol.* **2014**, *132*, 313–325. [CrossRef] [PubMed]

40. Sisler, I.; Koehler, E.; Koyama, T.; Domm, J.; Ryan, R.; Levine, J.; Pulsipher, M.; Haut, P.; Schultz, K.; Taylor, D.; *et al.* Impact of conditioning regimen in allogeneic hematopoetic stem cell transplantation for children with acute myelogenous leukemia beyond first complete remission: A pediatric blood and marrow transplant consortium (PBMTC) study. *Biol. Blood Marrow Transplant.* **2009**, *15*, 1620–1627. [CrossRef] [PubMed]

41. Aristei, C.; Santucci, A.; Corvò, R.; Gardani, G.; Ricardi, U.; Scarzello, G.; Magrini, S.M.; Donato, V.; Falcinelli, L.; Bacigalupo, A.; *et al.* In haematopoietic SCT for acute leukemia TBI impacts on relapse but not survival: Results of a multicentre observational study. *Bone Marrow Transplant.* **2013**, *48*, 908–914. [CrossRef] [PubMed]

42. Nemecek, E.R.; Gooley, T.A.; Woolfrey, A.E.; Carpenter, P.A.; Matthews, D.C.; Sanders, J.E. Outcome of allogeneic bone marrow transplantation for children with advanced acute myeloid leukemia. *Bone Marrow Transplant.* **2004**, *34*, 799–806. [CrossRef] [PubMed]

43. Kanate, A.; Pasquini, M.; Hari, P.; Hamadani, M. Allogeneic hematopoietic cell transplant for acute myeloid leukemia: Current state in 2013 and future directions. *World J. Stem Cells* **2014**, *6*, 69–81. [CrossRef] [PubMed]

44. Kelly, M.J.; Horan, J.T.; Alonzo, T.A.; Eapen, M.; Gerbing, R.B.; He, W.; Lange, B.J.; Parsons, S.K.; Woods, W.G. Comparable survival for pediatric acute myeloid leukemia with poor-risk cytogenetics following chemotherapy, matched related donor, or unrelated donor transplantation. *Pediatr. Blood Cancer* **2014**, *61*, 269–275. [CrossRef] [PubMed]

45. Ebihara, Y.; Takahashi, S.; Mochizuki, S.; Kato, S.; Kawakita, T.; Ooi, J.; Yokoyama, K.; Nagamura, F.; Tojo, A.; Asano, S.; *et al.* Unrelated cord blood transplantation after myeloablative conditioning regimen in adolescent and young adult patients with hematologic malignancies: A single institute analysis. *Leuk. Res.* **2012**, *36*, 128–131. [CrossRef] [PubMed]

46. González-Vicent, M.; Molina, B.; Andión, M.; Sevilla, J.; Ramirez, M.; Pérez, A.; Díaz, M.A. Allogeneic hematopoietic transplantation using haploidentical donor *vs.* unrelated cord blood donor in pediatric patients: A single-center retrospective study. *Eur. J. Haematol.* **2011**, *87*, 46–53. [CrossRef] [PubMed]

47. Aversa, F.; Tabilio, A.; Velardi, A.; Cunningham, I.; Terenzi, A.; Falzetti, F.; Ruggeri, L.; Barbabietola, G.; Aristei, C.; Latini, P.; *et al.* Treatment of high-risk acute leukemia with T-cell-depleted stem cells from related donors with one fully mismatched HLA haplotype. *N. Engl. J. Med.* **1998**, *339*, 1186–1193. [CrossRef] [PubMed]

48. Ciceri, F.; Labopin, M.; Aversa, F.; Rowe, J.M.; Bunjes, D.; Lewalle, P.; Nagler, A.; Di Bartolomeo, P.; Lacerda, J.F.; Lupo Stanghellini, M.T.; *et al.* A survey of fully haploidentical hematopoietic stem cell transplantation in adults with high-risk acute leukemia: A risk factor analysis of outcomes for patients in remission at transplantation. *Blood* **2008**, *112*, 3574–3581. [CrossRef] [PubMed]

49. Luznik, L.; O'Donnell, P.V.; Symons, H.J.; Chen, A.R.; Leffell, M.S.; Zahurak, M.; Gooley, T.A.; Piantadosi, S.; Kaup, M.; Ambinder, R.F.; *et al.* HLA-haploidentical bone marrow transplantation for hematologic malignancies using nonmyeloablative conditioning and high-dose, posttransplantation cyclophosphamide. *Biol. Blood Marrow Transplant.* **2008**, *14*, 641–650. [CrossRef] [PubMed]

50. Woods, W.G.; Neudorf, S.; Gold, S.; Sanders, J.; Buckley, J.D.; Barnard, D.R.; Dusenbery, K.; DeSwarte, J.; Arthur, D.C.; Lange, B.J.; *et al.* A comparison of allogeneic bone marrow transplantation, autologous bone marrow transplantation, and aggressive chemotherapy in children with acute myeloid leukemia in remission. *Blood* **2001**, *97*, 56–62. [CrossRef] [PubMed]

51. Suciu, S.; Mandelli, F.; de Witte, T.; Zittoun, R.; Gallo, E.; Labar, B.; de Rosa, G.; Belhabri, A.; Giustolisi, R.; Delarue, R.; *et al.* Allogeneic compared with autologous stem cell transplantation in the treatment of patients younger than 46 years with acute myeloid leukemia (AML) in first complete remission (CR1): An intention-to-treat analysis of the EORTC/GIMEMAAML-10 trial. *Blood* **2003**, *102*, 1232–1240. [CrossRef] [PubMed]

52. Pui, C.-H.; Sandlund, J.; Pei, D.; Campana, D.; Rivera, G.; Ribeiro, R.; Rubnitz, J.; Razzouk, B.; Howard, S.; Hudson, M.; *et al.* Improved outcome for children with acute lymphoblastic leukemia: Results of Total Therapy Study XIIIB at St Jude Children's Research Hospital. *Blood* **2004**, *104*, 2690–2696. [CrossRef] [PubMed]

53. Ofran, Y.; Rowe, J.M. Treatment for relapsed acute myeloid leukemia: What is new? *Curr. Opin. Hematol.* **2012**, *19*, 89–94. [CrossRef] [PubMed]

54. Larson, S.M.; Campbell, N.P.; Huo, D.; Artz, A.; Zhang, Y.; Gajria, D.; Green, M.; Weiner, H.; Daugherty, C.; Odenike, O.; *et al.* High dose cytarabine and mitoxantrone: An effective induction regimen for high-risk acute myeloid leukemia (AML). *Leuk. Lymphoma* **2012**, *53*, 445–450. [CrossRef] [PubMed]

55. Nakayama, H.; Tabuchi, K.; Tawa, A.; Tsukimoto, I.; Tsuchida, M.; Morimoto, A.; Yabe, H.; Horibe, K.; Hanada, R.; Imaizumi, M.; *et al.* Outcome of children with relapsed acute myeloid leukemia following initial therapy under the AML99 protocol. *Int. J. Hematol.* **2014**, *100*, 171–179. [CrossRef] [PubMed]

56. Zhu, X.; Ma, Y.; Liu, D. Novel agents and regimens for acute myeloid leukemia: 2009 ASH annual meeting highlights. *J. Hematol. Oncol.* **2010**, *3*. [CrossRef] [PubMed]

57. Kaspers, G.J.; Zimmermann, M.; Reinhardt, D.; Gibson, B.E.; Tamminga, R.Y.; Aleinikova, O.; Armendariz, H.; Dworzak, M.; Ha, S.-Y.Y.; Hasle, H.; *et al.* Improved outcome in pediatric relapsed acute myeloid leukemia: Results of a randomized trial on liposomal daunorubicin by the International BFM Study Group. *J. Clin. Oncol.* **2013**, *31*, 599–607. [CrossRef] [PubMed]

58. Malfuson, J.V.; Konopacki, J.; Thepenier, C.; Eddou, H.; Foissaud, V.; de Revel, T. Fractionated doses of gemtuzumab ozogamicin combined with 3 + 7 induction chemotherapy as salvage treatment for young patients with acute myeloid leukemia in first relapse. *Ann. Hematol.* **2012**, *91*, 1871–1877. [CrossRef] [PubMed]

59. Borthakur, G.; Cortes, J.E.; Estey, E.E.; Jabbour, E.; Faderl, S.; O'Brien, S.; Garcia-Manero, G.; Kadia, T.M.; Wang, X.; Patel, K.; *et al.* Gemtuzumab ozogamicin with fludarabine, cytarabine, and granulocyte colony stimulating factor (FLAG-GO) as front-line regimen in patients with core binding factor acute myelogenous leukemia. *Am. J. Hematol.* **2014**, *89*, 964–968. [CrossRef] [PubMed]

60. Mato, A.R.; Morgans, A.; Luger, S.M. Novel strategies for relapsed and refractory acute myeloid leukemia. *Curr. Opin. Hematol.* **2008**, *15*, 108–114. [CrossRef] [PubMed]

61. Faderl, S.; Ferrajoli, A.; Wierda, W.; Huang, X.; Verstovsek, S.; Ravandi, F.; Estrov, Z.; Borthakur, G.; Kwari, M.; Kantarjian, H.M. Clofarabine combinations as acute myeloid leukemia salvage therapy. *Cancer* **2008**, *113*, 2090–2096. [CrossRef] [PubMed]

62. Hijiya, N.; Gaynon, P.; Barry, E.; Silverman, L.; Thomson, B.; Chu, R.; Cooper, T.; Kadota, R.; Rytting, M.; Steinherz, P.; *et al.* A multi-center phase I study of clofarabine, etoposide and cyclophosphamide in combination in pediatric patients with refractory or relapsed acute leukemia. *Leukemia* **2009**, *23*, 2259–2264. [CrossRef] [PubMed]

63. Phillips, C.L.; Davies, S.M.; McMasters, R.; Absalon, M.; O'Brien, M.; Mo, J.; Broun, R.; Moscow, J.A.; Smolarek, T.; Garzon, R.; *et al.* Low dose decitabine in very high risk relapsed or refractory acute myeloid leukaemia in children and young adults. *Br. J. Haematol.* **2013**, *161*, 406–410. [CrossRef] [PubMed]

64. Watt, T.C.; Cooper, T. Sorafenib as treatment for relapsed or refractory pediatric acute myelogenous leukemia. *Pediatr. Blood Cancer* **2012**, *59*, 756–757. [CrossRef] [PubMed]

65. Ravandi, F.; Arana Yi, C.; Cortes, J.E.; Levis, M.; Faderl, S.; Garcia-Manero, G.; Jabbour, E.; Konopleva, M.; O'Brien, S.; Estrov, Z.; *et al.* Final report of phase II study of sorafenib, cytarabine and idarubicin for initial therapy in younger patients with acute myeloid leukemia. *Leukemia* **2014**, *28*, 1543–1545. [CrossRef] [PubMed]

66. Inaba, H.; Rubnitz, J.; Coustan-Smith, E.; Li, L.; Furmanski, B.; Mascara, G.; Heym, K.; Christensen, R.; Onciu, M.; Shurtleff, S.; *et al.* Phase I pharmacokinetic and pharmacodynamic study of the multikinase inhibitor sorafenib in combination with clofarabine and cytarabine in pediatric relapsed/refractory leukemia. *J. Clin. Oncol.* **2011**, *29*, 3293–3300. [CrossRef] [PubMed]

67. Levis, M.; Ravandi, F.; Wang, E.S.; Baer, M.R.; Perl, A.; Coutre, S.; Erba, H.; Stuart, R.K.; Baccarani, M.; Cripe, L.D.; *et al.* Results from a randomized trial of salvage chemotherapy followed by lestaurtinib for patients with FLT3 mutant AML in first relapse. *Blood* **2011**, *117*, 3294–3301. [CrossRef] [PubMed]

68. Fathi, A.; Levis, M. FLT3 inhibitors: A story of the old and the new. *Curr. Opin. Hematol.* **2011**, *18*, 71–76. [CrossRef] [PubMed]

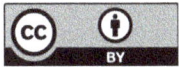

Journal of
Clinical Medicine

MDPI

Review

Pediatric AML: From Biology to Clinical Management

Jasmijn D. E. de Rooij, C. Michel Zwaan and Marry van den Heuvel-Eibrink *

Department of Pediatric Oncology, Erasmus MC-Sophia Children's Hospital, 3015CN Rotterdam, The Netherlands; j.d.e.derooij@erasmusmc.nl (J.D.E.R.); c.m.zwaan@erasmusmc.nl (C.M.Z.)
* Author to whom correspondence should be addressed; m.vandenheuvel@erasmusmc.nl; Tel.: +31-107-036-691.

Academic Editor: Celalettin Ustun
Received: 17 October 2014; Accepted: 28 November 2014; Published: 9 January 2015

Abstract: Pediatric acute myeloid leukemia (AML) represents 15%–20% of all pediatric acute leukemias. Survival rates have increased over the past few decades to ~70%, due to improved supportive care, optimized risk stratification and intensified chemotherapy. In most children, AML presents as a *de novo* entity, but in a minority, it is a secondary malignancy. The diagnostic classification of pediatric AML includes a combination of morphology, cytochemistry, immunophenotyping and molecular genetics. Outcome is mainly dependent on the initial response to treatment and molecular and cytogenetic aberrations. Treatment consists of a combination of intensive anthracycline- and cytarabine-containing chemotherapy and stem cell transplantation in selected genetic high-risk cases or slow responders. In general, ~30% of all pediatric AML patients will suffer from relapse, whereas 5%–10% of the patients will die due to disease complications or the side-effects of the treatment. Targeted therapy may enhance anti-leukemic efficacy and minimize treatment-related morbidity and mortality, but requires detailed knowledge of the genetic abnormalities and aberrant pathways involved in leukemogenesis. These efforts towards future personalized therapy in a rare disease, such as pediatric AML, require intensive international collaboration in order to enhance the survival rates of pediatric AML, while aiming to reduce long-term toxicity.

Keywords: pediatric AML; clinical management; cytogenetics; molecular aberrations

1. Clinical Introduction

1.1. Epidemiology of AML

In children, the most frequently occurring hematological malignancies include acute leukemias, of which 80% are classified as acute lymphoblastic leukemia (ALL) and 15%–20% as acute myeloid leukemia (AML). The incidence of AML in infants is 1.5 per 100,000 individuals per year, the incidence decreases to 0.9 per 100,000 individuals aged 1–4 and 0.4 per 100,000 individuals aged 5–9 years, after which it gradually increases into adulthood, up to an incidence of 16.2 per 100,000 individuals aged over 65 years [1]. The underlying cause of AML is unknown, and childhood AML generally occurs *de novo*. In adult and elderly patients, AML is often preceded by myelodysplastic syndrome (MDS), but in children, the occurrence of AML preceded by clonal evolution of preleukemic myeloproliferative diseases, such as MDS or juvenile myelomonocytic leukemia (JMML), is rare. Germline affected individuals, such as those with Fanconi anemia or Bloom syndrome, have an increased risk for developing AML as a secondary malignancy [2,3]. Recently, germ-line mutations in several genes, such as TP53, RUNX1, GATA2 and CEBPA, have been found in families with an unexplained high risk of AML, suggesting a familial predisposition to develop AML [4–8].

Children with Down syndrome classically present with a unique megakaryoblastic subtype of AML, classically following a transient myeloproliferative disorder in the neonatal period, which is characterized by somatic mutations in the *GATA1* gene. The leukemic cells of patients with

Down syndrome are usually highly sensitive to chemotherapy with an exceptional high survival rate, and therefore it is possible to treat these patients with adjusted treatment protocols [9]. In addition, AML may occur following previous radiotherapy or chemotherapy containing alkylating agents or epipodophyllotoxins, as secondary neoplasm. These are typically characterized by either MLL-rearrangements or by monosomy 7 [10,11].

1.2. Diagnostic Approach and Classification

AML is a heterogeneous disease with respect to morphology, immunophenotyping, cooperating underlying germline and somatic genetic abnormalities, as well as clinical behavior. The standard diagnostic process of AML is based on a combination of morphology, cytochemistry, immunophenotyping, cytogenetic and molecular characterization of the leukemic blasts derived from the bone marrow or peripheral blood [12]. Each AML patient can be risk-classified into a clinically relevant subgroup. The previously used morphology-based French-American-British (FAB) classification is nowadays replaced by the World Health Organization (WHO) classification, which also takes karyotype and molecular aberrations into account (Table 1) [13,14]. Cytochemistry and immunophenotyping is generally used to distinguish AML from ALL, which further classifies pediatric AML according to the cell lineage of origin and differentiation stage at which the differentiation arrest occurs. Especially for the diagnosis of FAB-types, M0 and M7 immunophenotyping is indispensable [12,15]. The majority of chromosomal abnormalities is detected by conventional karyotyping and complemented with FISH or reverse transcriptase PCR to detect relevant (cryptic) translocations, fusion genes or loss of chromosome material [16]. In young children under two years of age, it is important to search for specific pediatric AML translocations that are not yet acknowledged in the WHO classification as separate entities, such as t(7;12)(q36;p13), also known as *HLXB9-MNX1*, t(11;12)(p15;p13)/*NUP98-KDM5A* and t(1;22)(p13;q13)/*RBM15-MKL1* [12,17–19].

Table 1. The WHO classification of acute myeloid leukemia (AML) and related neoplasms [14].

WHO Classification of AML and Related Neoplasms	
Acute myeloid leukemia with recurrent genetic abnormalities	AML with t(8;21)(q22;q22); *RUNX1-RUNX1T1* AML with inv(16)(p13.1q22) or t(16;16)(p13.1;q22); *CBFB-MYH11* Acute promyelocytic leukemia with t(15;17)(q22;q12); *PML-RARA* AML with 11q23 (*MLL*) abnormalities AML with t(6;9)(p23;q34); *DEK-NUP214* AML with inv(3)(q21q26.2) or t(3;3)(q21;q26.2); *RPN1-EVI1* t(1;22)(p13;q13); *RBM15-MKL1* Provisional entity: AML with mutated *NPM1* Provisional entity: AML with mutated *CEBPA*
Acute myeloid leukemia with myelodysplasia-related changes	
Therapy-related myeloid neoplasms	
Acute myeloid leukemia, not otherwise specified	AML with minimal differentiation AML without maturation AML with maturation Acute myelomonocytic leukemia Acute monoblastic/monocytic leukemia Acute erythroid leukemia Pure erythroid leukemia Erythroleukemia, erythroid/myeloid Acute megakaryoblastic leukemia Acute basophilic leukemia Acute panmyelosis with myelofibrosis
Myeloid sarcoma	
Myeloid proliferations related to Down syndrome	Transient abnormal myelopoiesis Myeloid leukemia associated with Down syndrome
Blastic plasmacytoid dendritic cell neoplasm	

1.3. Treatment and Outcome

The clinical outcome of pediatric AML has improved significantly over the past few decades, with current long-term survival rates of ~70% (Table 2) [20–30]. This improvement is due to intensification of chemotherapeutic regimens, better risk-group stratification, better salvage at relapse and improved supportive care. Risk-group stratification is usually based on (cyto)genetic abnormalities present in the leukemic blasts in combination with early response to treatment, either specified as complete remission (CR) rate after one or two courses or applying minimal-residual disease measurements, which in AML is mainly based on flow-cytometry [31]. The chemotherapeutic regimens consist of 4–5 cycles of intensive chemotherapy, typically including cytarabine combined with an anthracycline. In younger adult patients, studies suggest that there is a benefit for outcome using high-dose cytarabine in induction, but from previous trials, a similar effect in pediatric AML patients could not be confirmed [26,32]. In randomized controlled trials, the anthracyclines, daunorubicin and mitoxantrone, resulted in similar overall survival, but mitoxantrone-based treatment eventually resulted in a lower relapse rate [33]. When comparing idarubicin and liposomal daunorubicin, survival was similar, whereas liposomal daunorubicin was more effective in *RUNX1/RUNX1T1* translocated cases and caused less treatment-related mortality [34].

The added value of hematopoietic stem cell transplantation (SCT) in newly-diagnosed pediatric AML is under discussion, as in general, the occurrence of procedure-related deaths needs to be counterbalanced by the reduction in relapse risk. The procedure-related deaths are dependent on the intensity of the prior induction chemotherapy. SCT in first CR is therefore currently only recommended for a selected subset of high risk cases in most European protocols. SCT plays a more prominent role in most North-American treatment protocols [35,36]. Recent studies show an increase in survival after SCT now that stricter risk stratification is improving. Currently, several trials include minimal residual disease (MRD) levels after Courses 1 or 2 in risk stratification for SCT [37–40]. Of note is that the excess in mortality and the burden of disease long after myeloablative therapy are not taken into account in the reported survival.

Despite intensive treatment, ~30% of the pediatric patients relapse, and outcome is poor, reflected by the ~30%–40% of patients surviving in the largest and most recent series reported to date [41,42]. Nevertheless, the high frequency of treatment-related deaths (5%–10%), both in treatment protocols for newly-diagnosed, as well as for relapsed disease, and the occurrence of long-term side effects, such as anthracycline-induced cardiomyopathy, illustrate that further intensification of chemotherapy seems no longer feasible [43]. Therefore, knowledge on the molecular and genetic background is of utmost relevance in order to detect novel, leukemia and patient-specific treatment targets.

1.4. Relevant Molecular and Genetic Aberrations in Pediatric AML

AML is thought to arise from at least two classes of cooperating genetic events [44]. Type I abnormalities result in increased, uncontrolled proliferation and/or survival of the leukemic cell and are often activating mutations of genes involved in signal transduction pathways, such as *FLT3*, *KIT*, *N-RAS*, *K-RAS* and *PTPN11*. Type II abnormalities impair differentiation and mainly result from genetic aberrations in hematopoietic transcription factors, due to, for instance, the AML-characteristic translocations t(8;21)(q22;q22)/*AML1-ETO* and 11q23/*MLL* rearrangements or from mutations in genes, such as *NPM1* and *CEBPA* [7,45–48]. The most common cytogenetic abnormalities (Type II) in children are t(8;21)(q22;q22), inv(16)(p13.1q22) (together referred to as core binding factor (CBF)-AML), t(15;17)(q22;q21) and 11q23/*MLL*-rearranged abnormalities (Figure 1A) [49–52]. Together, these account for approximately half of all pediatric AML cases, a much higher frequency than in adults. Some translocations, for example t(1;22)(p13;q13), t(7;12)(q36;p13) and t(11;12)(p15;p13), are specific for children and are rarely or never found in adults [17–19,53–57]. Translocations involving hematopoietic transcription factors often lead to dysregulated gene expression, either as a result of the fusion partner itself or the recruitment of different co-factors to the transcription complex. For example, the *MLL* gene has histone methyltransferase activity and is part of a chromatin modifying complex. More than 60 fusion partners have been identified in AML, but the breakpoint of the *MLL* gene is highly conserved [58,59]. Fusion proteins lead to a gain of function of the *MLL*-complex, resulting in inappropriate histone modification and increased expression of *MEIS1* and, specifically, *HOXA* genes, maintaining a stem-cell phenotype. In addition, the presence of DOT1L, which is recruited into the *MLL*-complex, is required for the leukemogenic activity of several *MLL* rearrangements and may be a target for treatment [60,61].

Only 20%–25% of pediatric AML cases are cytogenetically normal [48,62]. Of interest in these cases, specific Type II mutations and translocations are identified in ~70% of the cases, such as *NPM1* mutations, biallelic *CEBPA* mutations, as well as the cryptic translocations, *NUP98/NSD1*, all invisible with conventional karyotyping and, hence, requiring additional molecular diagnostics (Figure 1B) [17,46,57,63].

The combination of the Type I and Type II mutations does not seem to be completely random; specific combinations seem more prevalent, such as the Ras pathway mutations, which are often found in combination with *MLL*-rearrangements, *KIT* mutations, which are mainly found in CBF-AML, and *FLT3*-itd, which is often seen in combination with *PML/RARA* and *NUP98/NSD1* (Figure 1) [48,57].

Mutations in epigenetic regulators, such as *EZH2*, *ASXL1* and *DNMT3A*, add another level of complexity and contribute to both the maturation arrest and proliferative capacity, which are needed to develop AML (Figure 2) [63–71]. These mutations are rare in pediatric AML, but specific Type II subgroups present with an altered methylation (hypo- or hyper-methylation), which may indicate that these children could benefit from treatment with demethylating agents or histone modification inhibitors, as recently described for infants suffering from ALL [72].

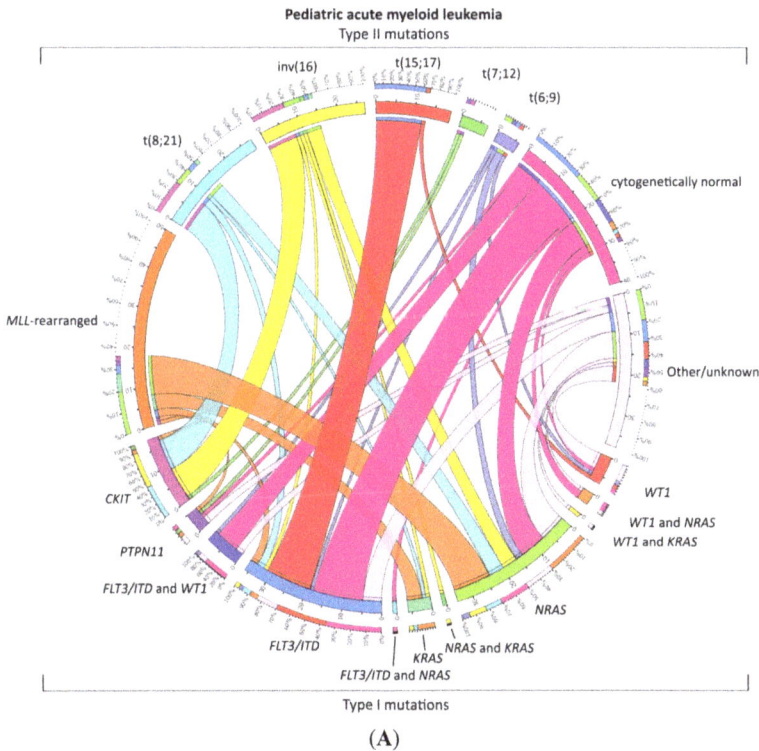

Figure 1. *Cont.*

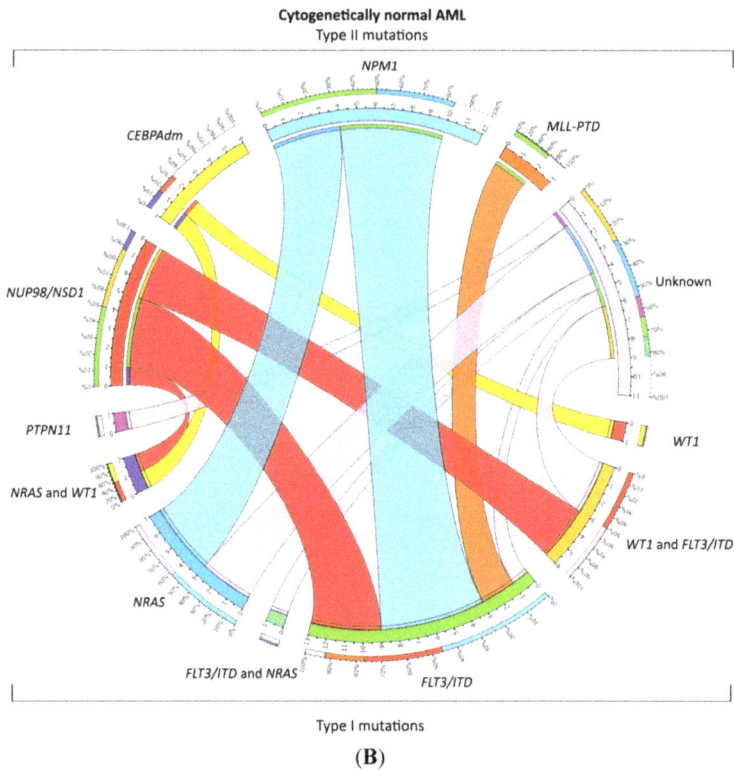

Figure 1. Distribution of Type I/II abnormalities in pediatric AML. (**A**) Cooperating Type I and Type II mutations in pediatric AML. The circos plot [73] depicts the frequency of the Type II mutations and co-occurrence of Type I mutations in patients with *de novo* pediatric AML. The length of the arch corresponds to the frequency of the Type II mutation and the width of the ribbon with the percentage of patients with a specific Type I mutation or a combination of Type I mutations. FLT3/ITD denotes FLT3 internal tandem duplication; (**B**) Cooperating Type I and Type II mutations in cytogenetically normal AML. The circos plot [73] depicts the frequency of the Type II mutations and co-occurrence of Type I mutations in patients with *de novo* pediatric cytogenetically normal AML. The length of the arch corresponds to the frequency of the Type II mutation, and the width of the ribbon with the percentage of patients with a specific Type I mutation or a combination of Type I mutations. FLT3/ITD denotes FLT3 internal tandem duplication.

Table 2. Survival of pediatric AML.

Study Group	Study and Inclusion Time (Calendar Years of Inclusion)	Patients (*n*)	Patients Treated with SCT (*n*)	EFS (%)	OS (%)	Relapse (%)	Source
BFM-SG	AML-BFM 2004 (2004–2010)	521	NA	5 years 55 ± 2	5 years 74 ± 2	29	Creutzig *et al.*, 2013 [34]
JACLS	AML99 (2003–2006)	146	22 (15%)	5 years 66.7 ± 4.0	5 years 77.7 ± 8.0	30.2	Imamura *et al.*, 2012 [74]
	AML99 (2000–2002)	240	Allo-SCT 41 (17%) Auto-SCT 5 (2%)	5 years 61.6 ± 6.5	5 years 75.6 ± 5.3	32.2	Tsukimoto *et al.*, 2009 [27]
AIEOP	AML2002/01 (2002–2011)	482	Allo-SCT 141 (29%) Auto-SCT 102 (21%)	8 years 55.0 ± 2.6	8 years 67.7 ± 2.4	24	Pession *et al.*, 2013 [9]
COG	AAML03P1 (2003–2005)	340	73 (21%)	3 years 53 ± 6	3 years 66 ± 5	33 ± 6	Cooper *et al.*, 2012 [75]
NOPHO	NOPHO AML 2004 (2004–2009)	151	22 (15%)	3 years 57 ± 5	3 years 69 ± 5	30	Abrahamsson *et al.*, 2011 [20]
MRC	MRC AML12 (1995–2002)	564	64 (11%)	10 years 54	10 years 63	32	Gibson *et al.*, 2011 [13]
SJCRH	AML02 (2002–2008)	216	59 (25%)	3 years 63	3 years 71	21	Rubnitz *et al.*, 2010 [26]
PPLLSG	PPLLSG AML-98 (1998–2002)	104	Allo-SCT 14 (13%) Auto-SCT 8 (8%)	5 years 47 ± 5	5 years 50 ± 5	24	Dluzniewska *et al.*, 2005 [76]

Abbreviations: *n*, indicates number; SCT, stem cell transplantation; EFS, event-free survival; OS, overall survival; BFM-SG, Berlin-Frankfurt-Munster-Study-Group (Germany); AML, acute myeloid leukemia; JACLS, Japan Association of Childhood Leukemia Study; Allo, allogeneic; Auto, autologous; AIEOP, Italian association of Pediatric Hematology and Oncology (Associazione Italiana Ematologia Oncologia Pediatrica); COG, Childhood Oncology Group (United States of America); NOPHO, Nordic Society of Pediatric Haematology and Oncology; MRC, Medical Research Council (United Kingdom); SJCRH, St. Jude Children's Research Hospital (United States of America); PPLLSG, Polish Pediatric Leukemia/Lymphoma Study Group.

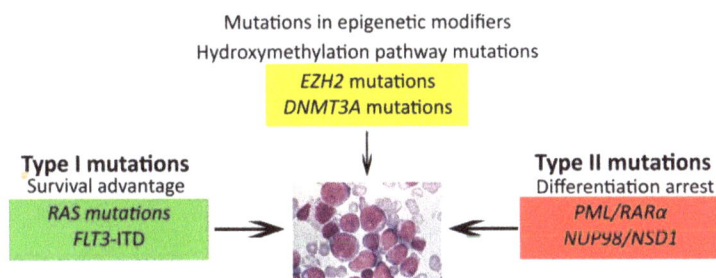

Figure 2. Model of cooperating genetic events in AML. Different types of genetic and epigenetic events collaborate in leukemogenesis.

1.5. Prognostic Factors and Risk Group Stratification

Most important prognostic factors for the survival of pediatric AML are the initial response to treatment and the underlying genetic and molecular aberrations [12,77,78]. CBF-AML is a favorable prognostic subgroup [48,52,79]. Outcome in *MLL*-rearranged AML is variable and depends on the translocation partner. For example, the *MLL*-translocation t(1;11)(q21;q23) is associated with a very favorable outcome in pediatric AML. In contrast, poor survival rates were reported in pediatric AML with translocations t(6;11)(q27;q23) and t(10;11)(p12;q23) [80,81]. The acute megakaryoblastic leukemias (AMKL, FABM7) in non-Down syndrome patients represent a subgroup with poor outcome, with the exception of AMKL harboring t(1;22)(p13;q13), which seems to confer a favorable prognostic group, in contrast to Down syndrome, where AMKL confers a favorable outcome [9,17]. Monosomy 7 is a well-known poor-prognostic factor and confers a worse outcome [52,82]. Deletion of 7q is described as an intermediate risk in the prognosis in adults, in contrast to the outcome of pediatric AML with a 7q deletion in children. In those pediatric patients, the outcome seems to be dependent on other cytogenetic abnormalities in the leukemic cell [52,82]. The described poor prognostic abnormalities in adult AML of chromosomes 3q and 5q and the monosomal karyotypes are rare in children [30,83–85]. Overexpression of *EVI1* caused by 3q26 abnormalities predicts an adverse outcome in adult AML, but *EVI1* overexpression is not an independent prognostic factor in pediatric AML [86,87]. The Type I mutations of *WT1* and *FLT3*-itd predict a poor outcome, the latter dependent on the allele ratio, and these mutations are described as events in clonal evolution towards relapse [88].

A special subtype of pediatric AML is the cytogenetically normal (CN) AML group, where clinical outcome is highly dependent on the presence of single-gene mutations or cryptic translocations. Of special interest are *NPM1* and bi-allelic *CEBPA* mutations, conferring a favorable prognosis, while the cryptic translocation *NUP98/NSD1* confers a poor prognosis, due to a poor response to treatment and a high risk for relapse, independent of the poor prognostic Type I *FLT3*-itd abnormality [46,57,89].

2. Future Strategies

2.1. Genomic Approaches to Unravel the Biology of Pediatric AML

In order to provide more insight into the heterogeneity and biology of AML, genome-wide approaches have been recently employed, although the success rate is variable. Array-based comparative genomic hybridization (array-CGH) and single-nucleotide polymorphism (SNP) arrays identified several regions with loss of heterozygosity and recurrent copy number variations (CNVs), albeit with low frequency in AML [90]. These CNVs included aberrations in *WT1*, *NF1* and *TET2*, the latter being more common in adults than in children [47,65,67,91].

Gene expression profiling could predict the cytogenetic subtypes of AML with high accuracy, although its value for diagnostic purposes remains limited, since most aberrations can be identified with conventional karyotyping [92–95]. Nevertheless, novel genes involved in the pathogenesis of pediatric AML subtypes were identified using this method, such as *BRE* and *IGSF4* [96,97].

In addition to discovering novel gene mutations, next generation sequencing has also proven to be a powerful tool in the study of the clonal evolution of both adult and pediatric AML [98,99]. By comparing the mutational spectrum of diagnosis-relapse pairs, it was shown that the founding clone gained novel mutations and evolved into the relapse clone. Moreover, minor subclones present at diagnosis can survive chemotherapy, gain mutations and present as dominant clones at relapse, illustrating their leukemia-driving capacity. Therapeutic targeting of novel identified mutations to prevent relapse may provide an improved outcome for selected patients [100,101].

Epigenetic profiling was able to distinguish cytogenetic subtypes of adult AML [102]. Differences in promoter hypermethylation of selected genes between pediatric and adult AML warrant the profiling of DNA methylation in pediatric AML [103]. These studies may point out subsets of patients eligible for treatment with demethylating agents or histone modification inhibitors, as was shown for pediatric ALL [72].

Differences in microRNA expression levels can classify several types of cancer [104]. Profiling studies in adult AML have shown that variations in microRNA expression patterns are associated with subtypes of AML and that specific microRNAs target genes of interest for the biology of AML [105–107]. In pediatric AML, microRNA expression patterns vary among subtypes of AML, as well, although some differences in the expression patterns of specific microRNAs were observed between children and adults [108].

2.2. Towards Optimized Therapy

The translation from molecular aberrations towards targeted therapy might be the solution to improve outcome in the next few decades. Since further intensification of current chemotherapy treatment seems not feasible in pediatric AML, due to high morbidity and mortality rates, new therapeutic approaches that are more tumor-specific and cause less severe side effects are urgently needed. Some new compounds directed at specific molecular targets have already been investigated in early clinical trials in pediatric AML.

Tyrosine kinase inhibitors directed at inhibiting the constitutive activation of the *FLT3* gene are among the best studied drugs in this respect in pediatric AML and include trials using PKC412, CEP701, AC220 and sorafenib [109–111]. Recent data suggest a potentially generic mechanism of drug resistance when combining these inhibitors with chemotherapy due to FLT3 ligand upregulation, which questions their use in this fashion, although novel, more potent inhibitors may overcome this [112,113]. In the AAML1031 study of the Childhood Oncology Group (COG), patients with a *FLT3* gene mutation are treated with sorafenib in addition to standard intensive chemotherapy [114]. However, there are no convincing randomized studies to date showing an increase in overall survival in *FLT3* mutated patients with such therapeutic regimens.

Other potential targets in AML include *KIT* and *RAS* gene mutations. Patients with *KIT* mutations include the imatinib-resistant patients with the *D816V/Y* mutation, who are sensitive to dasatinib [48,115]. A phase I study of dasatinib has been completed in children [116]. There is an ongoing trial in adults using dasatinib together with chemotherapy in CBF-AML [117]. No trials have been reported using small molecule RAS-pathway inhibitors, e.g., MEK-inhibitors, after studies using farnesyl transferase inhibitors failed to show a benefit in older patients with AML [118]. To inhibit signal transduction pathways, such as the Ras-pathway, which is notorious for escaping behavior, which makes the leukemic cell survives despite intensive chemotherapy, combinations of inhibitors may be more promising, and this approach is currently being further explored in synthetic lethality screens, which combines different inhibitors in order to find a lethal combination for the leukemic cells, for different types of cancer [119,120].

In *MLL*-rearranged AML, efforts are directed at developing targeted therapy, for instance by inhibiting DOT1L, which is part of the MLL-complex, with current clinical trials ongoing [60]. Interestingly, these DOT1L inhibitors also seem valuable in the treatment of t(6;11)(q27;q23)-positive cells, which lack DOT1L in the formed complex, indicating that this drug is able to target aberrant H3K79 methylation [121].

Gemtuzumab ozogamicin is a conjugated monoclonal antibody against CD33 and linked to a cytostatic agent, calicheamicin, an anti-tumor antibiotic. AML cells often express CD33 and are therefore targeted by this drug. The first phase III studies did not show an improvement in disease-free and overall survival in pediatric AML patients, but it was favorable in patients with refractory or relapsed disease and was effective at reducing MRD levels before SCT [75,122–125].

Clofarabine is a purine nucleoside antimetabolite, registered for relapsed or refractory pediatric ALL. Early trials in pediatric AML did not show convincing efficacy, probably due to the intensive pre-treatment in these cases [126]. However, in refractory or relapsed pediatric AML patients, the combination of clofarabine and cytarabine resulted in 48% responders, with a three-year overall survival of 46% [127]. In ongoing studies, fludarabine, used in the "FLAG"-therapy, consisting of fludarabine, cytarabine and G-CSF, is replaced by clofarabine, as well as clofarabine combined with cyclophosphamide and etoposide [128]. Another phase II study showed a beneficial outcome for patients treated with the combination of clofarabine, topotecan, vinorelbine and thiotepa in pediatric patients with refractory or relapsed AML [129].

In xenograft models, treatment of AML with a combination of decitabine, a hypomethylating agent, and cytarabine was more effective at reducing tumor burden in comparison to cytarabine alone [130]. Low-dose decitabine was administered to high-risk relapsed or refractory AML patients, and 3/8 patients responded to this therapy [131]. Azacitidine, another hypomethylating agent, and decitabine show comparable treatment efficacy, but azacitidine may result in less adverse events [132].

International collaboration, which has been pursued over the last few decades on the levels of the International Berlin-Frankfurt-Munster Study Group (IBFM-SG), Innovative Therapies for Children with Cancer (ITCC), European Network for Cancer Research in Children and Adolescents (ENCCA), Therapeutic Advances in Childhood Leukemia (TACL) and Childhood Oncology Group (COG), has been proven successful in clinical and biological studies and will speed up efforts to enhance therapeutic options and the availability of novel agents for individual pediatric AML patients [12,17,28,80–82].

3. Conclusions

Current survival of pediatric AML is ~70%, and a therapeutic plateau has been reached with current chemotherapy. Further intensification of treatment is not feasible because of toxicity. The heterogeneity of AML is illustrated by the various prognostically relevant non-randomly associated molecular and cytogenetic aberrations that were discovered in recent years. However, many cooperating events in leukemogenesis still remain unknown. The application of new techniques, especially next generation sequencing, will contribute to our understanding of the genetic landscape of AML and enable the development of more targeted and personalized therapy in the near future. To achieve such goals for such a rare disease as pediatric AML, international collaboration is crucial.

Acknowledgments: Jasmijn D. E. de Rooij was funded by Kinder Oncologisch Centrum Rotterdam (KOCR).

Author Contributions: Jasmijn D. E. de Rooij, C. Michel Zwaan and Marry M. van den Heuvel-Eibrink designed the study. Jasmijn D. E. de Rooij performed the literature search. C. Michel Zwaan and Marry M. van den Heuvel-Eibrink supervised and reviewed the study. Jasmijn D. E. de Rooij wrote the manuscript. C. Michel Zwaan and Marry M. van den Heuvel-Eibrink critically reviewed the manuscript.

Conflicts of Interest: The authors declare no conflict of interest.

References

1. Howlader, N.N.A.; Krapcho, M.; Garshell, J.; Miller, D.; Altekruse, S.F.; Kosary, C.L.; Yu, M.; Ruhl, J.; Tatalovich, Z.; Mariotto, A.; *et al.* *SEER Cancer Statistics Review, 1975–2011*; National Cancer Institute: Bethesda, MD, USA, 2012.

2. Seif, A.E. Pediatric leukemia predisposition syndromes: Clues to understanding leukemogenesis. *Cancer Genet.* **2011**, *204*, 227–244. [CrossRef] [PubMed]

3. Tonnies, H.; Huber, S.; Kuhl, J.S.; Gerlach, A.; Ebell, W.; Neitzel, H. Clonal chromosomal aberrations in bone marrow cells of Fanconi anemia patients: Gains of the chromosomal segment 3q26q29 as an adverse risk factor. *Blood* **2003**, *101*, 3872–3874. [CrossRef] [PubMed]

4. Hahn, C.N.; Chong, C.E.; Carmichael, C.L.; Wilkins, E.J.; Brautigan, P.J.; Li, X.C.; Babic, M.; Lin, M.; Carmagnac, A.; Lee, Y.K.; *et al.* Heritable *GATA2* mutations associated with familial myelodysplastic syndrome and acute myeloid leukemia. *Nat. Genet.* **2011**, *43*, 1012–1017. [CrossRef] [PubMed]

5. Link, D.C.; Schuettpelz, L.G.; Shen, D.; Wang, J.; Walter, M.J.; Kulkarni, S.; Payton, J.E.; Ivanovich, J.; Goodfellow, P.J.; Le Beau, M.; *et al.* Identification of a novel TP53 cancer susceptibility mutation through whole-genome sequencing of a patient with therapy-related AML. *JAMA* **2011**, *305*, 1568–1576. [CrossRef] [PubMed]

6. Owen, C.; Barnett, M.; Fitzgibbon, J. Familial myelodysplasia and acute myeloid leukaemia—A review. *Br. J. Haematol.* **2008**, *140*, 123–132. [CrossRef] [PubMed]

7. Smith, M.L.; Cavenagh, J.D.; Lister, T.A.; Fitzgibbon, J. Mutation of CEBPA in familial acute myeloid leukemia. *N. Engl. J. Med.* **2004**, *351*, 2403–2407. [CrossRef] [PubMed]

8. Song, W.J.; Sullivan, M.G.; Legare, R.D.; Hutchings, S.; Tan, X.; Kufrin, D.; Ratajczak, J.; Resende, I.C.; Haworth, C.; Hock, R.; *et al.* Haploinsufficiency of CBFA2 causes familial thrombocytopenia with propensity to develop acute myelogenous leukaemia. *Nat. Genet.* **1999**, *23*, 166–175. [CrossRef] [PubMed]

9. Zwaan, M.C.; Reinhardt, D.; Hitzler, J.; Vyas, P. Acute leukemias in children with Down syndrome. *Pediatr. Clin. North Am.* **2008**, *55*, 53–70. [CrossRef] [PubMed]

10. Sandler, E.S.; Friedman, D.J.; Mustafa, M.M.; Winick, N.J.; Bowman, W.P.; Buchanan, G.R. Treatment of children with epipodophyllotoxin-induced secondary acute myeloid leukemia. *Cancer* **1997**, *79*, 1049–1054. [CrossRef] [PubMed]

11. Weiss, B.; Vora, A.; Huberty, J.; Hawkins, R.A.; Matthay, K.K. Secondary myelodysplastic syndrome and leukemia following 131I-metaiodobenzylguanidine therapy for relapsed neuroblastoma. *J. Pediatr. Hematol. Oncol.* **2003**, *25*, 543–547. [CrossRef] [PubMed]

12. Creutzig, U.; van den Heuvel-Eibrink, M.M.; Gibson, B.; Dworzak, M.N.; Adachi, S.; de Bont, E.; Harbott, J.; Hasle, H.; Johnston, D.; Kinoshita, A.; *et al.* Diagnosis and management of acute myeloid leukemia in children and adolescents: Recommendations from an international expert panel. *Blood* **2012**, *120*, 3187–3205. [CrossRef] [PubMed]

13. Bennett, J.M.; Catovsky, D.; Daniel, M.T.; Flandrin, G.; Galton, D.A.; Gralnick, H.R.; Sultan, C. Proposals for the classification of the acute leukaemias. French-American-British (FAB) co-operative group. *Br. J. Haematol.* **1976**, *33*, 451–458. [CrossRef] [PubMed]

14. Vardiman, J.W.; Thiele, J.; Arber, D.A.; Brunning, R.D.; Borowitz, M.J.; Porwit, A.; Harris, N.L.; Le Beau, M.M.; Hellstrom-Lindberg, E.; Tefferi, A.; *et al.* The 2008 revision of the World Health Organization (WHO) classification of myeloid neoplasms and acute leukemia: Rationale and important changes. *Blood* **2009**, *114*, 937–951. [CrossRef] [PubMed]

15. Bennett, J.M.; Catovsky, D.; Daniel, M.T.; Flandrin, G.; Galton, D.A.; Gralnick, H.R.; Sultan, C. Criteria for the diagnosis of acute leukemia of megakaryocyte lineage (M7). A report of the French-American-British Cooperative Group. *Ann. Intern. Med.* **1985**, *103*, 460–462. [CrossRef] [PubMed]

16. Mrozek, K.; Heinonen, K.; Bloomfield, C.D. Clinical importance of cytogenetics in acute myeloid leukaemia. *Best Pract. Res. Clin. Haematol.* **2001**, *14*, 19–47. [CrossRef] [PubMed]

17. De Rooij, J.D.; Hollink, I.H.; Arentsen-Peters, S.T.; van Galen, J.F.; Berna Beverloo, H.; Baruchel, A.; Trka, J.; Reinhardt, D.; Sonneveld, E.; Zimmermann, M.; *et al.* NUP98/JARID1A is a novel recurrent abnormality in pediatric acute megakaryoblastic leukemia with a distinct *HOX* gene expression pattern. *Leukemia* **2013**, *27*, 2280–2288. [CrossRef] [PubMed]

18. Mercher, T.; Busson-Le Coniat, M.; Nguyen Khac, F.; Ballerini, P.; Mauchauffe, M.; Bui, H.; Pellegrino, B.; Radford, I.; Valensi, F.; Mugneret, F.; *et al.* Recurrence of OTT-MAL fusion in t(1;22) of infant AML-M7. *Genes Chromosomes Cancer* **2002**, *33*, 22–28. [CrossRef] [PubMed]

19. Von Bergh, A.R.; van Drunen, E.; van Wering, E.R.; van Zutven, L.J.; Hainmann, I.; Lonnerholm, G.; Meijerink, J.P.; Pieters, R.; Beverloo, H.B. High incidence of t(7;12)(q36;p13) in infant AML but not in infant ALL, with a dismal outcome and ectopic expression of HLXB9. *Genes Chromosomes Cancer* **2006**, *45*, 731–739. [CrossRef] [PubMed]

20. Abrahamsson, J.; Forestier, E.; Heldrup, J.; Jahnukainen, K.; Jonsson, O.G.; Lausen, B.; Palle, J.; Zeller, B.; Hasle, H. Response-guided induction therapy in pediatric acute myeloid leukemia with excellent remission rate. *J. Clin. Oncol.* **2011**, *29*, 310–315. [CrossRef] [PubMed]

21. Creutzig, U.Z.M.; Dworzak, M.; Bourquin, J.P.; Neuhoff, C.; Sander, A.; Stary, J.; Reinhardt, D. Study AML-BFM 2004: Improved Survival In Childhood Acute Myeloid Leukemia without Increased Toxicity. 2010. Available online: http://ash.confex.com/ash/2010/webprogram/Paper31036.html (accessed on 15 December 2014).

22. Entz-Werle, N.; Suciu, S.; van der Werff ten Bosch, J.; Vilmer, E.; Bertrand, Y.; Benoit, Y.; Margueritte, G.; Plouvier, E.; Boutard, P.; Vandecruys, E.; *et al.* Results of 58,872 and 58,921 trials in acute myeloblastic leukemia and relative value of chemotherapy *vs.* allogeneic bone marrow transplantation in first complete remission: The EORTC Children Leukemia Group report. *Leukemia* **2005**, *19*, 2072–2081. [CrossRef] [PubMed]

23. Gibson, B.E.; Wheatley, K.; Hann, I.M.; Stevens, R.F.; Webb, D.; Hills, R.K.; de Graaf, S.S.; Harrison, C.J. Treatment strategy and long-term results in paediatric patients treated in consecutive UK AML trials. *Leukemia* **2005**, *19*, 2130–2138. [CrossRef] [PubMed]

24. Perel, Y.; Auvrignon, A.; Leblanc, T.; Michel, G.; Reguerre, Y.; Vannier, J.P.; Dalle, J.H.; Gandemer, V.; Schmitt, C.; Mechinaud, F.; *et al.* Treatment of childhood acute myeloblastic leukemia: Dose intensification improves outcome and maintenance therapy is of no benefit—Multicenter studies of the French LAME (Leucemie Aigue Myeloblastique Enfant) Cooperative Group. *Leukemia* **2005**, *19*, 2082–2089. [CrossRef] [PubMed]

25. Pession, A.; Rondelli, R.; Basso, G.; Rizzari, C.; Testi, A.M.; Fagioli, F.; de Stefano, P.; Locatelli, F.; AML Strategy & Study Committee of the Associazione Italiana di Ematologia e Oncologia Pediatrica (AIEOP). Treatment and long-term results in children with acute myeloid leukaemia treated according to the AIEOP AML protocols. *Leukemia* **2005**, *19*, 2043–2053. [CrossRef] [PubMed]

26. Rubnitz, J.E.; Inaba, H.; Dahl, G.; Ribeiro, R.C.; Bowman, W.P.; Taub, J.; Pounds, S.; Razzouk, B.I.; Lacayo, N.J.; Cao, X.; *et al.* Minimal residual disease-directed therapy for childhood acute myeloid leukaemia: Results of the AML02 multicentre trial. *Lancet Oncol.* **2010**, *11*, 543–552. [CrossRef] [PubMed]

27. Tsukimoto, I.; Tawa, A.; Horibe, K.; Tabuchi, K.; Kigasawa, H.; Tsuchida, M.; Yabe, H.; Nakayama, H.; Kudo, K.; Kobayashi, R.; *et al.* Risk-stratified therapy and the intensive use of cytarabine improves the outcome in childhood acute myeloid leukemia: The AML99 trial from the Japanese Childhood AML Cooperative Study Group. *J. Clin. Oncol.* **2009**, *27*, 4007–4013. [CrossRef] [PubMed]
28. Creutzig, U.; Zimmermann, M.; Dworzak, M.N.; Ritter, J.; Schellong, G.; Reinhardt, D. Development of a curative treatment within the AML-BFM studies. *Klin. Padiatr.* **2013**, *225* (Suppl. S1), 79–86.
29. Horibe, K.; Saito, A.M.; Takimoto, T.; Tsuchida, M.; Manabe, A.; Shima, M.; Ohara, A.; Mizutani, S. Incidence and survival rates of hematological malignancies in Japanese children and adolescents (2006–2010): Based on registry data from the Japanese Society of Pediatric Hematology. *Int. J. Hematol.* **2013**, *98*, 74–88. [CrossRef] [PubMed]
30. Pession, A.; Masetti, R.; Rizzari, C.; Putti, M.C.; Casale, F.; Fagioli, F.; Luciani, M.; Lo Nigro, L.; Menna, G.; Micalizzi, C.; *et al.* Results of the AIEOP AML 2002/01 multicenter prospective trial for the treatment of children with acute myeloid leukemia. *Blood* **2013**, *122*, 170–178. [CrossRef] [PubMed]
31. Van der Velden, V.H.; van der Sluijs-Geling, A.; Gibson, B.E.; te Marvelde, J.G.; Hoogeveen, P.G.; Hop, W.C.; Wheatley, K.; Bierings, M.B.; Schuurhuis, G.J.; de Graaf, S.S.; *et al.* Clinical significance of flowcytometric minimal residual disease detection in pediatric acute myeloid leukemia patients treated according to the DCOG ANLL97/MRC AML12 protocol. *Leukemia* **2010**, *24*, 1599–1606. [CrossRef] [PubMed]
32. Becton, D.; Dahl, G.V.; Ravindranath, Y.; Chang, M.N.; Behm, F.G.; Raimondi, S.C.; Head, D.R.; Stine, K.C.; Lacayo, N.J.; Sikic, B.I.; *et al.* Randomized use of cyclosporin A (CsA) to modulate P-glycoprotein in children with AML in remission: Pediatric Oncology Group Study 9421. *Blood* **2006**, *107*, 1315–1324. [CrossRef] [PubMed]
33. Gibson, B.E.; Webb, D.K.; Howman, A.J.; de Graaf, S.S.; Harrison, C.J.; Wheatley, K.; United Kingdom Childhood Leukaemia Working Group; the Dutch Childhood Oncology Group. Results of a randomized trial in children with Acute Myeloid Leukaemia: Medical research council AML12 trial. *Br. J. Haematol.* **2011**, *155*, 366–376. [CrossRef] [PubMed]
34. Creutzig, U.; Zimmermann, M.; Bourquin, J.P.; Dworzak, M.N.; Fleischhack, G.; Graf, N.; Klingebiel, T.; Kremens, B.; Lehrnbecher, T.; von Neuhoff, C.; *et al.* Randomized trial comparing liposomal daunorubicin with idarubicin as induction for pediatric acute myeloid leukemia: Results from Study AML-BFM 2004. *Blood* **2013**, *122*, 37–43. [CrossRef] [PubMed]
35. Niewerth, D.; Creutzig, U.; Bierings, M.B.; Kaspers, G.J. A review on allogeneic stem cell transplantation for newly diagnosed pediatric acute myeloid leukemia. *Blood* **2010**, *116*, 2205–2214. [CrossRef] [PubMed]
36. Reinhardt, D.K.B.; Zimmermann, M.; Vormoor, J.; Dworzak, M.; Peters, C.; Creutzig, U.; Klingebiel, T. No Improvement of Overall-Survival in Children with High-Risk Acute Myeloid Leukemia by Stem Cell Transplantation in 1st Complete Remission. 2006. Available online: http://abstractshematologylibraryorg/cgi/content/short/108/11/320 (accessed on 15 December 2014).
37. Passweg, J.R.; Baldomero, H.; Peters, C.; Gaspar, H.B.; Cesaro, S.; Dreger, P.; Duarte, R.F.; Falkenburg, J.H.; Farge-Bancel, D.; Gennery, A.; *et al.* Hematopoietic SCT in Europe: Data and trends in 2012 with special consideration of pediatric transplantation. *Bone Marrow Transpl.* **2014**, *49*, 744–750. [CrossRef]
38. Bastos-Oreiro, M.; Perez-Corral, A.; Martinez-Laperche, C.; Bento, L.; Pascual, C.; Kwon, M.; Balsalobre, P.; Munoz, C.; Buces, E.; Serrano, D.; *et al.* Prognostic impact of minimal residual disease analysis by flow cytometry in patients with acute myeloid leukemia before and after allogeneic hemopoietic stem cell transplantation. *Eur. J. Haematol.* **2014**, *93*, 239–246. [PubMed]
39. Anthias, C.; Dignan, F.L.; Morilla, R.; Morilla, A.; Ethell, M.E.; Potter, M.N.; Shaw, B.E. Pre-transplant MRD predicts outcome following reduced-intensity and myeloablative allogeneic hemopoietic SCT in AML. *Bone Marrow Transpl.* **2014**, *49*, 679–683. [CrossRef]
40. Hasle, H. A critical review of which children with acute myeloid leukaemia need stem cell procedures. *Br. J. Haematol.* **2014**, *166*, 23–33. [CrossRef] [PubMed]
41. Sander, A.; Zimmermann, M.; Dworzak, M.; Fleischhack, G.; von Neuhoff, C.; Reinhardt, D.; Kaspers, G.J.; Creutzig, U. Consequent and intensified relapse therapy improved survival in pediatric AML: Results of relapse treatment in 379 patients of three consecutive AML-BFM trials. *Leukemia* **2010**, *24*, 1422–1428. [CrossRef] [PubMed]

42. Kaspers, G.J.; Zimmermann, M.; Reinhardt, D.; Gibson, B.E.; Tamminga, R.Y.; Aleinikova, O.; Armendariz, H.; Dworzak, M.; Ha, S.Y.; Hasle, H.; *et al.* Improved outcome in pediatric relapsed acute myeloid leukemia: Results of a randomized trial on liposomal daunorubicin by the International BFM Study Group. *J. Clin. Oncol.* **2013**, *31*, 599–607. [CrossRef] [PubMed]

43. Slats, A.M.; Egeler, R.M.; van der Does-van den Berg, A.; Korbijn, C.; Hahlen, K.; Kamps, W.A.; Veerman, A.J.; Zwaan, C.M. Causes of death—Other than progressive leukemia—In childhood acute lymphoblastic (ALL) and myeloid leukemia (AML): The Dutch Childhood Oncology Group experience. *Leukemia* **2005**, *19*, 537–544. [PubMed]

44. Kelly, L.M.; Gilliland, D.G. Genetics of myeloid leukemias. *Annu. Rev. Genomics Hum. Genet.* **2002**, *3*, 179–198. [CrossRef] [PubMed]

45. Ahmed, M.; Sternberg, A.; Hall, G.; Thomas, A.; Smith, O.; O'Marcaigh, A.; Wynn, R.; Stevens, R.; Addison, M.; King, D.; *et al.* Natural history of *GATA1* mutations in Down syndrome. *Blood* **2004**, *103*, 2480–2489. [CrossRef] [PubMed]

46. Hollink, I.H.; van den Heuvel-Eibrink, M.M.; Arentsen-Peters, S.T.; Zimmermann, M.; Peeters, J.K.; Valk, P.J.; Balgobind, B.V.; Sonneveld, E.; Kaspers, G.J.; de Bont, E.S.; *et al.* Characterization of CEBPA mutations and promoter hypermethylation in pediatric acute myeloid leukemia. *Haematologica* **2011**, *96*, 384–392. [CrossRef] [PubMed]

47. Hollink, I.H.; van den Heuvel-Eibrink, M.M.; Zimmermann, M.; Balgobind, B.V.; Arentsen-Peters, S.T.; Alders, M.; Willasch, A.; Kaspers, G.J.; Trka, J.; Baruchel, A.; *et al.* Clinical relevance of Wilms tumor 1 gene mutations in childhood acute myeloid leukemia. *Blood* **2009**, *113*, 5951–5960. [PubMed]

48. Balgobind, B.V.; Hollink, I.H.; Arentsen-Peters, S.T.; Zimmermann, M.; Harbott, J.; Beverloo, H.B.; von Bergh, A.R.; Cloos, J.; Kaspers, G.J.; de Haas, V.; *et al.* Integrative analysis of type-I and type-II aberrations underscores the genetic heterogeneity of pediatric acute myeloid leukemia. *Haematologica* **2011**, *96*, 1478–1487. [CrossRef] [PubMed]

49. Betts, D.R.; Ammann, R.A.; Hirt, A.; Hengartner, H.; Beck-Popovic, M.; Kuhne, T.; Nobile, L.; Caflisch, U.; Wacker, P.; Niggli, F.K. The prognostic significance of cytogenetic aberrations in childhood acute myeloid leukaemia. A study of the Swiss Paediatric Oncology Group (SPOG). *Eur. J. Haematol.* **2007**, *78*, 468–476. [CrossRef] [PubMed]

50. Grimwade, D. The clinical significance of cytogenetic abnormalities in acute myeloid leukaemia. *Best Pract. Res. Clin. Haematol.* **2001**, *14*, 497–529. [CrossRef] [PubMed]

51. Harrison, C.J.; Hills, R.K.; Moorman, A.V.; Grimwade, D.J.; Hann, I.; Webb, D.K.; Wheatley, K.; de Graaf, S.S.; van den Berg, E.; Burnett, A.K.; *et al.* Cytogenetics of childhood acute myeloid leukemia: United Kingdom Medical Research Council Treatment trials AML 10 and 12. *J. Clin. Oncol.* **2010**, *28*, 2674–2681. [CrossRef] [PubMed]

52. Von Neuhoff, C.; Reinhardt, D.; Sander, A.; Zimmermann, M.; Bradtke, J.; Betts, D.R.; Zemanova, Z.; Stary, J.; Bourquin, J.P.; Haas, O.A.; *et al.* Prognostic impact of specific chromosomal aberrations in a large group of pediatric patients with acute myeloid leukemia treated uniformly according to trial AML-BFM 98. *J. Clin. Oncol.* **2010**, *28*, 2682–2689.

53. Park, J.; Kim, M.; Lim, J.; Kim, Y.; Han, K.; Lee, J.; Chung, N.G.; Cho, B.; Kim, H.K. Three-way complex translocations in infant acute myeloid leukemia with t(7;12)(q36;p13): The incidence and correlation of a *HLXB9* overexpression. *Cancer Genet. Cytogenet.* **2009**, *191*, 102–105. [CrossRef] [PubMed]

54. Simmons, H.M.; Oseth, L.; Nguyen, P.; O'Leary, M.; Conklin, K.F.; Hirsch, B. Cytogenetic and molecular heterogeneity of 7q36/12p13 rearrangements in childhood AML. *Leukemia* **2002**, *16*, 2408–2416. [CrossRef] [PubMed]

55. Slater, R.M.; von Drunen, E.; Kroes, W.G.; Weghuis, D.O.; van den Berg, E.; Smit, E.M.; van der Does-van den Berg, A.; van Wering, E.; Hahlen, K.; Carroll, A.J.; *et al.* t(7;12)(q36;p13) and t(7;12)(q32;p13)—Translocations involving ETV6 in children 18 months of age or younger with myeloid disorders. *Leukemia* **2001**, *15*, 915–920. [CrossRef] [PubMed]

56. Torres, L.; Lisboa, S.; Vieira, J.; Cerveira, N.; Santos, J.; Pinheiro, M.; Correia, C.; Bizarro, S.; Almeida, M.; Teixeira, M.R. Acute megakaryoblastic leukemia with a four-way variant translocation originating the RBM15-MKL1 fusion gene. *Blood Cancer* **2011**, *56*, 846–849. [CrossRef]

57. Hollink, I.H.; van den Heuvel-Eibrink, M.M.; Arentsen-Peters, S.T.; Pratcorona, M.; Abbas, S.; Kuipers, J.E.; van Galen, J.F.; Beverloo, H.B.; Sonneveld, E.; Kaspers, G.J.; *et al.* NUP98/NSD1 characterizes a novel poor prognostic group in acute myeloid leukemia with a distinct *HOX* gene expression pattern. *Blood* **2011**, *118*, 3645–3656. [CrossRef] [PubMed]

58. Meyer, C.; Kowarz, E.; Hofmann, J.; Renneville, A.; Zuna, J.; Trka, J.; Ben Abdelali, R.; Macintyre, E.; De Braekeleer, E.; De Braekeleer, M.; *et al.* New insights to the MLL recombinome of acute leukemias. *Leukemia* **2009**, *23*, 1490–1499. [CrossRef] [PubMed]

59. Meyer, C.; Hofmann, J.; Burmeister, T.; Groger, D.; Park, T.S.; Emerenciano, M.; Pombo de Oliveira, M.; Renneville, A.; Villarese, P.; Macintyre, E.; *et al.* The MLL recombinome of acute leukemias in 2013. *Leukemia* **2013**, *27*, 2165–2176. [CrossRef] [PubMed]

60. Bernt, K.M.; Zhu, N.; Sinha, A.U.; Vempati, S.; Faber, J.; Krivtsov, A.V.; Feng, Z.; Punt, N.; Daigle, A.; Bullinger, L.; *et al.* MLL-rearranged leukemia is dependent on aberrant H3K79 methylation by DOT1L. *Cancer Cell* **2011**, *20*, 66–78. [CrossRef] [PubMed]

61. Marschalek, R. Mechanisms of leukemogenesis by MLL fusion proteins. *Br. J. Haematol.* **2011**, *152*, 141–154. [CrossRef] [PubMed]

62. Marcucci, G.; Haferlach, T.; Dohner, H. Molecular genetics of adult acute myeloid leukemia: Prognostic and therapeutic implications. *J. Clin. Oncol.* **2011**, *29*, 475–486. [CrossRef] [PubMed]

63. Ley, T.J.; Ding, L.; Walter, M.J.; McLellan, M.D.; Lamprecht, T.; Larson, D.E.; Kandoth, C.; Payton, J.E.; Baty, J.; Welch, J.; *et al.* DNMT3A mutations in acute myeloid leukemia. *N. Engl. J. Med.* **2010**, *363*, 2424–2433. [CrossRef] [PubMed]

64. Figueroa, M.E.; Abdel-Wahab, O.; Lu, C.; Ward, P.S.; Patel, J.; Shih, A.; Li, Y.; Bhagwat, N.; Vasanthakumar, A.; Fernandez, H.F.; *et al.* Leukemic *IDH1* and *IDH2* mutations result in a hypermethylation phenotype, disrupt TET2 function, and impair hematopoietic differentiation. *Cancer Cell* **2010**, *18*, 553–567. [CrossRef] [PubMed]

65. Delhommeau, F.; Dupont, S.; Della Valle, V.; James, C.; Trannoy, S.; Masse, A.; Kosmider, O.; Le Couedic, J.P.; Robert, F.; Alberdi, A.; *et al.* Mutation in TET2 in myeloid cancers. *N. Engl. J. Med.* **2009**, *360*, 2289–2301. [CrossRef] [PubMed]

66. Hollink, I.H.; Feng, Q.; Danen-van Oorschot, A.A.; Arentsen-Peters, S.T.; Verboon, L.J.; Zhang, P.; de Haas, V.; Reinhardt, D.; Creutzig, U.; Trka, J.; *et al.* Low frequency of *DNMT3A* mutations in pediatric AML, and the identification of the OCI-AML3 cell line as an *in vitro* model. *Leukemia* **2012**, *26*, 371–373. [CrossRef] [PubMed]

67. Langemeijer, S.M.; Jansen, J.H.; Hooijer, J.; van Hoogen, P.; Stevens-Linders, E.; Massop, M.; Waanders, E.; van Reijmersdal, S.V.; Stevens-Kroef, M.J.; Zwaan, C.M.; *et al.* TET2 mutations in childhood leukemia. *Leukemia* **2011**, *25*, 189–192. [CrossRef] [PubMed]

68. Ho, P.A.; Alonzo, T.A.; Kopecky, K.J.; Miller, K.L.; Kuhn, J.; Zeng, R.; Gerbing, R.B.; Raimondi, S.C.; Hirsch, B.A.; Oehler, V.; *et al.* Molecular alterations of the *IDH1* gene in AML: A Children's Oncology Group and Southwest Oncology Group study. *Leukemia* **2010**, *24*, 909–913. [CrossRef] [PubMed]

69. Yan, X.J.; Xu, J.; Gu, Z.H.; Pan, C.M.; Lu, G.; Shen, Y.; Shi, J.Y.; Zhu, Y.M.; Tang, L.; Zhang, X.W.; *et al.* Exome sequencing identifies somatic mutations of DNA methyltransferase gene *DNMT3A* in acute monocytic leukemia. *Nat. Genet.* **2011**, *43*, 309–315. [CrossRef] [PubMed]

70. Valerio, D.G.; Katsman-Kuipers, J.E.; Jansen, J.H.; Verboon, L.J.; de Haas, V.; Stary, J.; Baruchel, A.; Zimmermann, M.; Pieters, R.; Reinhardt, D.; *et al.* Mapping epigenetic regulator gene mutations in cytogenetically normal pediatric acute myeloid leukemia. *Haematologica* **2014**, *99*. [CrossRef]

71. Mardis, E.R.; Ding, L.; Dooling, D.J.; Larson, D.E.; McLellan, M.D.; Chen, K.; Koboldt, D.C.; Fulton, R.S.; Delehaunty, K.D.; McGrath, S.D.; *et al.* Recurring mutations found by sequencing an acute myeloid leukemia genome. *N. Engl. J. Med.* **2009**, *361*, 1058–1066. [CrossRef] [PubMed]

72. Stumpel, D.J.; Schneider, P.; van Roon, E.H.; Boer, J.M.; de Lorenzo, P.; Valsecchi, M.G.; de Menezes, R.X.; Pieters, R.; Stam, R.W. Specific promoter methylation identifies different subgroups of MLL-rearranged infant acute lymphoblastic leukemia, influences clinical outcome, and provides therapeutic options. *Blood* **2009**, *114*, 5490–5498. [CrossRef] [PubMed]

73. Krzywinski, M.; Schein, J.; Birol, I.; Connors, J.; Gascoyne, R.; Horsman, D.; Jones, S.J.; Marra, M.A. Circos: An information aesthetic for comparative genomics. *Genome Res.* **2009**, *19*, 1639–1645. [CrossRef] [PubMed]

74. Imamura, T.; Iwamoto, S.; Kanai, R.; Shimada, A.; Terui, K.; Osugi, Y.; Kobayashi, R.; Tawa, A.; Kosaka, Y.; Kato, K.; *et al.* Outcome in 146 patients with paediatric acute myeloid leukaemia treated according to the AML99 protocol in the period 2003–06 from the Japan Association of Childhood Leukaemia Study. *Br. J. Haematol.* **2012**, *159*, 204–210. [CrossRef] [PubMed]

75. Cooper, T.M.; Franklin, J.; Gerbing, R.B.; Alonzo, T.A.; Hurwitz, C.; Raimondi, S.C.; Hirsch, B.; Smith, F.O.; Mathew, P.; Arceci, R.J.; *et al.* AAML03P1, a pilot study of the safety of gemtuzumab ozogamicin in combination with chemotherapy for newly diagnosed childhood acute myeloid leukemia: A report from the Children's Oncology Group. *Cancer* **2012**, *118*, 761–769. [CrossRef] [PubMed]

76. Dluzniewska, A.; Balwierz, W.; Armata, J.; Balcerska, A.; Chybicka, A.; Kowalczyk, J.; Matysiak, M.; Ochocka, M.; Radwanska, U.; Rokicka-Milewska, R.; *et al.* Twenty years of Polish experience with three consecutive protocols for treatment of childhood acute myelogenous leukemia. *Leukemia* **2005**, *19*, 2117–2124. [CrossRef] [PubMed]

77. Bachas, C.; Schuurhuis, G.J.; Reinhardt, D.; Creutzig, U.; Kwidama, Z.J.; Zwaan, C.M.; van den Heuvel-Eibrink, M.M.; de Bont, E.S.; Elitzur, S.; Rizzari, C.; *et al.* Clinical relevance of molecular aberrations in paediatric acute myeloid leukaemia at first relapse. *Br. J. Haematol.* **2014**, *166*, 902–910. [CrossRef] [PubMed]

78. Creutzig, U.; Zimmermann, M.; Dworzak, M.N.; Gibson, B.; Tamminga, R.; Abrahamsson, J.; Ha, S.Y.; Hasle, H.; Maschan, A.; Bertrand, Y.; *et al.* The prognostic significance of early treatment response in pediatric relapsed acute myeloid leukemia: Results of the international study Relapsed AML 2001/01. *Haematologica* **2014**, *99*, 1472–1478. [CrossRef] [PubMed]

79. Rubnitz, J.E.; Raimondi, S.C.; Halbert, A.R.; Tong, X.; Srivastava, D.K.; Razzouk, B.I.; Pui, C.H.; Downing, J.R.; Ribeiro, R.C.; Behm, F.G. Characteristics and outcome of t(8;21)-positive childhood acute myeloid leukemia: A single institution's experience. *Leukemia* **2002**, *16*, 2072–2077. [CrossRef] [PubMed]

80. Balgobind, B.V.; Raimondi, S.C.; Harbott, J.; Zimmermann, M.; Alonzo, T.A.; Auvrignon, A.; Beverloo, H.B.; Chang, M.; Creutzig, U.; Dworzak, M.N.; *et al.* Novel prognostic subgroups in childhood 11q23/MLL-rearranged acute myeloid leukemia: Results of an international retrospective study. *Blood* **2009**, *114*, 2489–2496. [CrossRef] [PubMed]

81. Coenen, E.A.; Raimondi, S.C.; Harbott, J.; Zimmermann, M.; Alonzo, T.A.; Auvrignon, A.; Beverloo, H.B.; Chang, M.; Creutzig, U.; Dworzak, M.N.; *et al.* Prognostic significance of additional cytogenetic aberrations in 733 *de novo* pediatric 11q23/MLL-rearranged AML patients: Results of an international study. *Blood* **2011**, *117*, 7102–7111. [CrossRef] [PubMed]

82. Hasle, H.; Alonzo, T.A.; Auvrignon, A.; Behar, C.; Chang, M.; Creutzig, U.; Fischer, A.; Forestier, E.; Fynn, A.; Haas, O.A.; *et al.* Monosomy 7 and deletion 7q in children and adolescents with acute myeloid leukemia: An international retrospective study. *Blood* **2007**, *109*, 4641–4647. [CrossRef] [PubMed]

83. Johnston, D.L.; Alonzo, T.A.; Gerbing, R.B.; Hirsch, B.; Heerema, N.A.; Ravindranath, Y.; Woods, W.G.; Lange, B.J.; Gamis, A.S.; Raimondi, S.C. Outcome of pediatric patients with acute myeloid leukemia (AML) and -5/5q- abnormalities from five pediatric AML treatment protocols: A report from the Children's Oncology Group. *Pediatr. Blood Cancer* **2013**, *60*, 2073–2078. [PubMed]

84. Kelly, M.J.; Horan, J.T.; Alonzo, T.A.; Eapen, M.; Gerbing, R.B.; He, W.; Lange, B.J.; Parsons, S.K.; Woods, W.G. Comparable survival for pediatric acute myeloid leukemia with poor-risk cytogenetics following chemotherapy, matched related donor, or unrelated donor transplantation. *Pediatr. Blood Cancer* **2014**, *61*, 269–275. [CrossRef] [PubMed]

85. Manola, K.N.; Panitsas, F.; Polychronopoulou, S.; Daraki, A.; Karakosta, M.; Stavropoulou, C.; Avgerinou, G.; Hatzipantelis, E.; Pantelias, G.; Sambani, C.; *et al.* Cytogenetic abnormalities and monosomal karyotypes in children and adolescents with acute myeloid leukemia: Correlations with clinical characteristics and outcome. *Cancer Genet.* **2013**, *206*, 63–72. [CrossRef] [PubMed]

86. Balgobind, B.V.; Lugthart, S.; Hollink, I.H.; Arentsen-Peters, S.T.; van Wering, E.R.; de Graaf, S.S.; Reinhardt, D.; Creutzig, U.; Kaspers, G.J.; de Bont, E.S.; *et al.* EVI1 overexpression in distinct subtypes of pediatric acute myeloid leukemia. *Leukemia* **2010**, *24*, 942–949. [CrossRef] [PubMed]

87. Groschel, S.; Lugthart, S.; Schlenk, R.F.; Valk, P.J.; Eiwen, K.; Goudswaard, C.; van Putten, W.J.; Kayser, S.; Verdonck, L.F.; Lubbert, M.; *et al.* High EVI1 expression predicts outcome in younger adult patients with acute myeloid leukemia and is associated with distinct cytogenetic abnormalities. *J. Clin. Oncol.* **2010**, *28*, 2101–2107. [CrossRef] [PubMed]

88. Bachas, C.; Schuurhuis, G.J.; Hollink, I.H.; Kwidama, Z.J.; Goemans, B.F.; Zwaan, C.M.; van den Heuvel-Eibrink, M.M.; de Bont, E.S.; Reinhardt, D.; Creutzig, U.; *et al.* High-frequency type I/II mutational shifts between diagnosis and relapse are associated with outcome in pediatric AML: Implications for personalized medicine. *Blood* **2010**, *116*, 2752–2758. [CrossRef] [PubMed]

89. Hollink, I.H.; Zwaan, C.M.; Zimmermann, M.; Arentsen-Peters, T.C.; Pieters, R.; Cloos, J.; Kaspers, G.J.; de Graaf, S.S.; Harbott, J.; Creutzig, U.; *et al.* Favorable prognostic impact of *NPM1* gene mutations in childhood acute myeloid leukemia, with emphasis on cytogenetically normal AML. *Leukemia* **2009**, *23*, 262–270. [CrossRef] [PubMed]

90. Raghavan, M.; Lillington, D.M.; Skoulakis, S.; Debernardi, S.; Chaplin, T.; Foot, N.J.; Lister, T.A.; Young, B.D. Genome-wide single nucleotide polymorphism analysis reveals frequent partial uniparental disomy due to somatic recombination in acute myeloid leukemias. *Cancer Res.* **2005**, *65*, 375–378. [PubMed]

91. Balgobind, B.V.; van Vlierberghe, P.; van den Ouweland, A.M.; Beverloo, H.B.; Terlouw-Kromosoeto, J.N.; van Wering, E.R.; Reinhardt, D.; Horstmann, M.; Kaspers, G.J.; Pieters, R.; *et al.* Leukemia-associated NF1 inactivation in patients with pediatric T-ALL and AML lacking evidence for neurofibromatosis. *Blood* **2008**, *111*, 4322–4328. [CrossRef] [PubMed]

92. Balgobind, B.V.; Van den Heuvel-Eibrink, M.M.; De Menezes, R.X.; Reinhardt, D.; Hollink, I.H.; Arentsen-Peters, S.T.; van Wering, E.R.; Kaspers, G.J.; Cloos, J.; de Bont, E.S.; *et al.* Evaluation of gene expression signatures predictive of cytogenetic and molecular subtypes of pediatric acute myeloid leukemia. *Haematologica* **2011**, *96*, 221–230. [CrossRef] [PubMed]

93. Ross, M.E.; Mahfouz, R.; Onciu, M.; Liu, H.C.; Zhou, X.; Song, G.; Shurtleff, S.A.; Pounds, S.; Cheng, C.; Ma, J.; *et al.* Gene expression profiling of pediatric acute myelogenous leukemia. *Blood* **2004**, *104*, 3679–3687. [CrossRef] [PubMed]

94. Valk, P.J.; Verhaak, R.G.; Beijen, M.A.; Barjesteh van Waalwijk van Doorn-Khosrovani, S.; Erpelinck, C.A.; Boer, J.M.; Beverloo, H.B.; Moorhouse, M.J.; van der Spek, P.J.; Lowenberg, B.; *et al.* Prognostically useful gene-expression profiles in acute myeloid leukemia. *N. Engl. J. Med.* **2004**, *350*, 1617–1628. [CrossRef] [PubMed]

95. Wouters, B.J.; Jorda, M.A.; Keeshan, K.; Louwers, I.; Erpelinck-Verschueren, C.A.; Tielemans, D.; Langerak, A.W.; He, Y.; Yashiro-Ohtani, Y.; Zhang, P.; *et al.* Distinct gene expression profiles of acute myeloid/T-lymphoid leukemia with silenced CEBPA and mutations in NOTCH1. *Blood* **2007**, *110*, 3706–3714. [CrossRef] [PubMed]

96. Balgobind, B.V.; Zwaan, C.M.; Reinhardt, D.; Arentsen-Peters, T.J.; Hollink, I.H.; de Haas, V.; Kaspers, G.J.; de Bont, E.S.; Baruchel, A.; Stary, J.; *et al.* High BRE expression in pediatric MLL-rearranged AML is associated with favorable outcome. *Leukemia* **2010**, *24*, 2048–2055. [CrossRef] [PubMed]

97. Kuipers, J.E.; Coenen, E.A.; Balgobind, B.V.; Stary, J.; Baruchel, A.; de Haas, V.; de Bont, E.S.; Reinhardt, D.; Kaspers, G.J.; Cloos, J.; *et al.* High IGSF4 expression in pediatric M5 acute myeloid leukemia with t(9;11)(p22;q23). *Blood* **2011**, *117*, 928–935. [CrossRef] [PubMed]

98. Ding, L.; Ley, T.J.; Larson, D.E.; Miller, C.A.; Koboldt, D.C.; Welch, J.S.; Ritchey, J.K.; Young, M.A.; Lamprecht, T.; McLellan, M.D.; *et al.* Clonal evolution in relapsed acute myeloid leukaemia revealed by whole-genome sequencing. *Nature* **2012**, *481*, 506–510. [CrossRef] [PubMed]

99. Meshinchi, S.R.R.; Trevino, L.R.; Hampton, O.A.; Alonzo, T.A.; Farrar, J.E.; Guidry Auvil, J.M.; Davidsen, T.M.; Gesuwan, P.; Muzny, D.M.; Gamis, A.S.; *et al.* Identification of Novel Somatic Mutations, Regions of Recurrent Loss of Heterozygosity (LOH) and Significant Clonal Evolution From Diagnosis to Relapse in Childhood AML Determined by Exome Capture Sequencing-an NCI/COG Target AML Study. 2012. Available online: https://ash.confex.com/ash/2012/webprogram/Paper51517.html (accessed on 15 December 2014).

100. Kohlmann, A.M.G.; Hofmann, W.-K.; Kronnie, G.; Chiaretti, C.; Preudhomme, C.; Tagliafico, E.; Hernandez, J.; Gabriel, C.; Lion, T.; Vandenberghe, P.; *et al.* The Interlaboratory Robustness of Next-Generation Sequencing (IRON) Study Phase II: Deep-Sequencing Analyses of Hematological Malignancies Performed by an International Network Involving 26 Laboratories. 2012. Available online: https://ash.confex.com/ash/2012/webprogram/Paper49866.html (accessed on 15 December 2014).

101. Kohlmann, A.W.S.; Schoeck, U.; Grossmann, V.; Kern, W.; Haferlach, C.; Schnittger, S.; Haferlach, T. First Results of a 31-Gene Panel Targeted to Investigate Myeloid Malignancies by Next-Generation Amplicon Deep-Sequencing. 2012. Available online: https://ash.confex.com/ash/2012/webprogram/Paper48970.html (accessed on 15 December 2014).

102. Figueroa, M.E.; Lugthart, S.; Li, Y.; Erpelinck-Verschueren, C.; Deng, X.; Christos, P.J.; Schifano, E.; Booth, J.; van Putten, W.; Skrabanek, L.; *et al.* DNA methylation signatures identify biologically distinct subtypes in acute myeloid leukemia. *Cancer Cell* **2010**, *17*, 13–27. [CrossRef] [PubMed]

103. Juhl-Christensen, C.; Ommen, H.B.; Aggerholm, A.; Lausen, B.; Kjeldsen, E.; Hasle, H.; Hokland, P. Genetic and epigenetic similarities and differences between childhood and adult AML. *Pediatr Blood Cancer* **2012**, *58*, 525–531. [CrossRef] [PubMed]

104. Lu, J.; Getz, G.; Miska, E.A.; Alvarez-Saavedra, E.; Lamb, J.; Peck, D.; Sweet-Cordero, A.; Ebert, B.L.; Mak, R.H.; Ferrando, A.A.; *et al.* MicroRNA expression profiles classify human cancers. *Nature* **2005**, *435*, 834–838. [CrossRef] [PubMed]

105. Jongen-Lavrencic, M.; Sun, S.M.; Dijkstra, M.K.; Valk, P.J.; Lowenberg, B. MicroRNA expression profiling in relation to the genetic heterogeneity of acute myeloid leukemia. *Blood* **2008**, *111*, 5078–5085. [CrossRef] [PubMed]

106. Garzon, R.; Volinia, S.; Liu, C.G.; Fernandez-Cymering, C.; Palumbo, T.; Pichiorri, F.; Fabbri, M.; Coombes, K.; Alder, H.; Nakamura, T.; *et al.* MicroRNA signatures associated with cytogenetics and prognosis in acute myeloid leukemia. *Blood* **2008**, *111*, 3183–3189. [CrossRef] [PubMed]

107. Debernardi, S.; Skoulakis, S.; Molloy, G.; Chaplin, T.; Dixon-McIver, A.; Young, B.D. MicroRNA miR-181a correlates with morphological sub-class of acute myeloid leukaemia and the expression of its target genes in global genome-wide analysis. *Leukemia* **2007**, *21*, 912–916. [PubMed]

108. Danen-van Oorschot, A.A.; Kuipers, J.E.; Arentsen-Peters, S.; Schotte, D.; de Haas, V.; Trka, J.; Baruchel, A.; Reinhardt, D.; Pieters, R.; Zwaan, C.M.; *et al.* Differentially expressed miRNAs in cytogenetic and molecular subtypes of pediatric acute myeloid leukemia. *Pediatr. Blood Cancer* **2012**, *58*, 715–721. [CrossRef] [PubMed]

109. Zarrinkar, P.P.; Gunawardane, R.N.; Cramer, M.D.; Gardner, M.F.; Brigham, D.; Belli, B.; Karaman, M.W.; Pratz, K.W.; Pallares, G.; Chao, Q.; *et al.* AC220 is a uniquely potent and selective inhibitor of FLT3 for the treatment of acute myeloid leukemia (AML). *Blood* **2009**, *114*, 2984–2992. [CrossRef] [PubMed]

110. Inaba, H.; Rubnitz, J.E.; Coustan-Smith, E.; Li, L.; Furmanski, B.D.; Mascara, G.P.; Heym, K.M.; Christensen, R.; Onciu, M.; Shurtleff, S.A.; *et al.* Phase I pharmacokinetic and pharmacodynamic study of the multikinase inhibitor sorafenib in combination with clofarabine and cytarabine in pediatric relapsed/refractory leukemia. *J. Clin. Oncol.* **2011**, *29*, 3293–3300. [CrossRef] [PubMed]

111. Watt, T.C.; Cooper, T. Sorafenib as treatment for relapsed or refractory pediatric acute myelogenous leukemia. *Pediatr. Blood Cancer* **2012**, *59*, 756–757. [CrossRef] [PubMed]

112. Levis, M.; Ravandi, F.; Wang, E.S.; Baer, M.R.; Perl, A.; Coutre, S.; Erba, H.; Stuart, R.K.; Baccarani, M.; Cripe, L.D.; *et al.* Results from a randomized trial of salvage chemotherapy followed by lestaurtinib for patients with FLT3 mutant AML in first relapse. *Blood* **2011**, *117*, 3294–3301. [CrossRef] [PubMed]

113. Smith, C.C.; Wang, Q.; Chin, C.S.; Salerno, S.; Damon, L.E.; Levis, M.J.; Perl, A.E.; Travers, K.J.; Wang, S.; Hunt, J.P.; *et al.* Validation of *ITD* mutations in FLT3 as a therapeutic target in human acute myeloid leukaemia. *Nature* **2012**, *485*, 260–263. [CrossRef] [PubMed]

114. The world's chilhood cancer experts. Available online: http://www.childrensoncologygroup.org/index.php/aaml1031 (accessed on 15 December 2014).

115. Goemans, B.F.; Zwaan, C.M.; Miller, M.; Zimmermann, M.; Harlow, A.; Meshinchi, S.; Loonen, A.H.; Hahlen, K.; Reinhardt, D.; Creutzig, U.; *et al.* Mutations in KIT and RAS are frequent events in pediatric core-binding factor acute myeloid leukemia. *Leukemia* **2005**, *19*, 1536–1542. [CrossRef] [PubMed]

116. Zwaan, C.M.; Rizzari, C.; Mechinaud, F.; Lancaster, D.L.; Lehrnbecher, T.; van der Velden, V.H.; Beverloo, B.B.; den Boer, M.L.; Pieters, R.; Reinhardt, D.; *et al.* Dasatinib in children and adolescents with relapsed or refractory leukemia: Results of the CA180–018 phase I dose-escalation study of the Innovative Therapies for Children with Cancer Consortium. *J. Clin. Oncol.* **2013**, *31*, 2460–2468. [CrossRef] [PubMed]

117. Marcucci, G.G.S.; Zhao, J.; Carrol, A.J.; Bucci, D.; Vij, R.; Blum, W.; Pardee, T.; Wetzler, M.; Stock, W.; Bloomfield, C.D.; *et al.* Adding The KIT Inhibitor Dasatinib (DAS) To Standard Induction and Consolidation Therapy For Newly Diagnosed Patients (pts) With Core Binding Factor (CBF) Acute Myeloid Leukemia (AML): Initial Results Of The CALGB 10801 (Alliance) Study. 2013. Available online: https://ash.confex.com/ash/2013/webprogram/Paper63516.html (accessed on 15 December 2014).

118. Burnett, A.K.; Russell, N.H.; Culligan, D.; Cavanagh, J.; Kell, J.; Wheatley, K.; Virchis, A.; Hills, R.K.; Milligan, D.; Institute AMLWGotUNCR. The addition of the farnesyl transferase inhibitor, tipifarnib, to low dose cytarabine does not improve outcome for older patients with AML. *Br. J. Haematol.* **2012**, *158*, 519–522. [CrossRef] [PubMed]

119. Lamba, S.; Russo, M.; Sun, C.; Lazzari, L.; Cancelliere, C.; Grernrum, W.; Lieftink, C.; Bernards, R.; di Nicolantonio, F.; Bardelli, A. RAF Suppression Synergizes with MEK Inhibition in KRAS Mutant Cancer Cells. *Cell Rep.* **2014**, *8*, 1475–1483. [CrossRef] [PubMed]

120. Sun, C.; Hobor, S.; Bertotti, A.; Zecchin, D.; Huang, S.; Galimi, F.; Cottino, F.; Prahallad, A.; Grernrum, W.; Tzani, A.; *et al.* Intrinsic resistance to MEK inhibition in KRAS mutant lung and colon cancer through transcriptional induction of ERBB3. *Cell Rep.* **2014**, *7*, 86–93. [CrossRef] [PubMed]

121. Deshpande, A.J.; Chen, L.; Fazio, M.; Sinha, A.U.; Bernt, K.M.; Banka, D.; Dias, S.; Chang, J.; Olhava, E.J.; Daigle, S.R.; *et al.* Leukemic transformation by the MLL-AF6 fusion oncogene requires the H3K79 methyltransferase Dot1l. *Blood* **2013**, *121*, 2533–2541. [CrossRef] [PubMed]

122. O'Hear, C.; Inaba, H.; Pounds, S.; Shi, L.; Dahl, G.; Bowman, W.P.; Taub, J.W.; Pui, C.H.; Ribeiro, R.C.; Coustan-Smith, E.; *et al.* Gemtuzumab ozogamicin can reduce minimal residual disease in patients with childhood acute myeloid leukemia. *Cancer* **2013**, *119*, 4036–4043. [CrossRef] [PubMed]

123. Petersdorf, S.H.; Kopecky, K.J.; Slovak, M.; Willman, C.; Nevill, T.; Brandwein, J.; Larson, R.A.; Erba, H.P.; Stiff, P.J.; Stuart, R.K.; *et al.* A phase 3 study of gemtuzumab ozogamicin during induction and postconsolidation therapy in younger patients with acute myeloid leukemia. *Blood* **2013**, *121*, 4854–4860. [CrossRef] [PubMed]

124. Zwaan, C.M.; Reinhardt, D.; Zimmerman, M.; Hasle, H.; Stary, J.; Stark, B.; Dworzak, M.; Creutzig, U.; Kaspers, G.J.; International BFMSGoPAML. Salvage treatment for children with refractory first or second relapse of acute myeloid leukaemia with gemtuzumab ozogamicin: Results of a phase II study. *Br. J. Haematol.* **2010**, *148*, 768–776. [CrossRef] [PubMed]

125. Hasle, H.; Abrahamsson, J.; Forestier, E.; Ha, S.Y.; Heldrup, J.; Jahnukainen, K.; Jonsson, O.G.; Lausen, B.; Palle, J.; Zeller, B.; *et al.* Gemtuzumab ozogamicin as postconsolidation therapy does not prevent relapse in children with AML: Results from NOPHO-AML 2004. *Blood* **2012**, *120*, 978–984. [CrossRef] [PubMed]

126. Jeha, S.; Razzouk, B.; Rytting, M.; Rheingold, S.; Albano, E.; Kadota, R.; Luchtman-Jones, L.; Bomgaars, L.; Gaynon, P.; Goldman, S.; *et al.* Phase II study of clofarabine in pediatric patients with refractory or relapsed acute myeloid leukemia. *J. Clin. Oncol.* **2009**, *27*, 4392–4397. [CrossRef] [PubMed]

127. Cooper, T.M.; Alonzo, T.A.; Gerbing, R.B.; Perentesis, J.P.; Whitlock, J.A.; Taub, J.W.; Horton, T.M.; Gamis, A.S.; Meshinchi, S.; Loken, M.R.; *et al.* AAML0523: A report from the Children's Oncology Group on the efficacy of clofarabine in combination with cytarabine in pediatric patients with recurrent acute myeloid leukemia. *Cancer* **2014**, *120*, 2482–2489. [CrossRef] [PubMed]

128. Hijiya, N.; Thomson, B.; Isakoff, M.S.; Silverman, L.B.; Steinherz, P.G.; Borowitz, M.J.; Kadota, R.; Cooper, T.; Shen, V.; Dahl, G.; *et al.* Phase 2 trial of clofarabine in combination with etoposide and cyclophosphamide in pediatric patients with refractory or relapsed acute lymphoblastic leukemia. *Blood* **2011**, *118*, 6043–6049. [CrossRef] [PubMed]

129. Shukla, N.; Kobos, R.; Renaud, T.; Steinherz, L.J.; Steinherz, P.G. Phase II trial of clofarabine with topotecan, vinorelbine, and thiotepa in pediatric patients with relapsed or refractory acute leukemia. *Pediatr. Blood Cancer* **2014**, *61*, 431–435. [CrossRef] [PubMed]

130. Leonard, S.M.; Perry, T.; Woodman, C.B.; Kearns, P. Sequential treatment with cytarabine and decitabine has an increased anti-leukemia effect compared to cytarabine alone in xenograft models of childhood acute myeloid leukemia. *PLoS One* **2014**, *9*, e87475. [CrossRef] [PubMed]

131. Phillips, C.L.; Davies, S.M.; McMasters, R.; Absalon, M.; O'Brien, M.; Mo, J.; Broun, R.; Moscow, J.A.; Smolarek, T.; Garzon, R.; *et al.* Low dose decitabine in very high risk relapsed or refractory acute myeloid leukaemia in children and young adults. *Br. J. Haematol.* **2013**, *161*, 406–410. [CrossRef] [PubMed]

132. Lee, Y.G.; Kim, I.; Yoon, S.S.; Park, S.; Cheong, J.W.; Min, Y.H.; Lee, J.O.; Bang, S.M.; Yi, H.G.; Kim, C.S.; *et al.* Comparative analysis between azacitidine and decitabine for the treatment of myelodysplastic syndromes. *Br. J. Haematol.* **2013**, *161*, 339–347. [CrossRef] [PubMed]

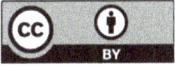

Journal of
Clinical Medicine

MDPI

Review

Effects of T-Cell Depletion on Allogeneic Hematopoietic Stem Cell Transplantation Outcomes in AML Patients

Gabriela Soriano Hobbs [1,2] and Miguel-Angel Perales [3,4,*]

1   Adult Leukemia Service, Massachusetts General Hospital, Boston, MA 02114 USA; ghobbs@partners.org
2   Harvard Medical School, Boston, MA 02115, USA
3   Adult Bone Marrow Transplantation Service, Memorial Sloan Kettering Cancer Center, New York, NY 10065, USA
4   Weill Cornell Medical College, New York, NY 10065, USA
*   Author to whom correspondence should be addressed; peralesm@mskcc.org; Tel.: +1-212-639-8682; Fax: +1-212-717-3500.

Academic Editor: Celalettin Ustun
Received: 7 September 2014; Accepted: 19 January 2015; Published: 19 March 2015

Abstract: Graft *versus* host disease (GVHD) remains one of the leading causes of morbidity and mortality associated with conventional allogeneic hematopoietic stem cell transplantation (HCT). The use of T-cell depletion significantly reduces this complication. Recent prospective and retrospective data suggest that, in patients with AML in first complete remission, CD34+ selected grafts afford overall and relapse-free survival comparable to those observed in recipients of conventional grafts, while significantly decreasing GVHD. In addition, CD34+ selected grafts allow older patients, and those with medical comorbidities or with only HLA-mismatched donors to successfully undergo transplantation. Prospective data are needed to further define which groups of patients with AML are most likely to benefit from CD34+ selected grafts. Here we review the history of T-cell depletion in AML, and techniques used. We then summarize the contemporary literature using CD34+ selection in recipients of matched or partially mismatched donors (7/8 or 8/8 HLA-matched), and provide a summary of the risks and benefits of using T-cell depletion.

Keywords: AML; CD34+ selection; T-cell depletion; graft-*versus*-host disease; hematopoietic stem cell transplantation

1. Introduction

Cytogenetic risk stratification in acute myelogenous leukemia (AML) allows clinicians to determine which patients are most likely to benefit from allogeneic hematopoietic stem cell transplantation (HCT), with evidence to support a survival advantage in patients with intermediate or high-risk cytogenetics [1]. In addition to more accurate patient selection based on cytogenetic risk factors, over the past decades, transplantation outcomes have also improved as a result of more accurate patient selection tools, such as the HCT Sorror comorbidity index [2], improvements in HLA matching techniques and supportive care.

Despite these improvements, graft-*versus*-host disease (GVHD) remains a leading cause of post-transplant morbidity and mortality. A variety of T-cell depletion (TCD) techniques have been developed and used over the years in an effort to reduce transplant-related mortality (TRM) due to GVHD (Table 1). In this chapter we will focus on outcomes of HCT using T cell depletion for the treatment of AML in recipients of matched or partially mismatched donors (7/8 or 8/8 HLA-matched), with a primary focus on *ex vivo* CD34+ selection of the graft. Other methods of T-cell depletion will be mentioned for historic context only.

J. Clin. Med. **2015**, *4*, 488–503

2. T-Cell Depletion Techniques

The goal of T-cell depleting a graft is to reduce GVHD while maintaining the graft-*versus*-leukemia or lymphoma (GVL) effect. A variety of TCD techniques have been used with mixed results. When reviewing reports utilizing TCD for transplantation it is critical to determine the following: (1) Which technique is being used? (2) Which cell population is being removed (*i.e.*, T, B, NK or all non-hematopoietic cells) and to what extent? Different techniques lead to both quantitative and qualitative differences in the cells being depleted with important clinical implications; (3) Is post-transplant GVHD prophylaxis utilized? and (4) What is the graft source and what is the degree of HLA matching? All of these factors significantly affect outcomes and therefore must be considered when interpreting published reports.

Early TCD techniques differed in the use of negative *vs.* positive selection. Negative selection can be achieved either through physical methods such as counterflow elutriation [3–5] or soybean lectin agglutination (SBA) and sheep red blood cell (sRBC)-rosette depletion (E-rosetting) [6–10], or immunological methods using monoclonal antibodies [5,11–29]. Monoclonal antibodies can be used with or without complement, or conjugated to toxins. Antibodies vary in their specificities, which can be narrow, such as T10B9 targeting the α/β T cell receptor (TCR), or broad, such as combination of antibodies targeting CD2, CD4 and CD8 [30].

Table 1. Results of T-cell depletion (TCD)-PBSCT in patients with acute myelogenous leukemia (AML) [1].

Method	Number of Patients	Patients With AML	Donor	Degree of Depletion	GVHD Prophylaxis	Acute GVHD	Graft Failure	EFS/DFS [2]	OS [2]	Reference
CD34+	50	29	HLA-MRD	NR	Cyclosporine or Cyclosporine + Steroids	16%	0	DFS 65%	Not reported	[31]
CD34+E−	52	21	HLA-MRD	5 logs	None	8%	0	NR	17% 1 year	[32]
CD34+E−	29	16	HLA-MRD HLA-MUD or HLA-MMUD	5 logs	None	9%	3%	57% at 4 years	59% at 4 years	[33]
CD34+	47	47	HLA-MRD	4.9 logs	None	22.7%	0	EFS 63% at 4 years	71% 4 years	[34]
CD3/CD19 depletion	29	16	Haplo	4.4 logs	None	48%	0	35% at 1 year	31% at 241 days	[35]
CD34+E− or CD34+	115	115	HLA-MUD or MRD	NR	None	5%		RFS 58% at 3 years	57% at 3 years	[36]

[1] Abbreviations: CD34: CD34-selection; CD34+E−: CD34-selection and E-rosetting; NR: not reported; [2] DFS and OS are reported for the entire patient population included in the studies.

Currently, the most common method for T cell depletion relies on positive selection of CD34+ hematopoietic stem cells from the graft [32–34,36,37]. CD34+ selection of peripheral blood stem cells (PBSCs) was performed in initial studies with the ISOLEX 300i magnetic cell selection system (Baxter, Deerfield, IL, USA), followed by E-rosetting [32,33,37]. The ISOLEX device is no longer being manufactured, and the most commonly used method in current studies uses immunomagnetic beads with the CliniMACS CD34 Reagent System (Miltenyi Biotech, Gladbach, Germany) for CD34+ selection [31,34,37]. The CliniMACS system can also be used to negatively select grafts through depletion of CD3+ and CD19+ cells or depletion of TCRαβ+ T cells [35,38–41]. The two CD34+ selection methods differ in the degree of TCD; for example, the CliniMACS CD34 Reagent System can achieve a 5-log reduction in T cells, whereas the ISOLEX 300i system achieves a 3.5-log reduction, requiring additional T-cell depletion through E-rosetting.

The cell dose and graft source also impact outcomes. In recipients of T-cell depleted marrow grafts from HLA-identical donors, the risk of GVHD was shown to increase if the graft contained >1 $\times 10^5$ T cells/kg [42]. Differences between TCD methods can have a significant impact on clinical outcomes, including the risk of graft failure, GVHD and relapse.

3. Outcomes in AML with T-Cell Depletion

One of the primary benefits of allogeneic HCT is derived from the GVL effect, driven by the recognition of tumor cells by donor T cells. Therefore, a concern in the utilization of TCD is the potentially negative impact on relapse resulting from reduced T-cell doses included in the graft. However, it is clear that certain diseases rely more on the GVL effect than others. For example, early studies with TCD in chronic myelogenous leukemia (CML) were associated with a significantly increased risk of relapse. In a retrospective study of 46 patients who received TCD grafts form HLA-identical siblings, relapse at 3-years was significantly higher in the TCD group (62% *vs.* 24%, $p = 0.0003$). However, a significant proportion of these patients were then salvaged with donor lymphocyte infusion (DLI), supporting the role of GVL for this disease [43].

On the other hand, studies utilizing TCD in AML and ALL have shown favorable outcomes in recipients of 7/8 or 8/8 HLA matched related or unrelated donors that are comparable to those seen in unmodified, conventional grafts, calling into question the contribution of GVL in those diseases [34,36,44,45].

4. TCD in AML—Early Studies

Studies using TCD done in the 1980's and 1990's mostly used bone marrow from sibling donors as the graft source and used a variety of techniques (lectin separation, elutriation, E-rosettes, antibodies against T and NK cells, antibodies with or without complement). These techniques were associated with a 1–2 log reduction in T cells in the graft, and patients were often given post-transplant cyclosporine for additional GVHD prophylaxis. These studies were also associated with increased graft failure [8,46]. The addition of antithymocyte globulin (ATG) and thiotepa to the conditioning regimens, which had traditionally included cyclophosphamide and total body irradiation (TBI) or busulfan, decreased the rate of graft failure and eliminated the need for post transplant GVHD prophylaxis. Favorable results were reported in recipients of HLA-identical donors using this approach along with sequential soybean lectin agglutination and sheep red blood cell-rosette depletion. A study by Papadopoulos *et al.* included 31 patients with AML in CR1 or CR2 and showed a disease-free survival (DFS) at 4 years of 70% with no GVHD or graft rejection [9]. Similar results were reported by Aversa *et al.* using the same regimen in 54 patients with acute leukemia, including 2 with HLA-DR mismatched donors [10]. No GVHD or graft rejection was observed and the event-free survival at 4.9 years was 74% in 30 patients with AML.

These early studies demonstrated the feasibility of TCD, and overcame graft rejection with the utilization of ATG, at the expense of added immunosuppression and ensuing delayed immune recovery.

5. TCD in AML—Contemporary Studies

Contemporary studies have utilized two main approaches of TCD by CD34+ selection described above, either the ISOLEX 300i Magnetic Cell Separator followed by sRBC-rosette depletion or, more recently, the Miltenyi CliniMACS CD34 Reagent System. In 2011, Devine *et al.* [34] reported the results of a Blood and Marrow Clinical Trials Network study (BMT CTN 0303) utilizing CD34+ selection with the Miltenyi CliniMACS CD34 Reagent System. The study included 44 patients with AML in CR1 or CR2 (excluding patients with *t*(15;17), and core binding factor leukemia) who received T cell depleted PBSCT from HLA-identical siblings after conditioning with hyperfractionated TBI (HFTBI), thiotepa, cyclophosphamide and ATG. No additional GVHD prophylaxis was given. All patients engrafted; the incidence of aGVHD (grades II–IV) was 22.7% and extensive cGVHD was 6.8% at 2 years. The relapse rate at three years for patients in CR1 was 17.4%, with a DFS for all patients at 6 months of 82% and a 2-year OS of 60%. Rates of infection were comparable to other studies; however EBV reactivation occurred in 18% of patients leading to 1 death from Epstein-Barr Virus (EBV) post-transplant lymphoproliferative disease (PTLD) [36,47,48]. In a second report, the outcomes of patients from the BMT CTN 0303 study were compared to a similar cohort of patients (AML in either CR1 or CR2, PBSCT from HLA-identical siblings) who received a conventional HCT on BMT CTN 0101 study (a study comparing fluconazole with voriconazole as antifungal prophylaxis after HCT) [44]. There were no differences in leukemia relapse (23% *vs.* 27% in the TCD and conventional graft groups, respectively) and 2-year OS (65% *vs.* 59% in the TCD and conventional graft groups, respectively). However rates of GVHD were higher in the conventional graft group (aGVHD 23% *vs.* 39%, *p* = 0.07 and cGVHD 19% *vs.* 50%, *p* < 0.001).

More recently, a retrospective study compared the use of TCD HCT to conventional grafts in patients with AML in CR1 by examining outcomes of 115 patients who received TCD grafts at Memorial Sloan Kettering Cancer Center (MSKCC) with a cohort of 181 patients at MD Anderson Cancer Center (MDACC) [36]. A hundred and seven patients in the MSKCC cohort received PBSC grafts, including 85 that were CD34-selected with the ISOLEX 300i Magnetic Cell Separator followed by sRBC-rosette depletion, and 22 with the Miltenyi CliniMACS CD34 Reagent System. Patients at both centers received myeloablative conditioning (MAC) and both cohorts included recipients of matched related, matched unrelated and mismatched donors. Patients at MSKCC were more likely to be recipients of a mismatched graft (27% *vs.* 14%, *p* < 0.001). Patients at MSKCC did not receive additional GVHD prophylaxis. Patients at MDACC received tacrolimus and mini-methotrexate for GVHD prophylaxis, and ATG for HLA-mismatched donors. There were no significant differences in the rate of relapse at 3 years between groups (18% *vs.* 25%, in the TCD *vs.* conventional grafts, respectively, *p* = 0.3). However, rates of GVHD were significantly lower in the TCD group (5% *vs.* 18% for aGVHD, *p* = 0.005, and 13% *vs.* 53% for cGVHD, *p* < 0.001).

Although contemporary studies that compare outcomes of conventional to TCD grafts are retrospective, the results suggest that TCD transplants offer similar DFS and OS with significantly lower rates of GVHD.

As noted above additional TCD approaches are being investigated beyond CD34 selection [35,38–41]. The potential advantages of negative selection by depletion of CD3+/CD19+ or TCRαβ+ T cells include the presence of additional cells in the graft such as natural killer (NK) cells or TCRγδ+ T cells, which may play a role in relapse or infection prevention. To date, the published studies of these approaches have been in recipients of haplo-identical grafts and there has been limited data on patients with AML. In a study by Bethge *et al.* [35], EFS was 35% at one year in 16 patients with AML who received a CD3/CD19 depleted transplant from a haplo-identical donor

Finally, an alternative GVHD prophylaxis approach that will be compared to CD34-selection in an upcoming phase 3 trial (BMT CTN 1301) relies on the use of post-transplant high dose cyclophosphamide after a T-replete bone marrow graft from a matched donor [49–51]. In a recently published study using this approach in 138 patients with AML, the 3-year DFS and OS were 43% (95% CI, 35% to 52%) and 53% (95% CI, 45% to 62%), respectively [50]. DFS (48% *vs.* 29% at 3 years) and OS (55% *vs.* 50% at 3 years) were higher in patients with AML in morphologic CR compared to those with active disease. The approach was associated with low rates of grade III to IV acute GVHD (11% at 100 days) and chronic GVHD (13% at 2 years).

6. Impact of T-Cell Depletion on Engraftment and Immune Reconstitution

Hematopoietic stem cell transplantation, regardless of donor source and manipulation, is associated with significant and prolonged immunosuppression and risk of severe and fatal infections [48,52], disease relapse and secondary malignancies [20,53]. The use of TCD, whether *in vivo* with agents such as alemtuzumab or ATG, or *ex vivo* with T-cell depletion considerably affects immune recovery. In early studies comparing immune reconstitution in TCD and unmodified grafts the rate of CD3+, CD4+ and CD8+ T cell reconstitution was significantly delayed in TCD recipients, correlating with increased risk of infections, including EBV-PTLD [48,54]. T-cell receptor (TCR) studies using 5′-RACE PCR with deep sequencing have confirmed these findings by showing more rapid recovery of TCR diversity in conventional graft recipients compared to TCD grafts [55]. Lower T-cell levels result from decreased thymic output, which can be quantified via measurements of T-cell receptor excision circles (TRECs). Studies have shown that older patients and recipients of TCD grafts have lower TRECs than unmodified graft recipients; however this difference abates beyond 9 months [56].

ATG plays an important role in TCD by reducing the risk of graft rejection. However it is associated with delayed immune recovery and an increased risk of opportunistic infections (OI), with approximately 15% of the patients in early TCD studies dying from OIs [9,10]. Furthermore, a study of immune reconstitution in patients receiving TCD grafts with or without ATG found delayed immune reconstitution with ATG, which was associated with increased OIs [54]. Although studies of TCD performed without ATG by substituting cyclophosphamide with fludarabine have demonstrated durable engraftment in recipients of matched related donors, there did not appear to be a significant effect on immune recovery or the risk of OIs [32].

It is important to note however that, in addition to age and TCD, the presence of GVHD also significantly hampers immune reconstitution via direct effects on the thymus [57–59], as well as the immunosuppressive drugs required for treatment of GVHD [60–64]. Although TCD impacts immune reconstitution leading to higher infection related deaths, GVHD in conventional grafts similarly leads to increased mortality. This is a potential explanation for the similar RFS and OS outcomes observed in patients with AML in the MSKCC/MDACC retrospective study and the BMT CTN study [36,44].

7. Strategies to Enhance Immune Recovery Post HCT

HCT affords a curative treatment option to many patients with otherwise incurable malignancies. However, the benefit of this therapy comes at the risk of significant complications, including infection, GVHD, relapse and secondary malignancies [20,48,52,53,65,66]. The rationale for TCD is to mitigate GVHD while preserving the benefit of GVL. TCD and HCT in general, are associated with prolonged immunosuppression. Therefore, strategies to optimize post transplant immunity, enhance GVL, while minimizing infectious complications are needed.

The addition of T cells post transplantation represents one such strategy. In one recent study, 19 pediatric patients (13 transplanted for malignant disease) received CD34+ selected matched unrelated donor (MUD) HCT with CD3+ T cells added back, at a dose of 1.0–2.5×10^5 CD3+/kg, and tacrolimus for GVHD prevention [67]. Rates of aGVHD, cGVHD and extensive cGVHD were 15.8%, 23.3% and 0%, respectively, which are low compared to conventional HCT. All patients on this study had neutrophil engraftment, and infection-related mortality at one year was 5%–6%, showing the feasibility of this approach. This approach has also been used in recipients of CD34-selected haplo-identical grafts [68]. The same group previously reported low rates of acute and chronic GVHD in a retrospective series of 16 patients who received DLI (up to 6×10^4 CD3+/kg) from haplo-identical donors to enhance immune recovery and/or treat infections [69]. One ongoing trial is evaluating the effect of serial DLI post TCD in patients with advanced multiple myeloma (NCT01131169).

Another strategy to boost immune reconstitution post-transplant is the use of Keratinocyte Growth Factor (KGF). KGF has been shown in pre-clinical models to play an important role in T cell homeostasis and immune recovery, as well as in thymic regeneration after radiation injury [70–72]. Based on these data, KGF along with sex steroid ablation is being studied in an ongoing phase II clinical trial (NCT01746849).

We recently published the results of a phase I study using recombinant human IL-7 (rhIL-7, CYT107, Cytheris) in recipients of TCD HCT and demonstrated enhanced immune recovery, with significant increases in CD4+ and CD8+ T cells along with increased T cell function, without causing significant GVHD or other serious toxicity [73].

8. Benefits of TCD HCT in AML

Although reduced intensity conditioning (RIC) regimens allow older patients to undergo HCT, they are associated with higher relapse rates in AML [74,75]. However, the combined toxicity of GVHD prophylaxis that usually includes a calineurin inhibitor (CNI) and methotrexate with myeloablative conditioning (MAC), makes this approach prohibitive in older patients. Unlike conventional grafts, CD34+ selected grafts do not require post-transplant GVHD prophylaxis, and as a result, older patients can be treated with MAC. In addition, patients with renal insufficiency can also successfully undergo transplantation by avoiding the use of CNIs.

The use of CD34+ selected grafts is associated with significant reductions in both acute and chronic GVHD. In addition to the obvious advantage of lowering GVHD, patients without fully matched donors are also able to undergo transplantation, therefore expanding the pool of potential donors.

Finally, CD34+ selected grafts are an ideal platform for post-transplant immunotherapy with adoptive cell therapy targeting both minimal residual disease and viral reactivation by CMV and EBV, among others [76–79]. The administration T cells specific for tumor or viral antigens post-transplant has the potential advantage of overcoming any loss of GVL or increased infectious risk associated with TCD without affecting the benefit of reduced GVHD.

9. Conclusions

After three decades of investigation, it is reasonable to consider CD34+ selected allografts for patients with AML in CR1 based on prospective data [34], and well conducted retrospective studies [36,44]. These contemporary studies are significantly more homogeneous in their methodology and patient inclusion than prior studies, mostly using the CliniMACS CD34 Reagent System for CD34+ selection, and reporting consistent favorable outcomes for patients with AML in CR. The use of CD34+ selected grafts overcomes the morbidity and mortality associated with GVHD, a significant contributor of transplant-related complications, without compromising the benefit of transplantation and affording the same overall survival as conventional transplantation.

TCD represents an important step in graft manipulation, allowing older patients, and those with comorbidities to successfully undergo transplantation. Ongoing research aims to continue to decrease morbidity and mortality associated with transplantation by improving immune reconstitution and the GVL effect.

As mentioned above, an ongoing national phase 3 trial will compare TCD with the CliniMACS CD34 Reagent System to post-transplant cyclophosphamide [49], and a control arm (tacrolimus and methotrexate) in patients with acute leukemia and MDS who are eligible for a MAC transplant from a matched related or unrelated donor (BMT CTN 1301).

Acknowledgments: This work was supported in part by PO1 CA23766 from the National Cancer Institute. The content is solely the responsibility of the authors and does not necessarily represent the official views of the National Institutes of Health. Gabriela Soriano Hobbs was supported in part by an American Society of Clinical Oncology Young Investigator Award.

Author Contributions: Gabriela Soriano Hobbs and Miguel-Angel Perales wrote reviewed the literature, wrote the manuscript and edited its contents.

Conflicts of Interest: The authors declare no conflict of interest.

References

1. Koreth, J.; Schlenk, R.; Kopecky, K.J.; Honda, S.; Sierra, J.; Djulbegovic, B.J.; Wadleigh, M.; DeAngelo, D.J.; Stone, R.M.; Sakamaki, H.; *et al.* Allogeneic stem cell transplantation for acute myeloid leukemia in first complete remission: Systematic review and meta-analysis of prospective clinical trials. *JAMA* **2009**, *301*, 2349–2361. [CrossRef] [PubMed]
2. Sorror, M.L.; Maris, M.B.; Storb, R.; Baron, F.; Sandmaier, B.M.; Maloney, D.G.; Storer, B. Hematopoietic cell transplantation (HCT)-specific comorbidity index: A new tool for risk assessment before allogeneic HCT. *Blood* **2005**, *106*, 2912–2919. [CrossRef] [PubMed]
3. De Witte, T.; Hoogenhout, J.; de Pauw, B.; Holdrinet, R.; Janssen, J.; Wessels, J.; van Daal, W.; Hustinx, T.; Haanen, C. Depletion of donor lymphocytes by counterflow centrifugation successfully prevents acute graft-*versus*-host disease in matched allogeneic marrow transplantation. *Blood* **1986**, *67*, 1302–1308. [PubMed]

4. Wagner, J.E.; Donnenberg, A.D.; Noga, S.J.; Cremo, C.A.; Gao, I.K.; Yin, H.J.; Vogelsang, G.B.; Rowley, S.; Saral, R.; Santos, G.W. Lymphocyte depletion of donor bone marrow by counterflow centrifugal elutriation: Results of a phase I clinical trial. *Blood* **1988**, *72*, 1168–1176. [PubMed]

5. Wagner, J.E.; Thompson, J.S.; Carter, S.L.; Kernan, N.A. Effect of graft-versus-host disease prophylaxis on 3-year disease-free survival in recipients of unrelated donor bone marrow (T-cell Depletion Trial): A multi-centre, randomised phase II-III trial. *Lancet* **2005**, *366*, 733–741. [CrossRef] [PubMed]

6. Reisner, Y.; Kapoor, N.; Kirkpatrick, D.; Pollack, M.S.; Cunningham-Rundles, S.; Dupont, B.; Hodes, M.Z.; Good, R.A.; O'Reilly, R.J. Transplantation for severe combined immunodeficiency with HLA-A,B,D,DR incompatible parental marrow cells fractionated by soybean agglutinin and sheep red blood cells. *Blood* **1983**, *61*, 341–348. [PubMed]

7. Reisner, Y.; Kapoor, N.; Kirkpatrick, D.; Pollack, M.S.; Dupont, B.; Good, R.A.; O'Reilly, R.J. Transplantation for acute leukaemia with HLA-A and B nonidentical parental marrow cells fractionated with soybean agglutinin and sheep red blood cells. *Lancet* **1981**, *2*, 327–331. [CrossRef] [PubMed]

8. Young, J.W.; Papadopoulos, E.B.; Cunningham, I.; Castro-Malaspina, H.; Flomenberg, N.; Carabasi, M.H.; Gulati, S.C.; Brochstein, J.A.; Heller, G.; Black, P.; *et al.* T-cell-depleted allogeneic bone marrow transplantation in adults with acute nonlymphocytic leukemia in first remission. *Blood* **1992**, *79*, 3380–3387. [PubMed]

9. Papadopoulos, E.B.; Carabasi, M.H.; Castro-Malaspina, H.; Childs, B.H.; Mackinnon, S.; Boulad, F.; Gillio, A.P.; Kernan, N.A.; Small, T.N.; Szabolcs, P.; *et al.* T-cell-depleted allogeneic bone marrow transplantation as postremission therapy for acute myelogenous leukemia: Freedom from relapse in the absence of graft-*versus*-host disease. *Blood* **1998**, *91*, 1083–1090. [PubMed]

10. Aversa, F.; Terenzi, A.; Carotti, A.; Felicini, R.; Jacucci, R.; Zei, T.; Latini, P.; Aristei, C.; Santucci, A.; Martelli, M.P.; *et al.* Improved outcome with T-cell-depleted bone marrow transplantation for acute leukemia. *J. Clin. Oncol.* **1999**, *17*, 1545–1550. [PubMed]

11. Prentice, H.G.; Blacklock, H.A.; Janossy, G.; Bradstock, K.F.; Skeggs, D.; Goldstein, G.; Hoffbrand, A.V. Use of anti-T-cell monoclonal antibody OKT3 to prevent acute graft-*versus*-host disease in allogeneic bone-marrow transplantation for acute leukaemia. *Lancet* **1982**, *1*, 700–703. [CrossRef] [PubMed]

12. Filipovich, A.H.; McGlave, P.B.; Ramsay, N.K.; Goldstein, G.; Warkentin, P.I.; Kesey, J.H. Pretreatment of donor bone marrow with monoclonal antibody OKT3 for prevention of acute graft-*versus*-host disease in allogeneic histocompatible bone-marrow transplantation. *Lancet* **1982**, *1*, 1266–1269. [CrossRef] [PubMed]

13. Prentice, H.G.; Blacklock, H.A.; Janossy, G.; Gilmore, M.J.; Price-Jones, L.; Tidman, N.; Trejdosiewicz, L.K.; Skeggs, D.B.; Panjwani, D.; Ball, S.; *et al.* Depletion of T lymphocytes in donor marrow prevents significant graft-*versus*-host disease in matched allogeneic leukaemic marrow transplant recipients. *Lancet* **1984**, *1*, 472–476. [CrossRef] [PubMed]

14. Martin, P.J.; Hansen, J.A.; Thomas, E.D. Preincubation of donor bone marrow cells with a combination of murine monoclonal anti-T-cell antibodies without complement does not prevent graft-*versus*-host disease after allogeneic marrow transplantation. *J. Clin. Immunol.* **1984**, *4*, 18–22. [CrossRef] [PubMed]

15. Martin, P.J.; Hansen, J.A.; Buckner, C.D.; Sanders, J.E.; Deeg, H.J.; Stewart, P.; Appelbaum, F.R.; Clift, R.; Fefer, A.; Witherspoon, R.P.; *et al.* Effects of *in vitro* depletion of T cells in HLA-identical allogeneic marrow grafts. *Blood* **1985**, *66*, 664–672. [PubMed]

16. Herve, P.; Flesch, M.; Cahn, J.Y.; Racadot, E.; Plouvier, E.; Lamy, B.; Rozenbaum, A.; Noir, A.; Des Floris, R.L.; Peters, A. Removal of marrow T cells with OKT3-OKT11 monoclonal antibodies and complement to prevent acute graft-*versus*-host disease. A pilot study in ten patients. *Transplantation* **1985**, *39*, 138–143. [CrossRef] [PubMed]

17. Trigg, M.E.; Billing, R.; Sondel, P.M.; Exten, R.; Hong, R.; Bozdech, M.J.; Horowitz, S.D.; Finlay, J.L.; Moen, R.; Longo, W.; *et al.* Clinical trial depleting T lymphocytes from donor marrow for matched and mismatched allogeneic bone marrow transplants. *Cancer Treat. Rep.* **1985**, *69*, 377–386. [PubMed]

18. Mitsuyasu, R.T.; Champlin, R.E.; Gale, R.P.; Ho, W.G.; Lenarsky, C.; Winston, D.; Selch, M.; Elashoff, R.; Giorgi, J.V.; Wells, J.; *et al.* Treatment of donor bone marrow with monoclonal anti-T-cell antibody and complement for the prevention of graft-*versus*-host disease. A prospective, randomized, double-blind trial. *Ann. Intern. Med.* **1986**, *105*, 20–26. [CrossRef] [PubMed]

19. Patterson, J.; Prentice, H.G.; Brenner, M.K.; Gilmore, M.; Janossy, G.; Ivory, K.; Skeggs, D.; Morgan, H.; Lord, J.; Blacklock, H.A.; *et al.* Graft rejection following HLA matched T-lymphocyte depleted bone marrow transplantation. *Br. J. Haematol.* **1986**, *63*, 221–230. [CrossRef] [PubMed]

20. Maraninchi, D.; Gluckman, E.; Blaise, D.; Guyotat, D.; Rio, B.; Pico, J.L.; Leblond, V.; Michallet, M.; Dreyfus, F.; Ifrah, N.; *et al.* Impact of T-cell depletion on outcome of allogeneic bone-marrow transplantation for standard-risk leukaemias. *Lancet* **1987**, *2*, 175–178. [CrossRef] [PubMed]

21. Cahn, J.Y.; Herve, P.; Flesch, M.; Plouvier, E.; Racadot, E.; Vuillier, J.; Montcuquet, P.; Noir, A.; Rozenbaum, A.; Leconte des Floris, R. Marrow transplantation from HLA non-identical family donors for the treatment of leukaemia: A pilot study of 15 patients using additional immunosuppression and T-cell depletion. *Br. J. Haematol.* **1988**, *69*, 345–349. [CrossRef] [PubMed]

22. Martin, P.J.; Hansen, J.A.; Torok-Storb, B.; Moretti, L.; Press, O.; Storb, R.; Thomas, E.D.; Weiden, P.L.; Vitetta, E.S. Effects of treating marrow with a CD3-specific immunotoxin for prevention of acute graft-*versus*-host disease. *Bone Marrow Transplant.* **1988**, *3*, 437–444. [PubMed]

23. Laurent, G.; Maraninchi, D.; Gluckman, E.; Vernant, J.P.; Derocq, J.M.; Gaspard, M.H.; Rio, B.; Michalet, M.; Reiffers, J.; Dreyfus, F.; *et al.* Donor bone marrow treatment with T101 Fab fragment-ricin A-chain immunotoxin prevents graft-*versus*-host disease. *Bone Marrow Transplant.* **1989**, *4*, 367–371. [PubMed]

24. Filipovich, A.H.; Vallera, D.; McGlave, P.; Polich, D.; Gajl-Peczalska, K.; Haake, R.; Lasky, L.; Blazar, B.; Ramsay, N.K.; Kersey, J.; *et al.* T cell depletion with anti-CD5 immunotoxin in histocompatible bone marrow transplantation. The correlation between residual CD5 negative T cells and subsequent graft-*versus*-host disease. *Transplantation* **1990**, *50*, 410–415. [CrossRef] [PubMed]

25. Antin, J.H.; Bierer, B.E.; Smith, B.R.; Ferrara, J.; Guinan, E.C.; Sieff, C.; Golan, D.E.; Macklis, R.M.; Tarbell, N.J.; Lynch, E.; *et al.* Selective depletion of bone marrow T lymphocytes with anti-CD5 monoclonal antibodies: Effective prophylaxis for graft-*versus*-host disease in patients with hematologic malignancies. *Blood* **1991**, *78*, 2139–2149. [PubMed]

26. Soiffer, R.J.; Fairclough, D.; Robertson, M.; Alyea, E.; Anderson, K.; Freedman, A.; Bartlett-Pandite, L.; Fisher, D.; Schlossman, R.L.; Stone, R.; *et al.* CD6-depleted allogeneic bone marrow transplantation for acute leukemia in first complete remission. *Blood* **1997**, *89*, 3039–3047. [PubMed]

27. Soiffer, R.J.; Freedman, A.S.; Neuberg, D.; Fisher, D.C.; Alyea, E.P.; Gribben, J.; Schlossman, R.L.; Bartlett-Pandite, L.; Kuhlman, C.; Murray, C.; Freeman, A.; *et al.* CD6+ T cell-depleted allogeneic bone marrow transplantation for non-Hodgkin's lymphoma. *Bone Marrow Transplant.* **1998**, *21*, 1177–1181. [CrossRef]

28. Alyea, E.P.; Weller, E.; Fisher, D.C.; Freedman, A.S.; Gribben, J.G.; Lee, S.; Schlossman, R.L.; Stone, R.M.; Friedberg, J.; DeAngelo, D.; *et al.* Comparable outcome with T-cell-depleted unrelated-donor *versus* related-donor allogeneic bone marrow transplantation. *Biol. Blood Marrow Transplant.* **2002**, *8*, 601–607. [CrossRef] [PubMed]

29. Lee, S.J.; Zahrieh, D.; Alyea, E.P.; Weller, E.; Ho, V.T.; Antin, J.H.; Soiffer, R.J. Comparison of T-cell-depleted and non-T-cell-depleted unrelated donor transplantation for hematologic diseases: Clinical outcomes, quality of life, and costs. *Blood* **2002**, *100*, 2697–2702. [CrossRef] [PubMed]

30. Champlin, R.E.; Passweg, J.R.; Zhang, M.J.; Rowlings, P.A.; Pelz, C.J.; Atkinson, K.A.; Barrett, A.J.; Cahn, J.Y.; Drobyski, W.R.; Gale, R.P.; *et al.* T-cell depletion of bone marrow transplants for leukemia from donors other than HLA-identical siblings: Advantage of T-cell antibodies with narrow specificities. *Blood* **2000**, *95*, 3996–4003. [PubMed]

31. Urbano-Ispizua, A.; Brunet, S.; Solano, C.; Moraleda, J.M.; Rovira, M.; Zuazu, J.; de La Rubia, J.; Bargay, J.; Caballero, D.; Diez-Martin, J.L.; *et al.* Allogeneic transplantation of CD34+-selected cells from peripheral blood in patients with myeloid malignancies in early phase: A case control comparison with unmodified peripheral blood transplantation. *Bone Marrow Transplant.* **2001**, *28*, 349–354. [CrossRef] [PubMed]

32. Jakubowski, A.A.; Small, T.N.; Young, J.W.; Kernan, N.A.; Castro-Malaspina, H.; Hsu, K.C.; Perales, M.A.; Collins, N.; Cisek, C.; Chiu, M.; *et al.* T cell depleted stem-cell transplantation for adults with hematologic malignancies: Sustained engraftment of HLA-matched related donor grafts without the use of antithymocyte globulin. *Blood* **2007**, *110*, 4552–4559. [CrossRef] [PubMed]

33. Jakubowski, A.A.; Small, T.N.; Kernan, N.A.; Castro-Malaspina, H.; Collins, N.; Koehne, G.; Hsu, K.C.; Perales, M.A.; Papanicolaou, G.; van den Brink, M.R.; *et al.* T Cell-Depleted Unrelated Donor Stem Cell Transplantation Provides Favorable Disease-Free Survival for Adults with Hematologic Malignancies. *Biol. Blood Marrow Transplant.* **2011**, *17*, 1335–1342. [CrossRef] [PubMed]

34. Devine, S.M.; Carter, S.; Soiffer, R.J.; Pasquini, M.C.; Hari, P.N.; Stein, A.; Lazarus, H.M.; Linker, C.; Stadtmauer, E.A.; Alyea, E.P., III; *et al.* Low risk of chronic graft-*versus*-host disease and relapse associated with T cell-depleted peripheral blood stem cell transplantation for acute myelogenous leukemia in first remission: Results of the blood and marrow transplant clinical trials network protocol 0303. *Biol. Blood Marrow Transplant.* **2011**, *17*, 1343–1351. [CrossRef] [PubMed]
35. Bethge, W.A.; Faul, C.; Bornhauser, M.; Stuhler, G.; Beelen, D.W.; Lang, P.; Stelljes, M.; Vogel, W.; Hagele, M.; Handgretinger, R.; *et al.* Haploidentical allogeneic hematopoietic cell transplantation in adults using CD3/CD19 depletion and reduced intensity conditioning: An update. *Blood Cells Mol. Dis.* **2008**, *40*, 13–19. [CrossRef] [PubMed]
36. Bayraktar, U.D.; de Lima, M.; Saliba, R.M.; Maloy, M.; Castro-Malaspina, H.R.; Chen, J.; Rondon, G.; Chiattone, A.; Jakubowski, A.A.; Boulad, F.; *et al.* Ex Vivo T Cell Depleted *versus* Unmodified Allografts in Patients with Acute Myeloid Leukemia in First Complete Remission. *Biol. Blood Marrow Transplant.* **2013**, *19*, 898–903. [CrossRef] [PubMed]
37. Aversa, F.; Terenzi, A.; Tabilio, A.; Falzetti, F.; Carotti, A.; Ballanti, S.; Felicini, R.; Falcinelli, F.; Velardi, A.; Ruggeri, L.; *et al.* Full haplotype-mismatched hematopoietic stem-cell transplantation: A phase II study in patients with acute leukemia at high risk of relapse. *J. Clin. Oncol.* **2005**, *23*, 3447–3454. [CrossRef] [PubMed]
38. Bertaina, A.; Merli, P.; Rutella, S.; Pagliara, D.; Bernardo, M.E.; Masetti, R.; Pende, D.; Falco, M.; Handgretinger, R.; Moretta, F.; *et al.* HLA-haploidentical stem cell transplantation after removal of alphabeta+ T and B cells in children with nonmalignant disorders. *Blood* **2014**, *124*, 822–826. [CrossRef] [PubMed]
39. Zecca, M.; Strocchio, L.; Pagliara, D.; Comoli, P.; Bertaina, A.; Giorgiani, G.; Perotti, C.; Corbella, F.; Brescia, L.; Locatelli, F. HLA-haploidentical T cell-depleted allogeneic hematopoietic stem cell transplantation in children with Fanconi anemia. *Biol. Blood Marrow Transplant.* **2014**, *20*, 571–576. [CrossRef] [PubMed]
40. Lang, P.; Teltschik, H.M.; Feuchtinger, T.; Muller, I.; Pfeiffer, M.; Schumm, M.; Ebinger, M.; Schwarze, C.P.; Gruhn, B.; Schrauder, A.; *et al.* Transplantation of CD3/CD19 depleted allografts from haploidentical family donors in paediatric leukaemia. *Br. J. Haematol.* **2014**, *165*, 688–698. [CrossRef] [PubMed]
41. Gonzalez-Llano, O.; Rodriguez-Romo, L.N.; Mancias-Guerra Mdel, C.; Tarin-Arzaga, L.; Jaime-Perez, J.C.; Herrera-Garza, J.L.; Cantu-Rodriguez, O.G.; Gutierrez-Aguirre, C.H.; Garcia-Sepulveda, R.D.; Garcia-Marin, A.Y.; *et al.* Feasibility of an outpatient HLA haploidentical stem cell transplantation program in children using a reduced-intensity conditioning regimen and CD3-CD19 depletion. *Hematology* **2014**, *19*, 10–17. [CrossRef] [PubMed]
42. Kernan, N.A.; Collins, N.H.; Juliano, L.; Cartagena, T.; Dupont, B.; O'Reilly, R.J. Clonable T lymphocytes in T cell-depleted bone marrow transplants correlate with development of graft-v-host disease. *Blood* **1986**, *68*, 770–773.
43. Sehn, L.H.; Alyea, E.P.; Weller, E.; Canning, C.; Lee, S.; Ritz, J.; Antin, J.H.; Soiffer, R.J. Comparative outcomes of T-cell-depleted and non-T-cell-depleted allogeneic bone marrow transplantation for chronic myelogenous leukemia: Impact of donor lymphocyte infusion. *J. Clin. Oncol.* **1999**, *17*, 561–568. [PubMed]
44. Pasquini, M.C.; Devine, S.; Mendizabal, A.; Baden, L.R.; Wingard, J.R.; Lazarus, H.M.; Appelbaum, F.R.; Keever-Taylor, C.A.; Horowitz, M.M.; Carter, S.; *et al.* Comparative outcomes of donor graft CD34+ selection and immune suppressive therapy as graft-*versus*-host disease prophylaxis for patients with acute myeloid leukemia in complete remission undergoing HLA-matched sibling allogeneic hematopoietic cell transplantation. *J. Clin. Oncol.* **2012**, *30*, 3194–3201. [CrossRef] [PubMed]
45. Hobbs, G.S.; Hilden, P.; Hamdi, A.; Goldberg, J.D.; Poon, M.; Ledesma, C.; Devlin, S.; Rondon, G.; Papadopoulos, E.B.; Jakubowski, A.A.; *et al.* Outcomes in Patients with Acute Lymphoblastic Leukemia in First or Second Complete Remission Receiving *Ex-Vivo* T-Cell Depleted or Unmodified Allografts: Comparison of Results At Two Institutions. *Blood* **2013**, *122*, 3370. [CrossRef]
46. Marmont, A.M.; Horowitz, M.M.; Gale, R.P.; Sobocinski, K.; Ash, R.C.; van Bekkum, D.W.; Champlin, R.E.; Dicke, K.A.; Goldman, J.M.; Good, R.A.; *et al.* T-cell depletion of HLA-identical transplants in leukemia. *Blood* **1991**, *78*, 2120–2130. [PubMed]
47. Small, T.N. Immunologic reconstitution following stem cell transplantation. *Curr. Opin. Hematol.* **1996**, *3*, 461–465. [CrossRef] [PubMed]

48. Small, T.N.; Papadopoulos, E.B.; Boulad, F.; Black, P.; Castro-Malaspina, H.; Childs, B.H.; Collins, N.; Gillio, A.; George, D.; Jakubowski, A.; *et al.* Comparison of immune reconstitution after unrelated and related T-cell-depleted bone marrow transplantation: Effect of patient age and donor leukocyte infusions. *Blood* **1999**, *93*, 467–480. [PubMed]

49. Luznik, L.; Bolanos-Meade, J.; Zahurak, M.; Chen, A.R.; Smith, B.D.; Brodsky, R.; Huff, C.A.; Borrello, I.; Matsui, W.; Powell, J.D.; *et al.* High-dose cyclophosphamide as single-agent, short-course prophylaxis of graft-*versus*-host disease. *Blood* **2010**, *115*, 3224–3230. [CrossRef] [PubMed]

50. Kanakry, C.G.; Tsai, H.L.; Bolanos-Meade, J.; Smith, B.D.; Gojo, I.; Kanakry, J.A.; Kasamon, Y.L.; Gladstone, D.E.; Matsui, W.; Borrello, I.; *et al.* Single-agent GVHD prophylaxis with posttransplantation cyclophosphamide after myeloablative, HLA-matched BMT for AML, ALL, and MDS. *Blood* **2014**, *124*, 3817–3827. [CrossRef] [PubMed]

51. Kanakry, C.G.; O'Donnell, P.V.; Furlong, T.; de Lima, M.J.; Wei, W.; Medeot, M.; Mielcarek, M.; Champlin, R.E.; Jones, R.J.; Thall, P.F.; *et al.* Multi-institutional study of post-transplantation cyclophosphamide as single-agent graft-*versus*-host disease prophylaxis after allogeneic bone marrow transplantation using myeloablative busulfan and fludarabine conditioning. *J. Clin. Oncol.* **2014**, *32*, 3497–3505. [CrossRef] [PubMed]

52. Storek, J.; Gooley, T.; Witherspoon, R.P.; Sullivan, K.M.; Storb, R. Infectious morbidity in long-term survivors of allogeneic marrow transplantation is associated with low CD4 T cell counts. *Am. J. Hematol.* **1997**, *54*, 131–138. [CrossRef] [PubMed]

53. Curtis, R.E.; Rowlings, P.A.; Deeg, H.J.; Shriner, D.A.; Socie, G.; Travis, L.B.; Horowitz, M.M.; Witherspoon, R.P.; Hoover, R.N.; Sobocinski, K.A.; *et al.* Solid cancers after bone marrow transplantation. *N. Engl. J. Med.* **1997**, *336*, 897–904. [CrossRef] [PubMed]

54. Small, T.N.; Avigan, D.; Dupont, B.; Smith, K.; Black, P.; Heller, G.; Polyak, T.; O'Reilly, R.J. Immune reconstitution following T-cell depleted bone marrow transplantation: Effect of age and posttransplant graft rejection prophylaxis. *Biol. Blood Marrow Transplant.* **1997**, *3*, 65–75. [PubMed]

55. Van Heijst, J.W.; Ceberio, I.; Lipuma, L.B.; Samilo, D.W.; Wasilewski, G.D.; Gonzales, A.M.; Nieves, J.L.; van den Brink, M.R.; Perales, M.A.; Pamer, E.G. Quantitative assessment of T cell repertoire recovery after hematopoietic stem cell transplantation. *Nat. Med.* **2013**, *19*, 372–377.

56. Lewin, S.R.; Heller, G.; Zhang, L.; Rodrigues, E.; Skulsky, E.; van den Brink, M.R.; Small, T.N.; Kernan, N.A.; O'Reilly, R.J.; Ho, D.D.; *et al.* Direct evidence for new T-cell generation by patients after either T-cell-depleted or unmodified allogeneic hematopoietic stem cell transplantations. *Blood* **2002**, *100*, 2235–2242. [PubMed]

57. Weinberg, K.; Blazar, B.R.; Wagner, J.E.; Agura, E.; Hill, B.J.; Smogorzewska, M.; Koup, R.A.; Betts, M.R.; Collins, R.H.; Douek, D.C. Factors affecting thymic function after allogeneic hematopoietic stem cell transplantation. *Blood* **2001**, *97*, 1458–1466. [CrossRef] [PubMed]

58. Clave, E.; Busson, M.; Douay, C.; Peffault de Latour, R.; Berrou, J.; Rabian, C.; Carmagnat, M.; Rocha, V.; Charron, D.; Socie, G.; *et al.* Acute graft-versus-host disease transiently impairs thymic output in young patients after allogeneic hematopoietic stem cell transplantation. *Blood* **2009**, *113*, 6477–6484. [CrossRef] [PubMed]

59. Olkinuora, H.; von Willebrand, E.; Kantele, J.M.; Vainio, O.; Talvensaari, K.; Saarinen-Pihkala, U.; Siitonen, S.; Vettenranta, K. The impact of early viral infections and graft-*versus*-host disease on immune reconstitution following paediatric stem cell transplantation. *Scand. J. Immunol.* **2011**, *73*, 586–593. [CrossRef] [PubMed]

60. Perales, M.A.; Ishill, N.; Lomazow, W.A.; Weinstock, D.M.; Papadopoulos, E.B.; Dastigir, H.; Chiu, M.; Boulad, F.; Castro-Malaspina, H.R.; Heller, G.; *et al.* Long-term follow-up of patients treated with daclizumab for steroid-refractory acute graft-*vs.*-host disease. *Bone Marrow Transplant.* **2007**, *40*, 481–486. [CrossRef] [PubMed]

61. Willenbacher, W.; Basara, N.; Blau, I.W.; Fauser, A.A.; Kiehl, M.G. Treatment of steroid refractory acute and chronic graft-*versus*-host disease with daclizumab. *Br. J. Haematol.* **2001**, *112*, 820–823. [CrossRef] [PubMed]

62. Arai, S.; Margolis, J.; Zahurak, M.; Anders, V.; Vogelsang, G.B. Poor outcome in steroid-refractory graft-*versus*-host disease with antithymocyte globulin treatment. *Biol. Blood Marrow Transplant.* **2002**, *8*, 155–160. [CrossRef] [PubMed]

63. McCaul, K.G.; Nevill, T.J.; Barnett, M.J.; Toze, C.L.; Currie, C.J.; Sutherland, H.J.; Conneally, E.A.; Shepherd, J.D.; Nantel, S.H.; Hogge, D.E.; *et al.* Treatment of steroid-resistant acute graft-*versus*-host disease with rabbit antithymocyte globulin. *J. Hematother. Stem Cell Res.* **2000**, *9*, 367–374. [CrossRef] [PubMed]

64. Khoury, H.; Kashyap, A.; Adkins, D.R.; Brown, R.A.; Miller, G.; Vij, R.; Westervelt, P.; Trinkaus, K.; Goodnough, L.T.; Hayashi, R.J.; *et al.* Treatment of steroid-resistant acute graft-*versus*-host disease with anti-thymocyte globulin. *Bone Marrow Transplant.* **2001**, *27*, 1059–1064. [CrossRef] [PubMed]

65. Storek, J.; Joseph, A.; Espino, G.; Dawson, M.A.; Douek, D.C.; Sullivan, K.M.; Flowers, M.E.; Martin, P.; Mathioudakis, G.; Nash, R.A.; *et al.* Immunity of patients surviving 20 to 30 years after allogeneic or syngeneic bone marrow transplantation. *Blood* **2001**, *98*, 3505–3512. [CrossRef] [PubMed]

66. Storek, J.; Witherspoon, R.P.; Storb, R. T cell reconstitution after bone marrow transplantation into adult patients does not resemble T cell development in early life. *Bone Marrow Transplant.* **1995**, *16*, 413–425.

67. Geyer, M.B.; Ricci, A.M.; Jacobson, J.S.; Majzner, R.; Duffy, D.; Van de Ven, C.; Ayello, J.; Bhatia, M.; Garvin, J.H., Jr.; George, D.; *et al.* T cell depletion utilizing CD34(+) stem cell selection and CD3(+) addback from unrelated adult donors in paediatric allogeneic stem cell transplantation recipients. *Br. J. Haematol.* **2012**, *157*, 205–219. [CrossRef] [PubMed]

68. Dvorak, C.C.; Gilman, A.L.; Horn, B.; Oon, C.Y.; Dunn, E.A.; Baxter-Lowe, L.A.; Cowan, M.J. Haploidentical related-donor hematopoietic cell transplantation in children using megadoses of CliniMACs-selected CD34(+) cells and a fixed CD3(+) dose. *Bone Marrow Transplant.* **2013**, *48*, 508–513. [CrossRef] [PubMed]

69. Dvorak, C.C.; Gilman, A.L.; Horn, B.; Jaroscak, J.; Dunn, E.A.; Baxter-Lowe, L.A.; Cowan, M.J. Clinical and immunologic outcomes following haplocompatible donor lymphocyte infusions. *Bone Marrow Transplant.* **2009**, *44*, 805–812. [CrossRef] [PubMed]

70. Alpdogan, O.; Hubbard, V.M.; Smith, O.M.; Patel, N.; Lu, S.; Goldberg, G.L.; Gray, D.H.; Feinman, J.; Kochman, A.A.; Eng, J.M.; *et al.* Keratinocyte growth factor (KGF) is required for postnatal thymic regeneration. *Blood* **2006**, *107*, 2453–2460. [CrossRef] [PubMed]

71. Jenq, R.R.; King, C.G.; Volk, C.; Suh, D.; Smith, O.M.; Rao, U.K.; Yim, N.L.; Holland, A.M.; Lu, S.X.; Zakrzewski, J.L.; *et al.* Keratinocyte growth factor enhances DNA plasmid tumor vaccine responses after murine allogeneic bone marrow transplantation. *Blood* **2009**, *113*, 1574–1580. [CrossRef] [PubMed]

72. Vadhan-Raj, S.; Goldberg, J.D.; Perales, M.A.; Berger, D.P.; van den Brink, M.R. Clinical applications of palifermin: Amelioration of oral mucositis and other potential indications. *J. Cell Mol. Med.* **2013**, *17*, 1371–1384. [CrossRef] [PubMed]

73. Perales, M.A.; Goldberg, J.D.; Yuan, J.; Koehne, G.; Lechner, L.; Papadopoulos, E.B.; Young, J.W.; Jakubowski, A.A.; Zaidi, B.; Gallardo, H.; *et al.* Recombinant human interleukin-7 (CYT107) promotes T-cell recovery after allogeneic stem cell transplantation. *Blood* **2012**, *120*, 4882–4891. [CrossRef] [PubMed]

74. Hegenbart, U.; Niederwieser, D.; Sandmaier, B.M.; Maris, M.B.; Shizuru, J.A.; Greinix, H.; Cordonnier, C.; Rio, B.; Gratwohl, A.; Lange, T.; *et al.* Treatment for acute myelogenous leukemia by low-dose, total-body, irradiation-based conditioning and hematopoietic cell transplantation from related and unrelated donors. *J. Clin. Oncol.* **2006**, *24*, 444–453. [CrossRef] [PubMed]

75. Aoudjhane, M.; Labopin, M.; Gorin, N.C.; Shimoni, A.; Ruutu, T.; Kolb, H.J.; Frassoni, F.; Boiron, J.M.; Yin, J.L.; Finke, J.; *et al.* Comparative outcome of reduced intensity and myeloablative conditioning regimen in HLA identical sibling allogeneic haematopoietic stem cell transplantation for patients older than 50 years of age with acute myeloblastic leukaemia: A retrospective survey from the Acute Leukemia Working Party (ALWP) of the European group for Blood and Marrow Transplantation (EBMT). *Leukemia* **2005**, *19*, 2304–2312. [CrossRef] [PubMed]

76. O'Reilly, R.J.; Doubrovina, E.; Trivedi, D.; Hasan, A.; Kollen, W.; Koehne, G. Adoptive transfer of antigen-specific T-cells of donor type for immunotherapy of viral infections following allogeneic hematopoietic cell transplants. *Immunol. Res.* **2007**, *38*, 237–250. [CrossRef] [PubMed]

77. Koehne, G.; Doubrovina, E.; Hasan, A.; Barker, J.N.; Castro-Malaspina, H.; Perales, M.A.; Jakubowski, A.; Papadopoulos, E.; Young, J.W.; Boulad, F.; *et al.* A Phase I Dose Escalation Trial of Donor T Cells Sensitized with Pentadecapeptides of the CMV-pp65 Protein for the Treatment of CMV Infections Following Allogeneic Hematopoietic Stem Cell Transplants. *Blood* **2009**, *114*, 2262.

78. Doubrovina, E.; Oflaz-Sozmen, B.; Prockop, S.E.; Kernan, N.A.; Abramson, S.; Teruya-Feldstein, J.; Hedvat, C.; Chou, J.F.; Heller, G.; Barker, J.N.; *et al.* Adoptive immunotherapy with unselected or EBV-specific T cells for biopsy-proven EBV+ lymphomas after allogeneic hematopoietic cell transplantation. *Blood* **2012**, *119*, 2644–2656. [CrossRef] [PubMed]

79. Blyth, E.; Clancy, L.; Simms, R.; Ma, C.K.; Burgess, J.; Deo, S.; Byth, K.; Dubosq, M.C.; Shaw, P.J.; Micklethwaite, K.P.; *et al.* Donor-derived CMV-specific T cells reduce the requirement for CMV-directed pharmacotherapy after allogeneic stem cell transplantation. *Blood* **2013**, *121*, 3745–3758. [CrossRef] [PubMed]

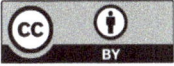

Journal of
Clinical Medicine

MDPI

Review

Alternative Donor Transplantation for Acute Myeloid Leukemia

Nelli Bejanyan [1],*, Housam Haddad [2] and Claudio Brunstein [1]

[1]   Division of Hematology, Oncology and Transplantation, University of Minnesota, 420 Delaware Street SE, Mayo Mail Code 480, Minneapolis, MN 55455, USA; bruns072@umn.edu

[2]   Hematology and Oncology Department, Staten Island University Hospital, 475 Seaview Ave, Staten Island, NY 10305, USA; husamhaddad@yahoo.com

*   Author to whom correspondence should be addressed; nbejanya@umn.edu; Tel.: +1-612-624-6982; Fax: +1-612-625-6919.

Academic Editors: Celalettin Ustun and Lucy A. Godley

Received: 14 April 2015; Accepted: 21 May 2015; Published: 9 June 2015

Abstract: Allogeneic hematopoietic cell transplantation (allo-HCT) is a potentially curative therapy for adult patients with acute myeloid leukemia (AML), but its use for consolidation therapy after first remission with induction chemotherapy used to be limited to younger patients and those with suitable donors. The median age of AML diagnosis is in the late 60s. With the introduction of reduced-intensity conditioning (RIC), many older adults are now eligible to receive allo-HCT, including those who are medically less fit to receive myeloablative conditioning. Furthermore, AML patients commonly have no human leukocyte antigen (HLA)-identical or medically suitable sibling donor available to proceed with allo-HCT. Technical advances in donor matching, suppression of alloreactivity, and supportive care have made it possible to use alternative donors, such as unrelated umbilical cord blood (UCB) and partially HLA-matched related (haploidentical) donors. Outcomes after alternative donor allo-HCT are now approaching the outcomes observed for conventional allo-HCT with matched related and unrelated donors. Thus, with both UCB and haploidentical donors available, lack of donor should rarely be a limiting factor in offering an allo-HCT to adults with AML.

Keywords: AML; alternative donor; UCB; Haploidentical; Transplantation

---

1. Introduction

Allogeneic hematopoietic cell transplantation (HCT) is widely used as a curative therapy for acute myeloid leukemia (AML). The use of reduced intensity conditioning (RIC) extended eligibility of HCT to older adults and those with comorbid conditions [1–4]. However, donor availability for many adults with AML still remains a significant challenge because HLA-identical matched sibling donors (MSD) or adult unrelated donors (MUD) are available for only about 60% of patients [5]. As the age cutoff for RIC HCT eligibility has increased, there has been a critical need for alternative donors for those who may not have a suitable HLA-matched MSD or MUD donor. Moreover, because high-risk AML is more common among the elderly, the time it takes to secure a MUD [1,2] increases the risk of leukemia relapse in this group who need to proceed to HCT promptly. Thus, in recent years unrelated umbilical cord blood (UCB) or haploidentical grafts have been studied as alternative donor types for adults with acute leukemia [1–4,6–10]. In this manuscript, we review the outcomes of HCT with these two alternative donor types in the management of adults with AML.

2. Umbilical Cord Blood Transplantation

UCB has been increasingly used for the past two decades as an alternative donor type given its rapid availability, less restrictive HLA-selection criteria, no donor risk, and relative low risk of graft-*versus*-host disease (GVHD). The introduction of double UCB (dUCB) transplantation extended access of UCB to most adults with hematological malignancies, including acute leukemia. However, barriers to UCB transplantation include limited stem cell content, delayed engraftment accompanied by increased risks of infectious complications, and cost. Several strategies have been used recently to improve the clinical outcome of UCB transplantation, such as achieving faster engraftment and further minimizing the incidence of GVHD without compromising immune reconstitution. Such promising strategies include the expansion of cord blood progenitor cells by various techniques [11–13], intra-bone marrow injection of cord blood cells [14–16] to improve hematopoietic engraftment, and use of Tregs to reduce risk of GVHD after UCB transplantation [17].

3. Myeloablative Single UCB Transplantation

Initial reports on the use of UCB as a donor type for hematopoietic cell transplantation (HCT) were based on the use of single UCB grafts and largely limited to pediatric patients [18–24]. At that time, the largest barrier to the use of UCB in adults was the weight of these patients relative to the limited cell dose available in individual UCB units. The first study to focus on UCB transplantation of adults reported on 68 patients [25] who were heavily pretreated and had high-risk hematological malignancies, 19 of whom had AML. The nucleated cell dose used in that study was inadequate considering today's standard; however, the cell dose used was based on available data largely from pediatric studies. Not unexpectedly, hematopoietic recovery was slow and treatment-related mortality (TRM) was high (47% at three months), resulting in poor leukemia-free survival (LFS) (26% at 40 months). That study found better outcomes among patients who received higher total nucleated (TNC) ($\geq$2.4 $\times$ 10^7/kg) and higher infused CD34+ ($\geq$1.2 $\times$ 10^5/kg) cell doses. In addition, the adult cohort of the Cord Blood Transplantation (COBLT) prospective study observed poor outcomes, mainly owing to inadequate TNC dose and the use of UCB as a "last resort" effort for very high-risk patients [26]. Despite limitations, these studies demonstrated the feasibility of UCB allografting in adults and set the stage for future studies seeking to improve outcomes among UCB recipients.

While many centers started using double UCB transplantation (reviewed below) to achieve an adequate cell dose for adult patients who are heavier than pediatric patients, many centers remained interested in single UCB transplantation either per institutional or country policy. Moreover, in recent years the availability of a larger inventory of UCB units has further improved the chances of finding adequate single-UCB unit grafts for adult transplantation. Takahashi *et al.* identified that, despite a delay in hematopoietic recovery, UCBT was associated with a markedly lower rate of chronic GVHD as compared to MRD transplantation [27]. More recently, the Valencia group reported their experience with single UCB transplantation after myeloablative conditioning in adults with higher-risk AML [28,29]. They used busulfan (BU)-based chemotherapy as a conditioning regimen and a UCB graft selection strategy based on improved cord blood banking standards that take into account the CD34+ cell count at the time of cryopreservation. They observed that median neutrophil engraftment occurred at 19 to 20 days and that disease-free survival (DFS) at five years was approximately 40%. Notably, patients with AML in first complete remission (CR1) who received a TNC dose $\geq$2 $\times$ 10^7/kg had a DFS at four years of 75%. In the most recent report, they also showed that patients receiving less well-HLA-matched UCB grafts had a lower risk of relapse and superior LFS [30]. Another important advance in single UCB transplantation is the strategy of delivering the graft, often with a TNC dose below current standards, directly into the bone marrow (known as intra-bone marrow infusion, IBMI) [14].

4. Myeloablative Double UCB Transplantation

The University of Minnesota pioneered the use of double UBC transplantation, which was developed to overcome the limitation of infused cell dose in adults and serve as a platform for graft manipulations [19]. The first series of double UCB recipients included 23 adult patients with high-risk leukemia using a myeloablative conditioning regimen consisting of cyclophosphamide (Cy; 120 mg/kg), fludarabine (Flu; 75 mg/m^2), and total body irradiation (TBI; 1320cGy) [31]. In this case series, double UCB transplantation led to improvements in median infused TNC dose (3.5 × 10^7/kg), sustained neutrophil engraftment (median of 23 days), and DFS at one year (57%). This success was in part due to no graft failure events and a low rate of TRM (22%). While the risk of acute GVHD (65%) with double UCB was higher than that seen in single UCB transplantation, it was largely due to an increase in grade II acute GVHD. The risk of chronic GVHD, however, was still low. Thus, the strategy of double UCB unit infusion became widely used, with other transplant centers investigating different preparative regimens and post-transplant immunosuppression [32–35]. While some preparative regimens were found not to support this treatment platform [32], variations of the myeloablative Cy/Flu/TBI regimen resulted in similar clinical outcomes, allowing many transplant centers worldwide to utilize double UCB transplantation for many adults with AML who required myeloablative conditioning [4,31,34,35]. The dissemination of this strategy, at least in part, was due to its simplicity, as any center technically able to thaw and infuse single UCB grafts was able to take advantage of the double UCB platform to extend transplantation to larger patients.

5. UCB Transplantation with Reduced Intensity Conditioning Regimen

The introduction of RIC extended the use of allogeneic HCT to older, less clinically fit, and extensively pre-treated patients, such as those who had previous autologous transplant. This transplant approach is particularly important for patients with AML as it typically presents in their late 60s, an age in which the morbidity and mortality of a conventional myeloablative regimen would be excessive. Furthermore, older patients may lack an HLA-matched sibling donor who is healthy enough to donate, making alternative donor transplantation necessary for this group of patients. Moreover, high-risk AML subtypes, such as secondary AML, for which allogeneic transplantation is the only potentially curative treatment option, is more frequent among older patients as well [36,37]; for such patients, long-term survival with chemotherapy alone is generally poor [37]. Thus, the advantage of RIC HCT using UCB for older patients is its rapid availability, which helps to avoid further delay in proceeding with a potentially curative HCT.

One of the most commonly used platforms for RIC HCT using UCB is the one developed at University of Minnesota that consists of Cy 50 mg/m^2, Flu 200 mg/m^2 divided in five days, and TBI 200 cGy with cyclosporine A (CSA) and mycophenolate mofetil (MMF) for immune suppression [38–43]. Variations on this platform, which have led to promising results, include the use of treosulfan by the Seattle group [44] and thiotepa (Thio) by the MSKCC group [45]. The backbone of the conditioning platform (Cy 50 mg/m^2, Flu 200 mg/m^2, TBI-200) has been used to support single and double UCB transplantation according to various institutional practice criteria and has been shown to result in sustained donor engraftment in >90% of recipients, TRM between 20%–30%, and long-term DFS in 25%–50% of patients depending on disease stage and the presence of co-morbid conditions prior to transplantation [4]. The Boston group has also reported on an equally promising regimen that includes the combination of Flu, melphalan (Mel), and rabbit ATG [3,46], and when sirolimus/tacrolimus was used for immune suppression, a very low risk of GVHD was observed [46]. In addition, these overall encouraging results of RIC UCB HCT have been recently reproduced by two multicenter phase II studies by the Blood and Marrow Transplant Clinical Trials Network (BMT-CTN) [7] and the Societé Française de Greffe de Moelle Osseuse et Therapie Cellulaire and Eurocord [47–49].

6. Double *versus* Single UCB Graft

Several reports demonstrate that clinical outcomes among recipients of double and single UCB grafts are similar [42,43,47,50]. A recent registry study in patients with acute leukemia (*n* = 409; 285 AML) compared adults who received an adequate single UCB graft defined as a TNC dose of $\geq$ 2.5×10^7/kg *vs.* double UCB grafts [42]. This study showed no difference in outcomes between one or two unit grafts. However, this conclusion has not been uniformly supported for relapse and acute GVHD. In some studies, a higher rate of AML relapse with single UCB transplantation was reported [43,51,52], but in other studies, no such association between number of infused UCB units and relapse or long-term treatment failure was observed [42,47,50,53,54]. In addition, although a higher risk of acute GVHD with double UCB was reported in one study [55], no difference in the risk of acute GVHD between single and double UCB transplantation was seen in other studies [53,54]. This discrepancy may in part be explained by differences in the patient population and use of ATG as part of the conditioning regimen. Additional evidence supporting the comparability of single and double UCB transplantation includes a recently reported prospective, multicenter, randomized, phase III study comparing single *vs.* double UCB grafts in children [56]. Outcomes were similar between the two groups. This study demonstrated that if a suitable single unit is available, there is no advantage in using a double UCB graft. However, an adequately dosed single-unit UCB graft cannot be frequently found for adults. Most double-unit UCB recipients would not have been eligible for UCB transplantation if an adequately dosed graft could not be generated with two UCB units. Thus, in adults who rarely have an adequate single UCB unit that meets the minimum cell dose criteria, a double UCB graft remains the standard of care.

7. UCB Grafts *versus* Other Donor Sources

Many retrospective studies have compared the outcomes of UCB to those of matched and mismatched URD in various settings including single [57] and double UCB [58] allografting and myeloablative [27,57–61] and RIC regimens [39,62–67] (Table 1). Notably, most studies have shown similar long-term outcomes between UCB and URD [27,58,61,67,68]. These studies demonstrated that UCB recipients had slower hematopoietic recovery [27,57–60,66], higher TRM [59,64–66,69], and often lower rates of acute grade II-IV and chronic GVHD than URD recipients [39,58,60]. Atsuta *et al.* reported higher TRM (30% *vs.* 19%, *p* = 0.004) and inferior survival (HR = 1.5; 95% CI 1.0–2.0; *p* = 0.028) among UCB recipients than URD recipients. As compared to other reports, this discrepancy can be explained in part by the majority of UCB recipients receiving a median TNC dose of 2.5×10^7/kg, an inadequately dosed UCB graft by today's standards [69]. In summary, the delay in hematological recovery and early TRM among UCB recipients observed in most studies was at least in part offset by lower risk of chronic GVHD and its complications and, in some series, remarkably lower risk of relapse, resulting in survival rates similar to other donor types. Novel strategies to improve the safety and efficacy of UCB transplantation are under way and have been reviewed elsewhere [70].

Table 1. Comparative allo-HCT studies of UCB with other donor types for acute leukemia in adults.

Reference	Malignancy	Donor Type	No of Patients	Median Age (range)	Median Time to ANC ≥500/μL	Median Time to Platelet >20 × 10^9/L	aGVHD (II-IV) CI (%)	cGVHD CI (%)	TRM	Relapse	DFS
Myeloablative conditioning											
Laughlin 2004	Hematologic Malignancy 200 AML	UCB	150	(16–60)	27 days	60 days	0.81	1.62	1.89	0.73	1.48
		URD (BM)	367	(16–60)	20 days	29 days	0.66 $p=0.17$	1.12 $p=0.02$	0.99 $p<0.001$	0.85 $p=0.16$	0.94 $p=0.001$
		MM URD (BM)	83	(16–60)	18 days $p<0.001$	29 days $p<0.001$	1.0 $p=0.04$	1.0 $p=0.69$	1.0 $p=0.96$	1.0 $p=0.65$	1.0 $p=0.69$
Rocha 2004	Hematologic Malignancy 362 AML	UCB	94	25 (15–55)	26 days	—	0.57	0.64	1.13	1.02	0.95
		URD BM	584	32 (15–59)	19 days $p<0.001$	—	1.0 $p=0.01$	1.0 $p=0.11$	1.0 $p=0.50$	1.0 $p=0.93$	1.0 $p=0.70$
Takahashi 2004	Hematologic Malignancy 54 AML	UCB	68	36 (16–53)	22 days	40 days	0.61	0.60	0.32	0.75	0.27
		URD BM	45	26 (16–50)	18 days $p=0.01$	22.5 days $p<0.01$	1.0 $p=0.05$	1.0 $p=0.18$	1.0 $p=0.02$	1.0 $p=0.73$	1.0 $p<0.01$
Takahashi 2007	Hematologic Malignancy 88 AML	UCB	92	38	22 days	40 days	1.09	0.49	0.49	0.72	0.74
		MRD	71	40 $p=0.083$	17 days $p<0.01$	22.5 days $p<0.01$	1.0 $p=0.69$	1.0 $p=0.01$	1.0 $p=0.13$	1.0 $p=0.26$	1.0 $p=0.26$
Gutman 2009	AML/ALL 53 AML	UCB	31	22	—	—	D100 80.6%	—	2yr 20.6%	2 yr 3.2%	2 yr 76.2%
		MUD	31	25	—	—	67.7% $p=$ NS	—	17% $p=0.78$	25.8% $p=0.018$	57.1% $p=0.17$
		MM URD	31	25	—	—	87.1% $p=$ NS	—	29.2% $p=0.41$	23% $p=0.019$	47.8% $p=0.041$
Atsuta 2009	AML	UCB	173	38	—	—	32%	28%	30%	31%	36%
		URD	311	38	—	—	35% $p=0.39$	32% $p=0.46$	19% $p=0.004$	24% $p=0.067$	54% $p<0.001$
Myeloablative conditioning											
Eapen 2010	AML/ALL 880 AML	UCB	165	28	24 days	52 days	1.0	1.0	1.0	1.0	1.0
		URD BM	332	39	19 days	28 days	0.78	0.63	1.69	0.85	1.15
		MM URD BM	140				0.59	0.59	1.06	0.84	0.93
		URD PB	632	33	14 days	19 days	0.57	0.38	1.62	0.85	1.12
		MM URD PB	256	$p<0.0001$	$p<0.0001$	—	0.49 $p<0.001$	0.46 $p<0.0001$	0.95 $p<0.0001$	0.91 $p=0.86$	0.91 $p=0.09$
Brunstein 2010	Hematologic Malignancy 476 acute leukemia	DUCB	128	25	26 days	53 days	1.0	1.0	1.0	1.0	1.0
		MRD	204	40	16 days	20 days	1.08	1.58 $p=0.03$	0.31 $p<0.01$	3.67 $p<0.01$	1.09
		URD	152	31	19 days	21 days	1.83 $p<0.01$	1.71 $p=0.01$	0.61	3.05 $p<0.01$	0.85
		MM URD	52	31 $p<0.01$	18.5 days $p<0.01$	21 days $p<0.01$	2.35 $p<0.01$	2.07 $p=0.01$	0.38 $p<0.01$	2.50 $p<0.01$	1.12 $p=$ NS

Table 1. *Cont.*

Reference	Malignancy	Donor Type	No of Patients	Median Age (range)	Median Time to ANC ≥500/μL	Median Time to Platelet >20 × 10^9/L	aGVHD (II-IV) CI (%)	cGVHD CI (%)	TRM	Relapse	DFS
					Myeloablative/Reduced intensity conditioning						
Ponce 2011	Hematologic Malignancy 133 AML	DUCB	75	37	MAC (RIC) 24 (10)	MAC (RIC) 51 (38)	D100 43%	1 yr 28%	D180 21%	2 yr 20%	2 yr 55%
		MRD	108	47	11 (11)	17 (12)	27%	31%	8%	19%	66%
		URD	184	48 *p* = 0.071	11 (10) *p* < 0.001 (*p* = 0.084)	18 (17) *p* < 0.001 (*p* < 0.001)	39% *p* = 0.33	44% *p* = 0.044	13% *p* = 0.017 *p* = 0.123	9% *p* = 0.813	55% *p* = 0.573
Raiola 2014	Hematologic, 232 acute leukemia 69% MAC	UCB	105	40 (18-64)	23 days	D50 (median) 40 days	D100 19%	4 yr 23%	D1000 35%	4 yr 30%	4 yr 33%
		MRD	176	47 (15-69)	18 days	160 days	31%	29%	24%	40%	32%
		8/8 URD	43	42 (19-66)	17 days	100 days	21%	22%	33%	23%	36%
		7/8 URD	43	47 (17-62)	16 days	110 days	42%	19%	35%	30%	34%
		Haplo	92	45 (17-69)	18 days *p* < 0.05	118 days *p* < 0.01	14% *p* < 0.001	15% *p* = 0.053	18% *p* = 0.10	35% *p* = 0.89	43% *p* = 0.20
					Reduced intensity conditioning						
Brunstein 2006	AML	UCB	43	53 (22-68)	88%	–	51%	–	1yr 28%	2yr 35%	2yr OS 31%
		Sib PBSC	21	54 (19-69)	100% *p* = 0.1	–	62% *p* = 0.85	–	38% *p* = 0.43	35% *p* = 0.72	32% *p* = 0.62
Majhail 2008	Hematologic malignancies 29 AML	UCB (88% DUCB)	43	59 (55-69)	–	–	D100 49%	3yr 17%	D180 28%	–	3yr 34%
		MRD	47	58 (65-70)	–	–	42% *p* = 0.20	40% *p* = 0.02	23% *p* = 0.23	–	30% *p* = 0.98
Majhail 2012	AML/MDS 70 AML	UCB (95% DUCB)	60	61 (55-69)	–	–	D100 45%	2yr 33%	2yr 25%	2yr 47%	2yr 22%
		MRD	38	63 (56-70)	–	–	38% *p* = 0.19	61% *p* = 0.04	25% *p* = 0.82	34% *p* = 0.19	34% *p* = 0.23
Brunstein 2012	AML/ALL 94% AML 90% AML	DUCBT-TCF 8/8 PBCT	121 313	56 (23-68) 59 (23-69)	1 0.21 *p* < 0.0001	–	D100 1 1.91 *p* < 0.001	2 yr 1 0.43 *p* < 0.001	2 yr 1 0.92	2 yr 1 1.26 *p* = 0.155	2 yr TF 1 1.13
	82% AML	7/8 PBCT	111	58 (21-69)	0.21 *p* = 0.013	–	1.44 *p* = 0.06	0.45 *p* < 0.001	0.72 0.57 *p* = 0.035	1.15 *p* = 0.495	0.37 0.88 *p* = 0.43
	75% AML	DUCB-other	40	48 (21-67)	–	–	–	–	–	–	–
Chen 2012	Hematologic malignancies, 95 AML	DUCBT	64	53 (19-67)	21.5	41	D200 14.1%	2yr 21.9%	3 yr 26.9%	3 yr 42.7%	3 yr 30%
		URD	221	58 (19-73)	13 *p* < 0.0001	19 *p* < 0.0001	20.3% *p* = 0.32	53.9% *p* < 0.0001	10.4% *p* = 0.0009	49.8% *p* = 0.09	40% *p* = 0.47

Table 1. *Cont.*

Reference	Malignancy	Donor Type	No of Patients	Median Age (range)	Median Time to ANC ≥500/uL	Median Time to Platelet >20 × 10⁹/L	aGVHD (II-IV) CI (%)	cGVHD CI (%)	TRM	Relapse	DFS
					Myeloablative conditioning						
					Reduced intensity conditioning						
Le Bourgeois 2013	Hematologic malignancies 38 AML	DUCB	39	56 (22–69)	16	38	26%	2yr 26%	2yr 26.5%	2yr 23%	2yr 50.5%
		PBSC	52	59 (22–70)	17	0	31% P = NS	35% p = 0.02	6% p = 0.02	35.5% p = 0.32	59% p = 0.43
Weisdorf 2014	AML	UCB 8/8 URD	205 441	59 (50–71) 58 (50–75)	D28 69% 97% p < 0.0001	D90 69% 91% p < 0.0001	D100 35% 36% p = 0.69	3 yr 28% 53% p < 0.0001	3 yr 35% 27% p = 0.05	3 yr 35% 35% p = 0.95	3 yr 28% 39% p = 0.01
		7/8 URD	94	58 (50–72)	91% p < 0.0001	89% p < 0.0001	44% p = 0.69	59% p < 0.0001	41% p = 0.01	26% at p = 0.13	34% at p = 0.39
Malard 2015	AML	UCB 10/10 URD	205 347	49 (19–69) 57 (19–70)	D42 75% 96% p < 0.001	>50K at D180 56% 84% p < 0.001	1 1.72 p = 0.08	1 2.15 p = 0.08	1 1.05 p = 0.85	1 0.60 p = 0.02	1 1.1 p = 0.49
		9/10 URD	99	55 (19–68)	95% p < 0.001	75% p < 0.001	2.61 p = 0.007	1.84 p = 0.23	1.58 p = 0.13	0.62 p = 0.07	1.17 p = 0.29

8. Haploidentical Transplantation

Allogenic HCT using a haploidentical (haplo) donor historically has been an attractive alternative approach given that donors are readily available for almost all patients. However, the initial experience with T-cell replete haplo-HCT was disappointing because of unacceptably high non-relapse mortality (NRM) and incidence of severe GVHD occurring in about half of patients [71–73]. In contrast, when *ex vivo* T-cell depletion platforms were utilized with the intention of minimizing GVHD, it led to an excessive increase in graft failure and infectious complication rates [74,75]. Novel strategies such as post-transplantation cyclophosphamide (PT-Cy), CD34+ "mega dose", and α/β+ T–cell depletion have improved clinical outcomes and broadened the use haplo-HCT in recent years. The advantages of this alternative donor type include immediate donor availability, motivation of family donors, simplicity of use (at least in the context of PT-Cy), and low cost [76–79]. This is particularly important in developing countries where ease of access to international unrelated donors and UCB may be limited by cost and local policies. The main limitation of haplo-HCT is still a high risk of disease relapse, which in part can be addressed by the use of more intensive conditioning regimens. Ongoing studies are investigating post-transplantation maintenance therapy methods. Delayed immune reconstitution has also been a major limitation in some haplo-HCT platforms. Thus, several strategies were undertaken to minimize GVHD after haplo-HCT without significantly affecting immune reconstitution. Most of these strategies are still in the developmental stage, including those directed towards augmentation of immune reconstitution after T-cell-depleted haplo-HCT, such as infusion of pathogen-specific T-cells [80–84], suicide-gene expressing T-cells [85–87], regulatory T-cells (Tregs) [88–90], or *ex vivo* photodepletion of alloreactive donor T-cells [91,92]. Selective allodepletion in T-cell replete haplo-HCT was another strategy explored that includes *ex vivo* T-cell tolerance induction via co-stimulation blockade [93,94], *ex vivo* selective depletion of T-cells [95–98], and use of PT-Cy [9,76,99–101].

9. T-Cell Depleted Haploidentical Graft

Infusion of a mega-dose (>10 × 10^6 cells/kg) of CD34+ selected cells is a strategy developed to overcome the poor hematopoietic engraftment of T-cell-depleted haploidentical grafts after myeloablative conditioning [8,102,103]. The Perugia group conducted a phase II trial of mega-dose infusion of CD34+ cells after intensive conditioning with Thio/Flu/TBI (8Gy) and rabbit ATG in 104 patients with acute leukemia [104]. Despite achievement of successful engraftment in over 90% of patients, the rate of NRM was still excessive (36.5%), mainly owing to infectious complications from delayed immune reconstitution. Similarly, EBMT reported unacceptable TRM (36%–61% ± 10% at two years) due to serious infections and poor immune reconstitution after T-cell-depleted myeloablative conditioning in 266 patients with acute leukemia [103]. However, this strategy led to a low incidence of GVHD and appeared promising. By using α/β/CD19+ T-cell depletion, Locatelli and colleagues recently reported that myeloablative haplo-HCT using Thio/Flu/TBI and ATG-based conditioning yielded acceptable engraftment, a low rate of GVHD, and faster immune reconstitution [98]. Although clinical outcomes of haplo-HCT appear to be improving with the use of these novel techniques, future studies will need to carefully weigh the cost and benefits of these approaches relative to other alternative donor choices.

10. Unmodified Haploidentical Graft with Post-Transplant Cyclophosphamide

The PT-Cy approach was pioneered by the John Hopkins group, and in recent years has become widely used at many transplant centers given its lower cost and ease of use. With this strategy, the bone marrow or peripheral blood stem cell graft is unmodified when it is infused into the patient, allowing alloreactive T-cells to proliferate until days +3 and +4 post-transplant. The patient then receives 50 mg/kg/day cyclophosphamide for *in vivo* T-cell depletion. As shown in animal models, and recently in humans, this dose of cyclophosphamide kills actively proliferating T-cells, but does not harm the hematopoietic progenitor and stem cells that are critical for blood count recovery and engraftment [78]. This strategy results in low risk of acute and chronic GVHD, which has been explained by the use of *in vivo* alloreactive T-cell depletion with high-dose Cy [78]. In addition, several recent studies suggest improvement of immune reconstitution with preserved memory T-cells when PT-Cy is used in T-cell-replete haplo-HCT [76,100]. Luznik and colleagues reported incidence rates of sustained engraftment, grades II-IV acute GVHD, and chronic GVHD of 87%, 34%, and <25%, respectively, among 67 RIC haplo-HCT recipients with hematological malignancies [105]. NRM at one year was acceptably low at 15%; however, the relapse rate was higher at 51%, resulting in two-year event-free survival (EFS) of only 26%. Similar results were observed in their most updated report of a phase II study involving 210 patients with hematological malignancies receiving RIC conditioning followed by bone marrow haplo-HCT and PT-Cy: the cumulative incidence rates of grade II-IV acute GVHD, chronic GVHD, five-year relapse, and EFS were 27%, 13%, 55%, and 27%, respectively [76]. Another recent study by Ciurea and colleagues compared the clinical outcomes of 65 haplo-HCT recipients with T-cell-replete haplo-HCT/PT-Cy *versus* T-cell-depleted peripheral blood HCT. They demonstrated the superiority of T-cell-replete haplo-HCT/PT-Cy in terms of one-year NRM (16% *vs.*42%, *p* = 0.03), chronic GVHD (8% *vs.* 18%, *p* = 0.03), PFS (45% *vs.* 21%, *p* = 0.03), and OS (66% *vs.* 30%, *p* = 0.02) [99]. Bashey and colleagues identified comparable rates of relapse, DFS, and OS between haplo-HCT/PT-Cy and MSD or adult URD HCT [9]. These results were reproduced by the Italian group in 459 allograft recipients of haplo-HCT/PT-Cy, MSD, matched URD, mismatched URD, and UCB [79]. Although in this study the UCB group had higher TRM and inferior survival compared to haplo-HCT, myeloablative conditioning with Thio/Bu/Flu or Bu/Cy was the most common regimen (83%) used for UCB allograft, which likely contributed to higher TRM and inferior survival in this group. A recent CIBMTR study examined the clinical outcomes of 2174 adults with AML receiving haplo-HCT/PT-Cy (*n* = 192) or matched URD (*n* = 1982) allograft and identified similar two-year survival rates for these two donor groups after both myeloablative conditioning and RIC [77]. The BMT-CTN conducted two parallel multicenter phase II trials of RIC haplo-HCT/PT-CY *versus* UCB HCT. Both of these alternative donor approaches produced comparable survival rates; however, a lower risk of TRM among recipients of RIC haplo-BMT/PT-CY was offset by a higher risk of relapse as compared to UCB HCT recipients [7]. A recent collaborative study by French and Italian groups retrospectively compared the clinical outcomes of haplo-HCT and UCB transplantation in 150 patients with various hematological malignancies [106]. While haplo-HCT in this study was mostly performed for a lymphoma diagnosis (84%), the UCB group in contrast was enriched with acute leukemia patients (63%) and those undergoing alloHCT with a significantly higher disease risk index (44% *vs.* 20%). These findings most likely contributed to a higher cumulative incidence of disease relapse and lower DFS after UCB transplantation as compared to haplo-HCT. However, these results had no impact on overall survival, and TRM was similar between the groups. A more recent and larger retrospective study by EBMT examined differences between haplo-HCT (32% PT-Cy-based) and UCB (49% Cy/Flu/TBI-based) allografts in 1446 patients with acute leukemia and identified delayed engraftment and a lower rate of chronic GVHD with UCB transplant, but otherwise similar long-term clinical outcomes with both donor types [107]. Newer strategies are being tested to further improve the outcomes of haplo-HCT/PT-Cy. Grosso and colleagues recently reported an encouraging two-year DFS of 74% among 30 patients with hematological malignancies who received myeloablative haplo-HCT with 1200 cGy TBI followed by infusion of fixed-dose donor T-cells, 48 hours later by high-dose Cy, and 24 hours later by selected donor CD34+ cell infusion [108]. In conclusion, clinical research to improve the outcomes of haplo-HCT has witnessed dramatic successes within the past decade (Table 2), allowing many adults with leukemia who do not have an available HLA-identical relative to receive allogenic HCT using readily available UCB or haploidentical donors.

Table 2. Haploidentical transplantation for acute leukemia in adults.

Reference	Malignancy	No of Patients	Conditioning Regimen	Median Age (range)	Median Time to ANC ≥500/µL	Median Time to Platelet >20 × 10⁹/L	aGVHD (II-IV) CI (%)	cGVHD CI (%)	TRM	Relapse	DFS
T-cell depleted haplo-HCT											
Aversa 2005	Acute leukemia 67 AML	104	Thio/Flu/TBI/ATG	33 (9-64)	11 days	15 days	8%	7%	36.5%	25% at 6mo	39% at median 22mo
Ciceri 2008	Hematologic Malignancy 173 AML	173	TBI-based: 74% CR1/CR2 71% advanced Mostly with ATG	37 (17-66) CR1/CR2 36 (16-63) advanced	12 days	–	5%	10%	36% CR1 54% CR2 66% advanced	16% CR1 23% CR2 32% advanced	48% CR1 21% CR2 1% advanced
Chang 2009	Hematologic Malignancy 43 AML	133	Bu/Cy +ATG	15 (2-18)	12 days	15 days	–	–	–	–	–
Chang BBMT 2009	Hematologic Malignancy 100 AML	348	Bu/Cy/cytarabine/ Semustine/rATG	24 (2-54)	13 days	16 days	–	–	–	–	–
Haplo-HCT with PT-Cy											
Luznik 2008	Hematologic Malignancy 27 AML	68	NMA Flu/Cy/TBI	46 (1-71)	15 days	24 days	34% at Day 200	5%-25% at 1-yr	15% at 1-yr	51% at 1-yr	26% at 2-yrs
Kazaman 2010	Hematologic Malignancy 49 AML	185	NMA Flu/Cy/TBI	50 (1-71)	–	–	31%	15%	15% at 1-yr	–	35% at 1-yr
Munchel 2011	Hematologic Malignancy 43 AML	210	NMA Flu/Cy/TBI	52 (1-73)	15 days	24 days	27%	13%	18% at 5-yr	55% at 5-yr	27% at 5-yr
Solomon 2012	Hematologic Malignancy 12 AML	20	MA Flu/Bu/Cy	44 (25-56)	16 days	27 days	30%	35%	10% at 1-yr	40% at 1-yr	50% at 1-yr
Haplo-HCT with PT-Cy											
Ciurea 2012	Hematologic Malignancy 42 AML/MDS	65	TCR-Haplo/PT-Cy: 26 MA & 6 NMA; TCD-Haplo/ATG: MA	45 (20-63); 36 (18-56)	18 days; 13 days	26 days; 12 days	20%; 11%	7%; 18%	16% at 1-yr; 42% at 1-yr	34% at 1-yr 36% at 1-yr	50% at 1-yr; 21% at 1-yr
Castagna 2014	Hematologic Malignancy 4 AML/MDS	46 BM 23 PB	NMA Flu/Cy/TBI	## (19-68) 54 (25-65)	21 days 20 days	29 days 27 days	25% 33%	13% 13%	22% at 2-yr 12% at 2-yr	–	62% at 2-yr 62% at 2-yr
Haplo-HCT with intensive immunosuppression											
Huang 2006	Hematologic Malignancy 51 AML	171	MA Bu/Cy/ARA-C/Semustine IS: ATG/CSA/MTX/MMF	25 (2-56)	12 days	15 days	55%	47% at 2-yr	19%-31% at 2-yr	12%-39% at 2-yr	42%-68% at 2-yr

Table 2. *Cont.*

Reference	Malignancy	Conditioning Regimen	No of Patients	Median Age (range)	Median Time to ANC ≥500/µL	Median Time to Platelet >20 × 10^9/L	aGVHD (II-IV) CI (%)	cGVHD CI (%)	TRM	Relapse	DFS
							T-cell depleted haplo-HCT				
Huang 2009	Acute leukemia 108 AML	MA Bu/Cy/ARA-C/ Semustine IS: ATG/CSA/MTX/ MMF	250	25 (2–56)	12 days	15 days	46%	23% at 3-yr	19%–51% at 3-yr	12%–49% at 3-yr	25%–71% at 3-yr
Di Bartolomeo 2013	Hematologic Malignancy 45 AML	80%MA /20%RIC Thio/Bu/Flu IS: ATG/CSA/MTX/ MMF/Basiliximab	80	37 (5–71)	21 days	28 days	24%	Extensive6% at 2-yr	36% at 1-yr	21% at 1-yr	38% at 3-yr
							Haplo-HCT with intensive immunosuppression				
Fu 2014	Hematologic Malignancy 34 AML	TBI/Cy/simustine/ATG Bu/Cy/simustine/ ARA-C/ATG	38 77	20 (13–46 24 (8–51))	13 days 12 days	19 days 16 days	32% 48%	61% at 1-yr 53% at 1-yr	13% at 1-yr 16% at 1-yr	27% at 2-yr 32% at 2-yr	58% at 2-yr 57% at 2-yr
							Comparative studies with Haplo-HCT				
Lu 2006	Hematologic malignancies 69 AML	MA Haplo (Bu/Cy/ATG) MRD (Bu/Cy)	135 158	24 (3–50) 37 (5–50)	12 days 15 days $p < 0.001$	15 days 15 days $p = NS$	D100 32% 40% $N = 0.13$	2-yr 55% 56% $p = 0.90$	2-yr 22% 14% $p = 0.10$	2-yr 18% 13% $p = 0.40$	2-yr 64% 71% $p = 0.27$
Brunstein 2011	Hematologic malignancies 51 AML	RIC Haplo PT-Cy dUCB	50 50	48 (7–70) 58 (16–69)	16 days 15 days	24 days 38 days	D100 32% 40% $p = 0.13$	1-yr 13% 25%	1-yr 7% 4%	1-yr 45% 31%	1-yr 48% 46%
Bashey 2013	Hematologic malignancies 91 AML	50% MA Haplo PT-Cy MRD 8/8 URD	46 50 51	59 (50–71) 58 (50–75) 58 (50–72)	---	---	D180 30% 38% 27% $p = NS$ 39% $p = NS$	2-yr 38% 54% $p < 0.05$ 54% $p < 0.05$	2-yr 7% 13% $p = NS$ 16% $p = NS$	2-yr 33% 34% $p = NS$ 34% $p = NS$	2-yr 60% 53% $p = NS$ 52% $p = NS$
							Comparative studies with Haplo-HCT				
Raiola 2014	Hematologic malignancies 232 acute leukemia	69% MA UCB MRD 8/8 URD 7/8 URD Haplo	105 176 43 43 92	40 (18–64) 47 (15–69) 42 (19–66) 47 (17–62) 45 (17–69)	23 days 18 days 17 days 16 days 18 days $p < 0.05$	D50 (median) 40 days 160 days 100 days 110 days 118 days $p < 0.01$	D100 19% 31% 21% 42% 14% $p < 0.001$	4 yr 23% 29% 22% 19% 15% $p = 0.053$	D100 35% 24% 33% 35% 18% $p = 0.10$	4 yr 30% 40% 23% 30% 35% $p = 0.89$	4 yr 33% 32% 36% 34% 43% $p = 0.20$

Table 2. *Cont.*

Reference	Malignancy	Conditioning Regimen	No of Patients	Median Age (range)	Median Time to ANC ≥500/µL	Median Time to Platelet >20 × 10⁹/L	aGVHD (II-IV) CI (%)	cGVHD CI (%)	TRM	Relapse	DFS
					T-cell depleted haplo-HCT						
Ciurea 2014 (ASH)	2174 AML	MA-Haplo PT-Cy MA-8/8 URD RIC-Haplo PT-Cy RIC-8/8 URD	104 125 88 737	21–70	D30 CI 90% 97% p = 0.01 93% 96% p = 0.25	– – – –	– – – –	– – – –	HR 1.0 1.07 p = 0.82 1.0 2.35 p = 0.03	HR 1.0 0.88 p = 0.40 1.0 0.76 p = 0.09	2-yr OS 47% 54% p = 0.22 53% 49% p = 0.25
Luo 2014	Hematologic malignancies 126 AML	TCR-Haplo MRD 8/8 URD	99 90 116	25 (9-55) 34 (16-56) 26 (10-50)	12 days 12 days 12 days	15 days 12 days 13 days	D90 42% 16% p < 0.05 40% p = NS	2-yr 41% 24% p = NS 42% p = NS	31% 5% p < 0.001 22% p = NS	5-yr 14% 34% p = 0.008 21% p = NS	5-yr 58% 64% p = NS 58% p = NS
Ruggeri 2015	AML	Haplo (32% PT-Cy) UCB (49% Cy/Flu/TBI)	360 558	44 (18-75) 48 (18-72) P = 0.62	23 days 17 days p < 0.01	– –	27% 31% p = 0.10	HR 1.0 0.63 p = 0.008	HR 1.0 1.16 p = 0.47	HR 1.0 0.95 p = 0.76	HR 1.0 0.78 p = 0.78

11. Unmodified Haploidentical Graft with Intensive Immune Suppression

Another approach to minimizing the rate of GVHD after haploidentical transplantation is the use intensive immunosuppression [109–111]. This strategy was first studied by Huang and colleagues, in which 250 patients with acute leukemia received a G-CSF-primed, unmanipulated, haploidentical, peripheral blood or bone marrow graft [111]. Myeloablative conditioning consisted of Bu/Cy/cytarabine/semustine and rabbit ATG, and the immunosuppression consisted of CSA, MMF, and methotrexate (MTX). Neutrophil engraftment was achieved in all except one patient, and the rates of grade II-IV acute GVHD, grade III-IV acute GVHD, and extensive chronic GVHD were 46%, 13%, and 23%, respectively. At three years, TRM and the relapse rate were higher for high-risk AML patients at 29% and 49%, respectively. In their most updated report Luo and colleagues compared their haplo-HCT experience with MRD and matched URD and identified higher TRM and lower relapse rate associated with haplo-HCT as compared to MRD graft; however, five-year LFS was similar in all three groups [112]. Most recently, the same group from China compared the TBI/Cy/simustine/ATG conditioning regimen with the Bu/Cy/simustine/cytarabine/ATG regimen in 115 patients with acute leukemia and reported similar clinical outcomes except for a higher rate of organ toxicities with the Bu-based regimen [113]. Another group from China reported their experience using T-cell-replete haplo-HCT with myeloablative conditioning consisting of Bu/Cy/cytarabine/lamustine and low-dose (10 mg/kg) ATG and immunosuppression consisting of CSA, MMF, and MTX [112]. They compared this haplo-HCT platform (*n* = 99) to MSD (*n* = 90) and URD (*n* = 116) allografts and identified comparable long-term DFS in all three groups. While there was no difference in other clinical outcomes between haplo-HCT and URD grafts, haplo-HCT recipients had a higher incidence of TRM and acute GVHD, but a lower relapse rate, than MRD recipients. In addition, a G-CSF-priming conditioning regimen in T-cell-replete haplo-HCT with intensive immunosuppression resulted in a lower relapse rate and superior LFS and OS as compared to non-G-CSF priming in a Southwest China multicenter randomized controlled study [114]. A similar strategy of intensive immunosuppression after T-cell-replete haplo-HCT has been evaluated in 80 patients with high-risk hematologic malignancies [115]. GVHD prophylaxis consisted of five drugs (ATG, CSA, MMF, MTX and basiliximab), and most patients (80%) received myeloablative conditioning consisting mainly of Thio/Bu/Flu. This therapeutic approach produced acceptable hematopoietic engraftment and low rates of acute and chronic GVHD, leading to a three-year LFS rate of 30% for high-risk patients. A calcineurin inhibitor-free, sirolimus-based immunosuppressive platform in combination with ATG, MMF, and rituximab was another modality that was used after trosulfan/Flu conditioning and T-cell-replete haplo-HCT; this approach demonstrated rapid T-cell immune reconstitution and promoted *in vivo* expansion of Tregs [116,117]. On the basis of these clinical investigations, it is reasonable to view T-cell-replete haplo-HCT in combination with intensive immunosuppression to be another promising haplo-HCT platform.

12. The Way Forward

Alternative donor transplantation is now a reality that allows almost every patient who requires alloHCT to proceed with this potentially curative treatment modality. Mismatched URD represents yet another alternative donor type, especially with our improved understanding of the HLA-system and HLA-matching, such as the identification of "permissive" mismatches [118]. Future advances in clinical care will require physicians to encourage their patients to participate in prospective clinical trials so that strategies to improve the clinical outcomes of HCT recipients using alternative donor types and platform options can be rigorously compared. One such clinical trial is the phase III, randomized, multicenter trial (BMT CTN protocol 1101) of RIC and double UCB HCT *versus* haplo-HCT with PT-Cy in adults with leukemia and lymphoma. This study will compare clinical outcomes as well as cost efficacy, quality of life, and immune reconstitution: important outcomes for defining the relative efficacy of the two donor types and helping to establish evidence-based standards of care.

Acknowledgments: We would like to acknowledge Michael Franklin, MS, for assistance in editing this manuscript.

Author Contributions: Nelli Bejanyan, Housam Haddad and Claudio Brunstein wrote the paper.

Conflicts of Interest: The authors declare no conflict of interest.

References

1. Grewal, S.S.; Barker, J.N.; Davies, S.M.; Wagner, J.E. Unrelated donor hematopoietic cell transplantation: Marrow or umbilical cord blood? *Blood* **2003**, *101*, 4233–4244. [CrossRef] [PubMed]
2. Confer, D.; Robinett, P. The US National Marrow Donor Program role in unrelated donor hematopoietic cell transplantation. *Bone Marrow Transplant.* **2008**, *42* (Suppl. 1), S3–S5. [CrossRef] [PubMed]
3. Ballen, K.K.; Spitzer, T.R.; Yeap, B.Y.; McAfee, S.; Dey, B.R.; Attar, E.; Haspel, R.; Kao, G.; Liney, D.; Alyea, E.; *et al.* Double unrelated reduced-intensity umbilical cord blood transplantation in adults. *Biol. Blood Marrow Transplant.* **2007**, *13*, 82–89. [CrossRef] [PubMed]
4. Brunstein, C.G.; Barker, J.N.; Weisdorf, D.J.; DeFor, T.E.; Miller, J.S.; Blazar, B.R.; McGlave, P.B.; Wagner, J.E. Umbilical cord blood transplantation after nonmyeloablative conditioning: Impact on transplantation outcomes in 110 adults with hematologic disease. *Blood* **2007**, *110*, 3064–3070. [CrossRef] [PubMed]
5. Gladstone, D.E.; Zachary, A.A.; Fuchs, E.J.; Luznik, L.; Kasamon, Y.L.; King, K.E.; Brodsky, R.A.; Jones, R.J.; Leffell, M.S. Partially mismatched transplantation and human leukocyte antigen donor-specific antibodies. *Biol. Blood Marrow Transplant.* **2013**, *19*, 647–652. [CrossRef] [PubMed]
6. Misawa, M.; Kai, S.; Okada, M.; Nakajima, T.; Nomura, K.; Wakae, T.; Toda, A.; Itoi, H.; Takatsuka, H.; Itsukuma, T. Reduced-intensity conditioning followed by unrelated umbilical cord blood transplantation for advanced hematologic malignancies: Rapid engraftment in bone marrow. *Int. J. Hematol.* **2006**, *83*, 74–79. [CrossRef] [PubMed]
7. Brunstein, C.G.; Fuchs, E.J.; Carter, S.L.; Karanes, C.; Costa, L.J.; Wu, J.; Devine, S.M.; Wingard, J.R.; Aljitawi, O.S.; Cutler, C.S.; *et al.* Alternative donor transplantation after reduced intensity conditioning: Results of parallel phase 2 trials using partially HLA-mismatched related bone marrow or unrelated double umbilical cord blood grafts. *Blood* **2011**, *118*, 282–288. [CrossRef] [PubMed]
8. Chang, Y.J.; Xu, L.P.; Liu, D.H.; Liu, K.Y.; Han, W.; Chen, Y.H.; Wang, Y.; Chen, H.; Wang, J.Z.; Zhang, X.H. Platelet engraftment in patients with hematologic malignancies following unmanipulated haploidentical blood and marrow transplantation: Effects of CD34+ cell dose and disease status. *Biol. Blood Marrow Transplant.* **2009**, *15*, 632–638. [CrossRef] [PubMed]
9. Bashey, A.; Zhang, X.; Sizemore, C.A.; Manion, K.; Brown, S.; Holland, H.K.; Morris, L.E.; Solomon, S.R. T-cell-replete HLA-haploidentical hematopoietic transplantation for hematologic malignancies using post-transplantation cyclophosphamide results in outcomes equivalent to those of contemporaneous HLA-matched related and unrelated donor transplantation. *J. Clin. Oncol.* **2013**, *31*, 1310–1316. [CrossRef] [PubMed]
10. Kasamon, Y.L.; Luznik, L.; Leffell, M.S.; Kowalski, J.; Tsai, H.L.; Bolanos-Meade, J.; Morris, L.E.; Crilley, P.A.; O'Donnell, P.V.; Rossiter, N.; *et al.* Nonmyeloablative HLA-haploidentical bone marrow transplantation with high-dose posttransplantation cyclophosphamide: Effect of HLA disparity on outcome. *Biol. Blood Marrow Transplant.* **2010**, *16*, 482–489. [CrossRef] [PubMed]
11. Delaney, C.; Varnum-Finney, B.; Aoyama, K.; Brashem-Stein, C.; Bernstein, I.D. Dose-dependent effects of the Notch ligand Delta1 on *ex vivo* differentiation and *in vivo* marrow repopulating ability of cord blood cells. *Blood* **2005**, *106*, 2693–2699. [CrossRef] [PubMed]
12. De Lima, M.; McNiece, I.; Robinson, S.N.; Munsell, M.; Eapen, M.; Horowitz, M.; Alousi, A.; Saliba, R.; McMannis, J.D.; Kaur, I. Cord-blood engraftment with *ex vivo* mesenchymal-cell coculture. *N. Engl. J. Med.* **2012**, *367*, 2305–2315. [CrossRef] [PubMed]
13. Wagner, J.E.; Brunstein, C.G.; McKenna, D.; Sumstad, D.; Maahs, S.; Boitano, A.E.; Cooke, M.P.; Bleul, C.C. Safety and Exploratory Efficacy of *Ex Vivo* Expanded Umbilical Cord Blood (UCB) Hematopoietic Stem and Progenitor Cells (HSPC) Using Cytokines and Stem-Regenin 1 (SR1): Interim Results of a Phase 1/2 Dose Escalation Clinical Study. *Blood (ASH Annu. Meet. Abstr.)* **2013**, *122*, 698.
14. Frassoni, F.; Gualandi, F.; Podesta, M.; Raiola, A.M.; Ibatici, A.; Piaggio, G.; Sessarego, M.; Sessarego, N.; Gobbi, M.; Sacchi, N. Direct intrabone transplant of unrelated cord-blood cells in acute leukaemia: A phase I/II study. *Lancet Oncol.* **2008**, *9*, 831–839. [CrossRef]

15. Frassoni, F.; Varaldo, R.; Gualandi, F.; Bacigalupo, A.; Sambuceti, G.; Sacchi, N.; Podestà, M. The intra-bone marrow injection of cord blood cells extends the possibility of transplantation to the majority of patients with malignant hematopoietic diseases. *Best Pract. Res. Clin. Haematol.* **2010**, *23*, 237–244. [CrossRef] [PubMed]

16. Brunstein, C.G.; Barker, J.N.; Weisdorf, D.J.; Defor, T.E.; McKenna, D.; Chong, S.Y.; Miller, J.S.; McGlave, P.B.; Wagner, J.E. Intra-BM injection to enhance engraftment after myeloablative umbilical cord blood transplantation with two partially HLA-matched units. *Bone Marrow Transplant.* **2009**, *43*, 935–940. [CrossRef] [PubMed]

17. Brunstein, C.G.; Miller, J.S.; Cao, Q.; McKenna, D.H.; Hippen, K.L.; Curtsinger, J.; Defor, T.; Levine, B.L.; June, C.H.; Rubinstein, P.; et al. Infusion of *ex vivo* expanded T regulatory cells in adults transplanted with umbilical cord blood: Safety profile and detection kinetics. *Blood* **2011**, *117*, 1061–1070. [CrossRef] [PubMed]

18. Locatelli, F.; Perotti, C.; Torretta, L.; Maccario, R.; Montagna, D.; Ravelli, A.; Giorgiani, G.; De Benedetti, F.; Giraldi, E.; Magnani, M.L.; et al. Mobilization and selection of peripheral blood hematopoietic progenitors in children with systemic sclerosis. *Haematologica* **1999**, *84*, 839–843. [PubMed]

19. Barker, J.N.; Weisdorf, D.J.; Wagner, J.E. Creation of a double chimera after the transplantation of umbilical-cord blood from two partially matched unrelated donors. *N. Engl. J. Med.* **2001**, *344*, 1870–1871. [CrossRef] [PubMed]

20. Rocha, V.; Cornish, J.; Sievers, E.L.; Filipovich, A.; Locatelli, F.; Peters, C.; Remberger, M.; Michel, G.; Arcese, W.; Dallorso, S.; et al. Comparison of outcomes of unrelated bone marrow and umbilical cord blood transplants in children with acute leukemia. *Blood* **2001**, *97*, 2962–2971. [CrossRef] [PubMed]

21. Wagner, J.E.; Barker, J.N.; DeFor, T.E.; Baker, K.S.; Blazar, B.R.; Eide, C.; Goldman, A.; Kersey, J.; Krivit, W.; MacMillan, M.L.; et al. Transplantation of unrelated donor umbilical cord blood in 102 patients with malignant and nonmalignant diseases: Influence of CD34 cell dose and HLA disparity on treatment-related mortality and survival. *Blood* **2002**, *100*, 1611–1618. [PubMed]

22. Michel, G.; Rocha, V.; Chevret, S.; Arcese, W.; Chan, K.W.; Filipovich, A.; Takahashi, T.A.; Vowels, M.; Ortega, J.; Bordigoni, P.; et al. Unrelated cord blood transplantation for childhood acute myeloid leukemia: A Eurocord Group analysis. *Blood* **2003**, *102*, 4290–4297. [CrossRef] [PubMed]

23. Gluckman, E.; Rocha, V. Cord blood transplantation for children with acute leukaemia: A Eurocord registry analysis. *Blood Cells Mol. Dis.* **2004**, *33*, 271–273. [CrossRef] [PubMed]

24. Escolar, M.L.; Poe, M.D.; Provenzale, J.M.; Richards, K.C.; Allison, J.; Wood, S.; Wenger, D.A.; Pietryga, D.; Wall, D.; Champagne, M.; et al. Transplantation of umbilical-cord blood in babies with infantile Krabbe's disease. *N. Engl. J. Med.* **2005**, *352*, 2069–2081. [CrossRef] [PubMed]

25. Laughlin, M.J.; Barker, J.; Bambach, B.; Koc, O.N.; Rizzieri, D.A.; Wagner, J.E.; Gerson, S.L.; Lazarus, H.M.; Cairo, M.; Stevens, C.E.; et al. Hematopoietic engraftment and survival in adult recipients of umbilical-cord blood from unrelated donors. *N. Engl. J. Med.* **2001**, *344*, 1815–1822. [CrossRef] [PubMed]

26. Cornetta, K.; Laughlin, M.; Carter, S.; Wall, D.; Weinthal, J.; Delaney, C.; Wagner, J.; Sweetman, R.; McCarthy, P.; Chao, N. Umbilical cord blood transplantation in adults: Results of the prospective Cord Blood Transplantation (COBLT). *Biol. Blood Marrow Transplant.* **2005**, *11*, 149–160. [CrossRef] [PubMed]

27. Takahashi, S.; Ooi, J.; Tomonari, A.; Konuma, T.; Tsukada, N.; Oiwa-Monna, M.; Fukuno, K.; Uchiyama, M.; Takasugi, K.; Iseki, T.; et al. Comparative single-institute analysis of cord blood transplantation from unrelated donors with bone marrow or peripheral blood stem-cell transplants from related donors in adult patients with hematologic malignancies after myeloablative conditioning regimen. *Blood* **2007**, *109*, 1322–1330. [PubMed]

28. Sanz, J.; Sanz, M.A.; Saavedra, S.; Lorenzo, I.; Montesinos, P.; Senent, L.; Planelles, D.; Larrea, L.; Martín, G.; Palau, J.; et al. Cord blood transplantation from unrelated donors in adults with high-risk acute myeloid leukemia. *Biol. Blood Marrow Transplant.* **2010**, *16*, 86–94. [CrossRef] [PubMed]

29. Sanz, J.; Boluda, J.C.; Martin, C.; Gonzalez, M.; Ferra, C.; Serrano, D.; de Heredia, C.D.; Barrenetxea, C.; Martinez, A.M.; Solano, C.; et al. Single-unit umbilical cord blood transplantation from unrelated donors in patients with hematological malignancy using busulfan, thiotepa, fludarabine and ATG as myeloablative conditioning regimen. *Bone Marrow Transplant.* **2012**, *47*, 1287–1293. [CrossRef] [PubMed]

30. Sanz, J.; Jaramillo, F.J.; Planelles, D.; Montesinos, P.; Lorenzo, I.; Moscardo, F.; Martin, G.; López, F.; Martínez, J.; Jarque, I.; et al. Impact on outcomes of human leukocyte antigen matching by allele-level typing in adults with acute myeloid leukemia undergoing umbilical cord blood transplantation. *Biol. Blood Marrow Transplant.* **2014**, *20*, 106–110. [CrossRef] [PubMed]

31. Barker, J.N.; Weisdorf, D.J.; DeFor, T.E.; Blazar, B.R.; McGlave, P.B.; Miller, J.S.; Verfaillie, C.M.; Wagner, J.E. Transplantation of 2 partially HLA-matched umbilical cord blood units to enhance engraftment in adults with hematologic malignancy. *Blood* **2005**, *105*, 1343–1347. [CrossRef] [PubMed]

32. Horwitz, M.E.; Morris, A.; Gasparetto, C.; Sullivan, K.; Long, G.; Chute, J.; Verfaillie, C.M.; Wagner, J.E. Myeloablative intravenous busulfan/fludarabine conditioning does not facilitate reliable engraftment of dual umbilical cord blood grafts in adult recipients. *Biol. Blood Marrow Transplant.* **2008**, *14*, 591–594. [CrossRef] [PubMed]

33. Bradstock, K.; Hertzberg, M.; Kerridge, I.; Svennilson, J.; George, B.; McGurgan, M.; Huang, G.; Antonenas, V.; Gottlieb, D. Single *versus* double unrelated umbilical cord blood units for allogeneic transplantation in adults with advanced haematological malignancies: A retrospective comparison of outcomes. *Intern. Med. J.* **2009**, *39*, 744–751. [CrossRef] [PubMed]

34. Kanda, J.; Rizzieri, D.A.; Gasparetto, C.; Long, G.D.; Chute, J.P.; Sullivan, K.M.; Morris, A.; Smith, C.A.; Hogge, D.E.; Nitta, J.; *et al.* Adult dual umbilical cord blood transplantation using myeloablative total body irradiation (1350 cGy) and fludarabine conditioning. *Biol. Blood Marrow Transplant.* **2011**, *17*, 867–874. [CrossRef] [PubMed]

35. Kai, S.; Wake, A.; Okada, M.; Kurata, M.; Atsuta, Y.; Ishikawa, J.; Nakamae, H.; Aotsuka, N.; Kasai, M.; Misawa, M.; *et al.* Double-unit cord blood transplantation after myeloablative conditioning for patients with hematologic malignancies: A multicenter phase II study in Japan. *Biol. Blood Marrow Transplant.* **2013**, *19*, 812–819. [CrossRef] [PubMed]

36. Hulegardh, E.; Nilsson, C.; Lazarevic, V.; Garelius, H.; Antunovic, P.; Rangert Derolf, A.; Möllgård, L.; Uggla, B.; Wennström, L.; Wahlin, A.; *et al.* Characterization and prognostic features of secondary acute myeloid leukemia in a population-based setting: A report from the Swedish Acute Leukemia Registry. *Am. J. Hematol.* **2015**, *90*, 208–214. [CrossRef] [PubMed]

37. Shin, S.H.; Yahng, S.A.; Yoon, J.H.; Lee, S.E.; Cho, B.S.; Eom, K.S.; Lee, S.; Min, C.K.; Kim, H.J.; Cho, S.G.; *et al.* Survival benefits with transplantation in secondary AML evolving from myelodysplastic syndrome with hypomethylating treatment failure. *Bone Marrow Transplant.* **2013**, *48*, 678–683. [CrossRef] [PubMed]

38. Barker, J.N.; Weisdorf, D.J.; DeFor, T.E.; Blazar, B.R.; Miller, J.S.; Wagner, J.E. Rapid and complete donor chimerism in adult recipients of unrelated donor umbilical cord blood transplantation after reduced-intensity conditioning. *Blood* **2003**, *102*, 1915–1919. [CrossRef] [PubMed]

39. Brunstein, C.G.; Eapen, M.; Ahn, K.W.; Appelbaum, F.R.; Ballen, K.K.; Champlin, R.E.; Cutler, C.; Kan, F.; Laughlin, M.J.; Soiffer, R.J.; *et al.* Reduced-intensity conditioning transplantation in acute leukemia: The effect of source of unrelated donor stem cells on outcomes. *Blood* **2012**, *119*, 5591–5598. [CrossRef] [PubMed]

40. Rocha, V.; Crotta, A.; Ruggeri, A.; Purtill, D.; Boudjedir, K.; Herr, A.L.; Ionescu, I.; Gluckman, E.; Eurocord Registry. Double cord blood transplantation: Extending the use of unrelated umbilical cord blood cells for patients with hematological diseases. *Best Pract. Res. Clin. Haematol.* **2010**, *23*, 223–229. [CrossRef] [PubMed]

41. Robin, M.; Ruggeri, A.; Labopin, M.; Niederwieser, D.; Tabrizi, R.; Sanz, G.; Bourhis, J.H.; van Biezen, A.; Koenecke, C.; Blaise, D.; *et al.* Comparison of Unrelated Cord Blood and Peripheral Blood Stem Cell Transplantation in Adults with Myelodysplastic Syndrome after Reduced-Intensity Conditioning Regimen: A Collaborative Study from Eurocord (Cord blood Committee of Cellular Therapy & Immunobiology Working Party of EBMT) and Chronic Malignancies Working Party. *Biol. Blood Marrow Transplant.* **2015**, *21*, 489–495. [PubMed]

42. Scaradavou, A.; Brunstein, C.G.; Eapen, M.; Le-Rademacher, J.; Barker, J.N.; Chao, N.; Cutler, C.; Delaney, C.; Kan, F.; Isola, L.; *et al.* Double unit grafts successfully extend the application of umbilical cord blood transplantation in adults with acute leukemia. *Blood* **2013**, *121*, 752–758. [CrossRef] [PubMed]

43. Kindwall-Keller, T.L.; Hegerfeldt, Y.; Meyerson, H.J.; Margevicius, S.; Fu, P.; van Heeckeren, W.; Lazarus, H.M.; Cooper, B.W.; Gerson, S.L.; Barr, P.; *et al.* Prospective study of one- *vs.* two-unit umbilical cord blood transplantation following reduced intensity conditioning in adults with hematological malignancies. *Bone Marrow Transplant.* **2012**, *47*, 924–933. [CrossRef] [PubMed]

44. Newell, L.F.; Milano, F.; Gutman, J.A.; Riffkin, I.; Lopez, M.; Ziegler, D.; Nemecek, E.R.; Delaney, C. Treosulfan-Based Conditioning Is Sufficient to Promote Engraftment in Cord Blood Transplantation. *Biol. Blood Marrow Transplant.* **2011**, *17*, S227–S228. [CrossRef]

45. Ponce, D.M.; Sauter, C.; Devlin, S.; Lubin, M.; Gonzales, A.M.; Kernan, N.A.; Scaradavou, A.; Giralt, S.; Goldberg, J.D.; Koehne, G.; *et al.* A novel reduced-intensity conditioning regimen induces a high incidence of

sustained donor-derived neutrophil and platelet engraftment after double-unit cord blood transplantation. *Biol. Blood Marrow Transplant.* **2013**, *19*, 799–803. [CrossRef] [PubMed]

46. Cutler, C.; Stevenson, K.; Kim, H.T.; Brown, J.; McDonough, S.; Herrera, M.; Reynolds, C.; Liney, D.; Kao, G.; Ho, V.; *et al.* Double umbilical cord blood transplantation with reduced intensity conditioning and sirolimus-based GVHD prophylaxis. *Bone Marrow Transplant.* **2011**, *46*, 659–667. [CrossRef] [PubMed]

47. Rio, B.; Chevret, S.; Vigouroux, S.; Chevallier, P.; Furst, S.; Sirvent, A.; Bay, J.O.; Socie, G.; Ceballos, P.; Huynh, A.; *et al.* Reduced Intensity Conditioning Regimen Prior to Unrelated Cord Blood Transplantation in Patients with Acute Myeloid leukemia: Preliminary Analysis of a Prospective Phase II Multicentric Trial on Behalf of Societe Française De Greffe De Moelle Osseuse Et Therapie Cellulaire (SFGM-TC) and Eurocord. *Blood (ASH Annu. Meet. Abstr.)* **2010**, *116*, 911.

48. Wallet, H.L.; Sobh, M.; Morisset, S.; Robin, M.; Fegueux, N.; Furst, S.; Mohty, M.; Deconinck, E.; Fouillard, L.; Bordigoni, P.; *et al.* Double umbilical cord blood transplantation for hematological malignancies: A long-term analysis from the SFGM-TC registry. *Exp. Hematol.* **2013**, *41*, 924–933. [CrossRef] [PubMed]

49. Rio, B.; Chevret, S.; Vigouroux, S.; Chevallier, P.; Furst, S.; Sirvent, A.; Bay, J.O.; Socié, G.; Ceballos, P.; Huynh, A.; *et al.* Decreased Nonrelapse Mortality after Unrelated Cord Blood Transplantation for Acute Myeloid Leukemia Using Reduced-Intensity Conditioning: A Prospective Phase II Multicenter Trial. *Biol. Blood Marrow Transplant.* **2015**, *21*, 445–453. [CrossRef] [PubMed]

50. Robin, M.; Sanz, G.F.; Ionescu, I.; Rio, B.; Sirvent, A.; Renaud, M.; Carreras, E.; Milpied, N.; Mohty, M.; Beguin, Y.; *et al.* Unrelated cord blood transplantation in adults with myelodysplasia or secondary acute myeloblastic leukemia: A survey on behalf of Eurocord and CLWP of EBMT. *Leukemia* **2011**, *25*, 75–81. [CrossRef] [PubMed]

51. Rocha, V.; Labopin, M.; Ruggeri, A.; Podestà, M.; Caballero, D.; Bonifazi, F.; Montserrat, R.; Gallamini, A.; Fagioli, F.; Socié, G.; *et al.* Unrelated Cord Blood Transplantation: Comparison After Single Unit Cord Blood Intrabone Injection and Double Unit Cord Blood Transplantation In Patients with Hematological Malignant Disorders. A Eurocord-EBMT Analysis. *Blood (ASH Annu. Meet. Abstr.)* **2010**, *116*, 223. [CrossRef] [PubMed]

52. Verneris, M.R.; Brunstein, C.G.; Barker, J.; MacMillan, M.L.; DeFor, T.; McKenna, D.H.; Burke, M.J.; Blazar, B.R.; Miller, J.S.; McGlave, P.B.; *et al.* Relapse risk after umbilical cord blood transplantation: Enhanced graft-versus-leukemia effect in recipients of 2 units. *Blood* **2009**, *114*, 4293–4299. [CrossRef] [PubMed]

53. Sanz, J.; Wagner, J.E.; Sanz, M.A.; DeFor, T.; Montesinos, P.; Bachanova, V.; Lorenzo, I.; Warlick, E.; Sanz, G.F.; Brunstein, C. Myeloablative cord blood transplantation in adults with acute leukemia: Comparison of two different transplant platforms. *Biol. Blood Marrow Transplant.* **2013**, *19*, 1725–1730. [CrossRef] [PubMed]

54. Ruggeri, A.; Sanz, G.; Bittencourt, H.; Sanz, J.; Rambaldi, A.; Volt, F.; Yakoub-Agha, I.; Ribera, J.M.; Mannone, L.; Sierra, J.; Mohty, M.; *et al.* Comparison of outcomes after single or double cord blood transplantation in adults with acute leukemia using different types of myeloablative conditioning regimen, a retrospective study on behalf of Eurocord and the Acute Leukemia Working Party of EBMT. *Leukemia* **2014**, *28*, 779–786. [CrossRef] [PubMed]

55. MacMillan, M.L.; Weisdorf, D.J.; Brunstein, C.G.; Cao, Q.; DeFor, T.E.; Verneris, M.R.; Blazar, B.R.; Wagner, J.E. Acute graft-versus-host disease after unrelated donor umbilical cord blood transplantation: Analysis of risk factors. *Blood* **2009**, *113*, 2410–2415. [CrossRef] [PubMed]

56. Wagner, J.E., Jr.; Eapen, M.; Carter, S.; Wang, Y.; Schultz, K.R.; Wall, D.A.; Bunin, N.; Delaney, C.; Haut, P.; Margolis, D.; *et al.* One-unit *versus* two-unit cord-blood transplantation for hematologic cancers. *N. Engl. J. Med.* **2014**, *371*, 1685–1694. [CrossRef] [PubMed]

57. Eapen, M.; Rocha, V.; Sanz, G.; Scaradavou, A.; Zhang, M.J.; Arcese, W.; Sirvent, A.; Champlin, R.E.; Chao, N.; Gee, A.P.; *et al.* Effect of graft source on unrelated donor haemopoietic stem-cell transplantation in adults with acute leukaemia: A retrospective analysis. *Lancet Oncol.* **2010**, *11*, 653–660. [CrossRef]

58. Brunstein, C.G.; Gutman, J.A.; Weisdorf, D.J.; Woolfrey, A.E.; Defor, T.E.; Gooley, T.A.; Verneris, M.R.; Appelbaum, F.R.; Wagner, J.E.; Delaney, C. Allogeneic hematopoietic cell transplantation for hematologic malignancy: Relative risks and benefits of double umbilical cord blood. *Blood* **2010**, *116*, 4693–4699. [CrossRef] [PubMed]

59. Laughlin, M.J.; Eapen, M.; Rubinstein, P.; Wagner, J.E.; Zhang, M.J.; Champlin, R.E.; Stevens, C.; Barker, J.N.; Gale, R.P.; Lazarus, H.M.; *et al.* Outcomes after transplantation of cord blood or bone marrow from unrelated donors in adults with leukemia. *N. Engl. J. Med.* **2004**, *351*, 2265–2275. [CrossRef] [PubMed]

J. Clin. Med. **2015**, *4*, 1240–1268

60. Rocha, V.; Labopin, M.; Sanz, G.; Arcese, W.; Schwerdtfeger, R.; Bosi, A.; Jacobsen, N.; Ruutu, T.; de Lima, M.; Finke, J.; *et al.* Transplants of umbilical-cord blood or bone marrow from unrelated donors in adults with acute leukemia. *N. Engl. J. Med.* **2004**, *351*, 2276–2285. [CrossRef] [PubMed]

61. Gutman, J.A.; Leisenring, W.; Appelbaum, F.R.; Woolfrey, A.E.; Delaney, C. Low relapse without excessive transplant-related mortality following myeloablative cord blood transplantation for acute leukemia in complete remission: A matched cohort analysis. *Biol. Blood Marrow Transplant.* **2009**, *15*, 1122–1129. [CrossRef] [PubMed]

62. Majhail, N.S.; Brunstein, C.G.; Tomblyn, M.; Thomas, A.J.; Miller, J.S.; Arora, M.; Kaufman, D.S.; Burns, L.J.; Slungaard, A.; McGlave, P.B.; *et al.* Reduced-intensity allogeneic transplant in patients older than 55 years: Unrelated umbilical cord blood is safe and effective for patients without a matched related donor. *Biol. Blood Marrow Transplant.* **2008**, *14*, 282–289. [CrossRef] [PubMed]

63. Majhail, N.S.; Brunstein, C.G.; Shanley, R.; Sandhu, K.; McClune, B.; Oran, B.; Warlick, E.D.; Wagner, J.E.; Weisdorf, D.J. Reduced-intensity hematopoietic cell transplantation in older patients with AML/MDS: Umbilical cord blood is a feasible option for patients without HLA-matched sibling donors. *Bone Marrow Transplant.* **2012**, *47*, 494–498. [CrossRef] [PubMed]

64. Chen, Y.B.; Aldridge, J.; Kim, H.T.; Ballen, K.K.; Cutler, C.; Kao, G.; Liney, D.; Bourdeau, G.; Alyea, E.P.; Armand, P.; *et al.* Reduced-intensity conditioning stem cell transplantation: Comparison of double umbilical cord blood and unrelated donor grafts. *Biol. Blood Marrow Transplant.* **2012**, *18*, 805–812. [CrossRef] [PubMed]

65. Le Bourgeois, A.; Mohr, C.; Guillaume, T.; Delaunay, J.; Malard, F.; Loirat, M.; Peterlin, P.; Blin, N.; Dubruille, V.; Mahe, B.; *et al.* Comparison of outcomes after two standards-of-care reduced-intensity conditioning regimens and two different graft sources for allogeneic stem cell transplantation in adults with hematologic diseases: A single-center analysis. *Biol. Blood Marrow Transplant.* **2013**, *19*, 934–939. [CrossRef] [PubMed]

66. Weisdorf, D.; Eapen, M.; Ruggeri, A.; Zhang, M.J.; Zhong, X.; Brunstein, C.; Ustun, C.; Rocha, V.; Gluckman, E. Alternative donor transplantation for older patients with acute myeloid leukemia in first complete remission: A center for international blood and marrow transplant research-eurocord analysis. *Biol. Blood Marrow Transplant.* **2014**, *20*, 816–822. [CrossRef] [PubMed]

67. Malard, F.; Milpied, N.; Blaise, D.; Chevallier, P.; Michallet, M.; Lioure, B.; Clément, L.; Hicheri, Y.; Cordonnier, C.; Huynh, A.; *et al.* Effect of graft source on unrelated donor hemopoietic stem cell transplantation in adults with acute myeloid leukaemia after reduced intensity or non-myeloablative conditioning: A study from the Societe Francaise de Greffe de Moelle et de Therapie Cellulaire. *Biol. Blood Marrow Transplant.* **2015**, *21*, 1059–1067. [PubMed]

68. Ponce, D.M.; Zheng, J.; Gonzales, A.M.; Lubin, M.; Heller, G.; Castro-Malaspina, H.; Giralt, S.; Hsu, K.; Jakubowski, A.A.; Jenq, R.R. Reduced late mortality risk contributes to similar survival after double-unit cord blood transplantation compared with related and unrelated donor hematopoietic stem cell transplantation. *Biol. Blood Marrow Transplant.* **2011**, *17*, 1316–1326. [CrossRef] [PubMed]

69. Atsuta, Y.; Suzuki, R.; Nagamura-Inoue, T.; Taniguchi, S.; Takahashi, S.; Kai, S.; Sakamaki, H.; Kouzai, Y.; Kasai, M.; Fukuda, T.; *et al.* Disease-specific analyses of unrelated cord blood transplantation compared with unrelated bone marrow transplantation in adult patients with acute leukemia. *Blood* **2009**, *113*, 1631–1638. [CrossRef] [PubMed]

70. Appelbaum, F.R.; Anasetti, C.; Antin, J.H.; Atkins, H.; Davies, S.; Devine, S.; Giralt, S.; Heslop, H.; Laport, G.; Lee, S.J.; *et al.* Blood and marrow transplant clinical trials network state of the Science Symposium 2014. *Biol. Blood Marrow Transplant.* **2015**, *21*, 202–224. [CrossRef] [PubMed]

71. Powles, R.L.; Morgenstern, G.R.; Kay, H.E.; McElwain, T.J.; Clink, H.M.; Dady, P.J.; Barrett, A.; Jameson, B.; Depledge, M.H.; Watson, J.G.; *et al.* Mismatched family donors for bone-marrow transplantation as treatment for acute leukaemia. *Lancet* **1983**, *1*, 612–615. [CrossRef]

72. Szydlo, R.; Goldman, J.M.; Klein, J.P.; Gale, R.P.; Ash, R.C.; Bach, F.H.; Bradley, B.A.; Casper, J.T.; Flomenberg, N.; Gajewski, J.L.; *et al.* Results of allogeneic bone marrow transplants for leukemia using donors other than HLA-identical siblings. *J. Clin. Oncol.* **1997**, *15*, 1767–1777. [PubMed]

73. Beatty, P.G.; Clift, R.A.; Mickelson, E.M.; Nisperos, B.B.; Flournoy, N.; Martin, P.J.; Sanders, J.E.; Stewart, P.; Buckner, C.D.; Storb, R. Marrow transplantation from related donors other than HLA-identical siblings. *N. Engl. J. Med.* **1985**, *313*, 765–771. [CrossRef] [PubMed]

74. O'Reilly, R.J.; Keever, C.; Kernan, N.A.; Brochstein, J.; Collins, N.; Flomenberg, N.; Laver, J.; Emanuel, D.; Dupont, B.; Cunningham, I.; *et al.* HLA nonidentical T cell depleted marrow transplants: A comparison of results in patients treated for leukemia and severe combined immunodeficiency disease. *Transplant. Proc.* **1987**, *19* (6 Suppl. 7), 55–60. [PubMed]

75. Ash, R.C.; Horowitz, M.M.; Gale, R.P.; van Bekkum, D.W.; Casper, J.T.; Gordon-Smith, E.C.; Henslee, P.J.; Kolb, H.J.; Lowenberg, B.; Masaoka, T. Bone marrow transplantation from related donors other than HLA-identical siblings: Effect of T cell depletion. *Bone Marrow Transplant.* **1991**, *7*, 443–452. [PubMed]

76. Munchel, A.; Kesserwan, C.; Symons, H.J.; Luznik, L.; Kasamon, Y.L.; Jones, R.J.; Fuchs, E.J. Nonmyeloablative, HLA-haploidentical bone marrow transplantation with high dose, post-transplantation cyclophosphamide. *Pediatr. Rep.* **2011**, *3* (Suppl. 2), e15. [CrossRef] [PubMed]

77. Ciurea, S.O.; Zhang, M.J.; Bacigalupo, A.; Bashey, A.; Appelbaum, F.R.; Antin, J.H.; Chen, J.; Devine, S.M.; Fowler, D.H.; Nakamura, R.; *et al.* Survival after T-Cell Replete Haplo-Identical Related Donor Transplant Using Post-Transplant Cyclophosphamide Compared with Matched Unrelated Donor Transplant for Acute Myeloid Leukemia. *Blood (ASH Annu. Meet. Abstr.)* **2014**, *124*, 679.

78. Luznik, L.; Fuchs, E.J. High-dose, post-transplantation cyclophosphamide to promote graft-host tolerance after allogeneic hematopoietic stem cell transplantation. *Immunol. Res.* **2010**, *47*, 65–77. [CrossRef] [PubMed]

79. Raiola, A.M.; Dominietto, A.; di Grazia, C.; Lamparelli, T.; Gualandi, F.; Ibatici, A.; Bregante, S.; Van Lint, M.T.; Varaldo, R.; Ghiso, A.; *et al.* Unmanipulated haploidentical transplants compared with other alternative donors and matched sibling grafts. *Biol. Blood Marrow Transplant.* **2014**, *20*, 1573–1579. [CrossRef] [PubMed]

80. Perruccio, K.; Tosti, A.; Burchielli, E.; Topini, F.; Ruggeri, L.; Carotti, A.; Capanni, M.; Urbani, E.; Mancusi, A.; Aversa, F.; *et al.* Transferring functional immune responses to pathogens after haploidentical hematopoietic transplantation. *Blood* **2005**, *106*, 4397–4406. [CrossRef] [PubMed]

81. Feuchtinger, T.; Opherk, K.; Bethge, W.A.; Topp, M.S.; Schuster, F.R.; Weissinger, E.M.; Mohty, M.; Or, R.; Maschan, M.; Schumm, M.; *et al.* Adoptive transfer of pp65-specific T cells for the treatment of chemorefractory cytomegalovirus disease or reactivation after haploidentical and matched unrelated stem cell transplantation. *Blood* **2010**, *116*, 4360–4367. [CrossRef] [PubMed]

82. Comoli, P.; Basso, S.; Zecca, M.; Pagliara, D.; Baldanti, F.; Bernardo, M.E.; Barberi, W.; Moretta, A.; Labirio, M.; Paulli, M.; *et al.* Preemptive therapy of EBV-related lymphoproliferative disease after pediatric haploidentical stem cell transplantation. *Am. J. Transplant.* **2007**, *7*, 1648–1655. [CrossRef] [PubMed]

83. Comoli, P.; Schilham, M.W.; Basso, S.; van Vreeswijk, T.; Bernardo, M.E.; Maccario, R.; van Tol, M.J.; Locatelli, F.; Veltrop-Duits, L.A. T-cell lines specific for peptides of adenovirus hexon protein and devoid of alloreactivity against recipient cells can be obtained from HLA-haploidentical donors. *J. Immunother.* **2008**, *31*, 529–536. [CrossRef] [PubMed]

84. Leen, A.M.; Christin, A.; Myers, G.D.; Liu, H.; Cruz, C.R.; Hanley, P.J.; Kennedy-Nasser, A.A.; Leung, K.S.; Gee, A.P.; Krance, R.A.; *et al.* Cytotoxic T lymphocyte therapy with donor T cells prevents and treats adenovirus and Epstein-Barr virus infections after haploidentical and matched unrelated stem cell transplantation. *Blood* **2009**, *114*, 4283–4292. [CrossRef] [PubMed]

85. Ciceri, F.; Bonini, C.; Stanghellini, M.T.; Bondanza, A.; Traversari, C.; Salomoni, M.; Turchetto, L.; Colombi, S.; Bernardi, M.; Peccatori, J.; *et al.* Infusion of suicide-gene-engineered donor lymphocytes after family haploidentical haemopoietic stem-cell transplantation for leukaemia (the TK007 trial): A non-randomised phase I-II study. *Lancet Oncol.* **2009**, *10*, 489–500. [CrossRef]

86. Vago, L.; Oliveira, G.; Bondanza, A.; Noviello, M.; Soldati, C.; Ghio, D.; Brigida, I.; Greco, R.; Lupo Stanghellini, M.T.; Peccatori, J.; *et al.* T-cell suicide gene therapy prompts thymic renewal in adults after hematopoietic stem cell transplantation. *Blood* **2012**, *120*, 1820–1830. [CrossRef] [PubMed]

87. Di Stasi, A.; Tey, S.K.; Dotti, G.; Fujita, Y.; Kennedy-Nasser, A.; Martinez, C.; Straathof, K.; Liu, E.; Durett, A.G.; Grilley, B.; *et al.* Inducible apoptosis as a safety switch for adoptive cell therapy. *N. Engl. J. Med.* **2011**, *365*, 1673–1683. [CrossRef] [PubMed]

88. Nguyen, V.H.; Shashidhar, S.; Chang, D.S.; Ho, L.; Kambham, N.; Bachmann, M.; Brown, J.M.; Negrin, R.S. The impact of regulatory T cells on T-cell immunity following hematopoietic cell transplantation. *Blood* **2008**, *111*, 945–953. [CrossRef] [PubMed]

89. Di Ianni, M.; Falzetti, F.; Carotti, A.; Terenzi, A.; Castellino, F.; Bonifacio, E.; Del Papa, B.; Zei, T.; Ostini, R.I.; Cecchini, D.; *et al.* Tregs prevent GVHD and promote immune reconstitution in HLA-haploidentical transplantation. *Blood* **2011**, *117*, 3921–3928. [CrossRef] [PubMed]

90. Martelli, M.F.; Di Ianni, M.; Ruggeri, L.; Falzetti, F.; Carotti, A.; Terenzi, A.; Pierini, A.; Massei, M.S.; Amico, L.; Urbani, E.; *et al.* HLA-haploidentical transplantation with regulatory and conventional T-cell adoptive immunotherapy prevents acute leukemia relapse. *Blood* **2014**, *124*, 638–644. [CrossRef] [PubMed]

91. Mielke, S.; Nunes, R.; Rezvani, K.; Fellowes, V.S.; Venne, A.; Solomon, S.R.; Fan, Y.; Gostick, E.; Price, D.A.; Scotto, C.; *et al.* A clinical-scale selective allodepletion approach for the treatment of HLA-mismatched and matched donor-recipient pairs using expanded T lymphocytes as antigen-presenting cells and a TH9402-based photodepletion technique. *Blood* **2008**, *111*, 4392–4402. [CrossRef] [PubMed]

92. Bastien, J.P.; Krosl, G.; Therien, C.; Rashkovan, M.; Scotto, C.; Cohen, S.; Allan, D.S.; Hogge, D.; Egeler, R.M.; Perreault, C.; *et al.* Photodepletion differentially affects CD4+ Tregs *versus* CD4+ effector T cells from patients with chronic graft-versus-host disease. *Blood* **2010**, *116*, 4859–4869. [CrossRef] [PubMed]

93. Lafferty, K.J.; Cunningham, A.J. A new analysis of allogeneic interactions. *Aust. J. Exp. Biol. Med. Sci.* **1975**, *53*, 27–42. [CrossRef] [PubMed]

94. Guinan, E.C.; Boussiotis, V.A.; Neuberg, D.; Brennan, L.L.; Hirano, N.; Nadler, L.M.; Fan, Y.; Gostick, E.; Price, D.A.; Scotto, C.; *et al.* Transplantation of anergic histoincompatible bone marrow allografts. *N. Engl. J. Med.* **1999**, *340*, 1704–1714. [CrossRef] [PubMed]

95. Federmann, B.; Bornhauser, M.; Meisner, C.; Kordelas, L.; Beelen, D.W.; Stuhler, G.; Stelljes, M.; Schwerdtfeger, R.; Christopeit, M.; Behre, G.; *et al.* Haploidentical allogeneic hematopoietic cell transplantation in adults using CD3/CD19 depletion and reduced intensity conditioning: A phase II study. *Haematologica* **2012**, *97*, 1523–1531. [CrossRef] [PubMed]

96. Godder, K.T.; Henslee-Downey, P.J.; Mehta, J.; Park, B.S.; Chiang, K.Y.; Abhyankar, S.; Lamb, L.S. Long term disease-free survival in acute leukemia patients recovering with increased gammadelta T cells after partially mismatched related donor bone marrow transplantation. *Bone Marrow Transplant.* **2007**, *39*, 751–757. [CrossRef] [PubMed]

97. Federmann, B.; Hagele, M.; Pfeiffer, M.; Wirths, S.; Schumm, M.; Faul, C.; Vogel, W.; Handgretinger, R.; Kanz, L.; Bethge, W.A. Immune reconstitution after haploidentical hematopoietic cell transplantation: Impact of reduced intensity conditioning and CD3/CD19 depleted grafts. *Leukemia* **2011**, *25*, 121–129. [CrossRef] [PubMed]

98. Locatelli, F.; Bauquet, A.; Palumbo, G.; Moretta, F.; Bertaina, A. Negative depletion of alpha/beta+ T cells and of CD19+ B lymphocytes: A novel frontier to optimize the effect of innate immunity in HLA-mismatched hematopoietic stem cell transplantation. *Immunol. Lett.* **2013**, *155*, 21–23. [CrossRef] [PubMed]

99. Ciurea, S.O.; Mulanovich, V.; Saliba, R.M.; Bayraktar, U.D.; Jiang, Y.; Bassett, R.; Wang, S.A.; Konopleva, M.; Fernandez-Vina, M.; Montes, N.; *et al.* Improved early outcomes using a T cell replete graft compared with T cell depleted haploidentical hematopoietic stem cell transplantation. *Biol. Blood Marrow Transplant.* **2012**, *18*, 1835–1844. [CrossRef] [PubMed]

100. Raiola, A.M.; Dominietto, A.; Ghiso, A.; Di Grazia, C.; Lamparelli, T.; Gualandi, F.; Bregante, S.; Van Lint, M.T.; Geroldi, S.; Luchetti, S.; *et al.* Unmanipulated haploidentical bone marrow transplantation and posttransplantation cyclophosphamide for hematologic malignancies after myeloablative conditioning. *Biol. Blood Marrow Transplant.* **2013**, *19*, 117–122. [CrossRef] [PubMed]

101. Solomon, S.R.; Sizemore, C.A.; Sanacore, M.; Zhang, X.; Brown, S.; Holland, H.K.; Morris, L.E.; Bashey, A. Haploidentical transplantation using T cell replete peripheral blood stem cells and myeloablative conditioning in patients with high-risk hematologic malignancies who lack conventional donors is well tolerated and produces excellent relapse-free survival: Results of a prospective phase II trial. *Biol. Blood Marrow Transplant.* **2012**, *18*, 1859–1866. [PubMed]

102. Chang, Y.J.; Xu, L.P.; Liu, D.H.; Liu, K.Y.; Han, W.; Chen, Y.H.; Wang, Y.; Chen, H.; Wang, J.Z.; Zhang, X.H.; *et al.* The impact of CD34+ cell dose on platelet engraftment in pediatric patients following unmanipulated haploidentical blood and marrow transplantation. *Pediatr. Blood Cancer* **2009**, *53*, 1100–1106. [CrossRef] [PubMed]

103. Ciceri, F.; Labopin, M.; Aversa, F.; Rowe, J.M.; Bunjes, D.; Lewalle, P.; Nagler, A.; Di Bartolomeo, P.; Lacerda, J.F.; Lupo Stanghellini, M.T.; *et al.* A survey of fully haploidentical hematopoietic stem cell transplantation in adults with high-risk acute leukemia: A risk factor analysis of outcomes for patients in remission at transplantation. *Blood* **2008**, *112*, 3574–3581. [CrossRef] [PubMed]

104. Aversa, F.; Terenzi, A.; Tabilio, A.; Falzetti, F.; Carotti, A.; Ballanti, S.; Falcinelli, F.; Velardi, A.; Ruggeri, L.; Aloisi, T.; *et al.* Full haplotype-mismatched hematopoietic stem-cell transplantation: A phase II study in patients with acute leukemia at high risk of relapse. *J. Clin. Oncol.* **2005**, *23*, 3447–3454. [CrossRef] [PubMed]
105. Luznik, L.; O'Donnell, P.V.; Symons, H.J.; Chen, A.R.; Leffell, M.S.; Zahurak, M.; Gooley, T.A.; Piantadosi, S.; Kaup, M.; Ambinder, R.F.; *et al.* HLA-haploidentical bone marrow transplantation for hematologic malignancies using nonmyeloablative conditioning and high-dose, posttransplantation cyclophosphamide. *Biol. Blood Marrow Transplant.* **2008**, *14*, 641–650. [CrossRef] [PubMed]
106. El-Cheikh, J.; Crocchiolo, R.; Furst, S.; Bramanti, S.; Sarina, B.; Granata, A.; Vai, A.; Lemarie, C.; Faucher, C.; Mohty, B.; *et al.* Unrelated cord blood compared with haploidentical grafts in patients with hematological malignancies. *Cancer* **2015**, *121*, 1809–1816. [CrossRef] [PubMed]
107. Ruggeri, A.; Labopin, M.; Sanz, G.; Piemontese, S.; Arcese, W.; Bacigalupo, A.; Blaise, D.; Bosi, A.; Huang, H.; Karakasis, D.; *et al.* Comparison of outcomes after unrelated cord blood and unmanipulated haploidentical stem cell transplantation in adults with acute leukemia. *Leukemia* **2015**. [CrossRef]
108. Grosso, D.; Gaballa, S.; Alpdogan, O.; Carabasi, M.; Filicko-O'Hara, J.; Kasner, M.; Martinez-Outschoorn, U.; Wagner, J.L.; O'Hara, W.; Rudolph, S.; *et al.* A Two-Step Approach to Myeloablative Haploidentical Transplantation: Low Nonrelapse Mortality and High Survival Confirmed in Patients with Earlier Stage Disease. *Biol. Blood Marrow Transplant.* **2015**, *21*, 646–652. [CrossRef] [PubMed]
109. Huang, X.J.; Liu, D.H.; Liu, K.Y.; Xu, L.P.; Chen, H.; Han, W.; Chen, Y.H.; Wang, J.Z.; Gao, Z.Y.; Zhang, Y.C.; *et al.* Haploidentical hematopoietic stem cell transplantation without *in vitro* T-cell depletion for the treatment of hematological malignancies. *Bone Marrow Transplant.* **2006**, *38*, 291–297. [CrossRef] [PubMed]
110. Lu, D.P.; Dong, L.; Wu, T.; Huang, X.J.; Zhang, M.J.; Han, W.; Chen, H.; Liu, D.H.; Gao, Z.Y.; Chen, Y.H.; *et al.* Conditioning including antithymocyte globulin followed by unmanipulated HLA-mismatched/haploidentical blood and marrow transplantation can achieve comparable outcomes with HLA-identical sibling transplantation. *Blood* **2006**, *107*, 3065–3073. [CrossRef] [PubMed]
111. Huang, X.J.; Liu, D.H.; Liu, K.Y.; Xu, L.P.; Chen, H.; Han, W.; Chen, Y.H.; Zhang, X.H.; Lu, D.P. Treatment of acute leukemia with unmanipulated HLA-mismatched/haploidentical blood and bone marrow transplantation. *Biol. Blood Marrow Transplant.* **2009**, *15*, 257–265. [CrossRef] [PubMed]
112. Luo, Y.; Xiao, H.; Lai, X.; Shi, J.; Tan, Y.; He, J.; Xie, W.; Zheng, W.; Zhu, Y.; Ye, X.; *et al.* T-cell-replete haploidentical HSCT with low-dose anti-T-lymphocyte globulin compared with matched sibling HSCT and unrelated HSCT. *Blood* **2014**, *124*, 2735–2743. [CrossRef] [PubMed]
113. Fu, H.; Xu, L.; Liu, D.; Liu, K.; Zhang, X.; Chen, H.; Chen, Y.; Han, W.; Wang, Y.; Wang, J.; *et al.* Total body irradiation and cyclophosphamide plus antithymocyte globulin regimen is well tolerated and promotes stable engraftment as a preparative regimen before T cell-replete haploidentical transplantation for acute leukemia. *Biol. Blood Marrow Transplant.* **2014**, *20*, 1176–1182. [CrossRef] [PubMed]
114. Gao, L.; Wen, Q.; Chen, X.; Liu, Y.; Zhang, C.; Gao, L.; Kong, P.; Zhang, Y.; Li, Y.; Liu, J.; *et al.* Effects of priming with recombinant human granulocyte colony-stimulating factor on conditioning regimen for high-risk acute myeloid leukemia patients undergoing human leukocyte antigen-haploidentical hematopoietic stem cell transplantation: A multicenter randomized controlled study in southwest China. *Biol. Blood Marrow Transplant.* **2014**, *20*, 1932–1939. [PubMed]
115. Di Bartolomeo, P.; Santarone, S.; De Angelis, G.; Picardi, A.; Cudillo, L.; Cerretti, R.; Adorno, G.; Angelini, S.; Andreani, M.; De Felice, L.; *et al.* Haploidentical, unmanipulated, G-CSF-primed bone marrow transplantation for patients with high-risk hematologic malignancies. *Blood* **2013**, *121*, 849–857. [CrossRef] [PubMed]
116. Peccatori, J.; Forcina, A.; Clerici, D.; Crocchiolo, R.; Vago, L.; Stanghellini, M.T.; Noviello, M.; Messina, C.; Crotta, A.; Assanelli, A.; *et al.* Sirolimus-based graft-versus-host disease prophylaxis promotes the *in vivo* expansion of regulatory T cells and permits peripheral blood stem cell transplantation from haploidentical donors. *Leukemia* **2015**, *29*, 396–405. [CrossRef] [PubMed]

117. Ciceri, F.; Bregni, M.; Peccatori, J. Innovative platforms for haploidentical stem cell transplantation: The role of unmanipulated donor graft. *J. Cancer* **2011**, *2*, 339–340. [CrossRef] [PubMed]
118. Pidala, J.; Lee, S.J.; Ahn, K.W.; Spellman, S.; Wang, H.L.; Aljurf, M.; Askar, M.; Dehn, J.; Fernandez Viña, M.; Gratwohl, A.; *et al.* Nonpermissive HLA-DPB1 mismatch increases mortality after myeloablative unrelated allogeneic hematopoietic cell transplantation. *Blood* **2014**, *124*, 2596–2606. [CrossRef] [PubMed]

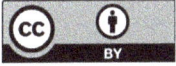

Journal of
Clinical Medicine

MDPI

Review

Current Approaches in the Treatment of Relapsed and Refractory Acute Myeloid Leukemia

Nestor R. Ramos [1,2], Clifton C. Mo [2], Judith E. Karp [3] and Christopher S. Hourigan [1,*]

[1] Myeloid Malignancies Section, Hematology Branch, National Heart, Lung and Blood Institute, National Institutes of Health, Bethesda, MD 20892-1583, USA; nestor.r.ramos.mil@mail.mil
[2] Department of Hematology-Oncology, John P. Murtha Cancer Center, Walter Reed National Military Medical Center, Bethesda, MD 20889, USA; clifton.c.mo.mil@mail.mil
[3] Division of Hematologic Malignancies, Sidney Kimmel Comprehensive Cancer Center, Johns Hopkins School of Medicine, Baltimore, MD 21205, USA; jkarp2@jhmi.edu
* Author to whom correspondence should be addressed; hourigan@nih.gov.

Academic Editors: Celalettin Ustun and Lucy A. Godley
Received: 16 January 2015; Accepted: 20 March 2015; Published: 10 April 2015

Abstract: The limited sensitivity of the historical treatment response criteria for acute myeloid leukemia (AML) has resulted in a different paradigm for treatment compared with most other cancers presenting with widely disseminated disease. Initial cytotoxic induction chemotherapy is often able to reduce tumor burden to a level sufficient to meet the current criteria for "complete" remission. Nevertheless, most AML patients ultimately die from their disease, most commonly as clinically evident relapsed AML. Despite a variety of available salvage therapy options, prognosis in patients with relapsed or refractory AML is generally poor. In this review, we outline the commonly utilized salvage cytotoxic therapy interventions and then highlight novel investigational efforts currently in clinical trials using both pathway-targeted agents and immunotherapy based approaches. We conclude that there is no current standard of care for adult relapsed or refractory AML other than offering referral to an appropriate clinical trial.

Keywords: salvage therapy; leukemia; neoplasm metastasis; AML; relapse

1. Introduction

Approximately 20,000 patients will be diagnosed with acute myeloid leukemia (AML) with greater than 10,000 AML patient deaths in the United States during 2015 [1]. While complete response rates can be as high as 80% in patients undergoing initial induction cytotoxic chemotherapy, the majority of AML patients will ultimately be diagnosed with relapsed or refractory disease [2,3]. Patients with relapsed or refractory AML (RR-AML) have, in general, a poor prognosis [4,5]. While several factors have been associated with worse outcomes at relapse, including unfavorable cytogenetics at diagnosis, duration of first complete response (CR) less than 12 months, older age, and prior history of hematopoietic stem cell transplant (HSCT) [5–7] even a patient without such adverse factors faces a formidable challenge in achieving and maintaining a second remission.

It is now clear that AML is a diagnosis encompassing a wide range of myeloid malignancies with heterogeneous genetic etiology [8]. It is also clear that AML is an oligoclonal disease even within a single patient, such that the predominant clone at initial presentation is not necessarily identical to the clone ultimately responsible for clinical relapse and death [9,10]. AML presenting as clinical relapse may be from three underlying sources: (1) chemo-sensitive disease that was only partially treated and returns, perhaps with additional mutations; (2) a subclone, derived from the same founder clone as the predominant clone, initially present at low frequency but given a clonal advantage during treatment due to decreased chemotherapy sensitivity; and (3) *de novo* generation of AML due to toxicity from treatment. Experimental evidence to date suggests the first two mechanisms are the most common [9,10], although the last may be operable in late relapses that occur three or more years after achieving initial CR.

While a variety of different treatment regimens have been studied in an effort to improve outcomes of patients with RR-AML, there appears to be no single superior approach. We therefore believe that the only current standard of care for a patient with relapsed AML is to offer enrollment in a clinical trial [11]. This article will review combinatorial chemotherapy regimens (both traditional and investigational) used in the AML (non-APL) salvage setting (Table 1), and will then discuss novel single agent approaches, including targeted small molecule drugs for known AML mutations and/or pathways (Table 2), as well as immunomodulatory drugs and antibody-based, vaccine-based, and adoptive cellular immunotherapies (Table 3).

2. Cytotoxic Chemotherapy

While most patients able to undergo initial cytotoxic induction therapy will initially achieve a CR, the most common cause of death is subsequent relapse of disease. Treatment options in this setting include aggressive therapy geared towards providing a bridge to an allogeneic hematopoietic stem cell transplantation (alloHSCT), which is often considered the only potentially curative option for patients with RR-AML, or best supportive care with palliative intent in patients who are not candidates for an aggressive approach. Patients must have a suitable donor, good performance status, minimal comorbidities, and generally should be in at least a CR prior to undergoing alloHSCT.

Table 1. Conventional and novel cytotoxic salvage chemotherapy regimens utilized in patients with relapsed/refractory acute myeloid leukemia (AML).

Regimen	Agents	CR	TRM or 30 Day Mortality	Reference
HIDAC	Cytarabine 3 g/m^2 every 12 h days 1–6	32%–47%	12%–15%	[12,13]
FLAG FLAG-IDA	Fludarabine 30 mg/m^2 days 1–5 Cytarabine 2 g/m^2 days 1–5 G-CSF 5 mcg/kg day 0 until ANC recovery	48%–55%	10%–11%	[14,15]
	Fludarabine 30 mg/m^2 days 1–5 Cytarabine 2 g/m^2 days 1–5 G-CSF 300 mcg day 0 until ANC recovery Idarubicin 8 mg/m^2 days 1–3	63%	17%	[16]
FLA	Fludarabine 30 mg/m^2 days 1–5 Cytarabine 2 g/m^2 days 1–5	61%	7%	[17]
CLAG CLAG-M	Cladribine 5 mg/m^2 days 2–6 Cytarabine 2 g/m^2 days 2–6 G-CSF 300 mcg days 1–6	38%–50%	0%–17%	[18–20]
	Cladribine 5 mg/m^2 days 1–5 Cytarabine 2 g/m^2 days 1–5 G-CSF 300 mcg days 0–5 Mitoxantrone 10 mg/m^2 days 1–3	50%–58% (53% after first course)	0%–7%	[18,21]
	Mitoxantrone 6 mg/m^2 days 1–6 Etoposide 80 mg/m^2 days 1–6 Cytarabine 1 g/m^2 days 1–6	59%–66%	3%–6%	[22,23]
MEC	Mitoxantrone 8 mg/m^2 days 1–5 Etoposide 100 mg/m^2 days 1–5 Cytarabine 1 mg/m^2 days 1–5	18%–24%	7%–11%	[20,24,25]
MEC/Decitabine	Decitabine 20 mg/m^2 days 1–10 Mitoxantrone 8 mg/m^2 days 16–20 Etoposide 100 mg/m^2 days 16–20 Cytarabine 1 mg/m^2 days 16–20	30% (CR + CRp + CRi = 50%)	20%	[26]

Table 1. *Cont.*

Regimen	Agents	CR	TRM or 30 Day Mortality	Reference
EMA-86	Mitoxantrone 12 mg/m^2 days 1–3 Cytarabine 500 mg/m^2 CI days 1–3 & 8–10 Etoposide 200 mg/m^2 CI days 8–10	60%	11%	[27]
MAV	Mitoxantrone 10 mg/m^2 days 4–8 Cytarabine 100 mg/m^2 CI days 1–8 Etoposide 100–120 mg/m^2 days 4–8	58%	11%	[28]
FLAD	Fludarabine 30 mg/m^2 days 1–3 Cytarabine 2 g/m^2 days 1–3 Liposomal daunorubicin 100 mg/m^2 days 1–3	53%	7.5%	[29]
FLAM	Flavopiridol 50 mg/m^2 days 1–3 Cytarabine 2 g/m^2/72 h starting day 6 Mitoxantrone 40 mg/m^2 day 9	28%–43%	5%–28%	[30,31]
Hybrid FLAM	Flavopiridol 30mg/m^2 bolus, 60 mg/m^2 over 4 h days 1–3 Cytarabine 2 g/m^2/72 h starting day 6 Mitoxantrone 40 mg/m^2 day 9	40%	9%	[32]
Clofarabine Cytarabine	Clofarabine 40 mg/m^2 days 2–6 Cytarabine 1 g/m^2 days 1–5	28%–51%	6.2%–13%	[33]
	Clofarabine 40 mg/m^2 days 1–5; Cytarabine 1 g/m^2 days 1–5			[34,35]
	Clofarabine 22.5 mg/m^2 days 1–5; Cytarabine 1 g/m^2 days 1–5			
GCLAC	Clofarabine 25 mg/m^2 days 1–5; Cytarabine 2 g/m^2 days 1–5; G-CSF 5 mcg/kg day 0 until ANC recovery	46%, (CR + CRp 61%)	13%	[36,37]
HAA	Homoharringtonine 4 mg/m^2 days 1–3 Cytarabine 150 mg/m^2 days 1–7 Aclarubicin 12 mg/m^2 days 1–7	76%–80%	0%	[38]
CPX 351	CPX 351 101 units/m^2 days 1, 3, and 5	23%–37% (CR + CRi = 49%)	7%–13%	[39]
	CPX 351 100 units/m^2 days 1, 3, 5 (first induction) and days 1 and 3 (second induction and consolidation)			[40]

Abbreviations: complete response (CR), complete response with incomplete platelet recovery (CRp), complete response with incomplete blood count recovery (CRi), treatment-related mortality (TRM), High-dose arabinoside cytarabine (HIDAC), granulocyte colony stimulating factor (G-CSF), continuous infusion (CI), cyclin-dependent kinase (CDK).

Table 2. Targeted agents under evaluation for treatment of patients with relapsed/refractory AML (RR-AML). *Ongoing clinical trials (either enrolling new patients with RR-AML or active but no longer enrolling patients).*

Agent	Mechanism of Action	Ongoing Clinical Trial	Reference
Ruxolitinib	JAK1 and JAK2 inhibitor	NCT02257138, NCT00674479, NCT01251965	[41,42]
Rapamycin	mTOR inhibitor	NCT01184898, NCT01869114, NCT00634244, NCT02109744	[43,44]
Everolimus	mTOR inhibitor	NCT00819546	[45]
Tosedostat	Aminopeptidase activity inhibitor	NCT01636609	[46,47]
Vorinostat	Histone deacetylase inhibitor	NCT01130506, NCT01534260, NCT01550224, NCT01617226, NCT02083250	[48–50]

Table 2. *Cont.*

Agent	Mechanism of Action	Ongoing Clinical Trial	Reference
AG-120	IDH1 inhibitor	NCT02074839	NCT02074839
AG-221	IDH2 inhibitor	NCT01915498	[51]
Elacytarabine	Elaidic acid ester of cytarabine	No active studies found	[52]
Vosaroxin	Anticancer quinolone derivative	NCT01191801	[53,54]
Pravastatin	HMG-CoA reductase inhibitor	NCT00840177	[55,56]
Bortezomib	Proteasome inhibitor	NCT01174888, NCT01127009, NCT01736943, NCT01861314, NCT01534260, NCT01075425, NCT00410423	[57]
Lenalidomide	Immunomodulatory agent	NCT01681537, NCT01904643, NCT01629082, NCT01132586, NCT01246622, NCT01743859, NCT01016600, NCT00466895, NCT01615042	[58]
CPI-613	Lipoate derivative	NCT01768897	[59]
ABT-199	BCL-2 inhibitor	NCT01994837	[60]
Erismodegib	Hedgehog inhibitor	NCT02129101	NCT02129101
PF-04449913	Hedgehog inhibitor	NCT02038777	NCT02038777

Source: www.clinicaltrials.gov.

Table 3. Immunotherapeutic agents under evaluation for treatment of patients with relapsed/refractory AML.

Agent	Mechanism of Action	Ongoing Clinical Trial	Reference
Gemtuzumab ozogamicin	Conjugated Antibody targeting CD33	NCT01869803, NCT00766116, NCT02221310	[61–63]
SGN-CD33A	Conjugated Antibody targeting CD33	NCT01902329	[64,65]
Lintuzumab	Unconjugated Antibody targeting CD33	No active studies found	[66]
CSL362	Unconjugated Antibody targeting CD123	No active studies found	[67,68]
AMG330	Bispecific T-cell Engaging Antibody targeting CD33 and CD3	No active studies found	[69,70]
MGD006	Dual Affinity Re-Targeting Antibody targeting CD123 and CD3	NCT02152956	[71]
CD16x33 BiKE	Bispecific Killer Cell Engager Antibody against CD16 and CD33	No active studies found	[72]
CART33	Chimeric Antigen Receptor-Transduced T Cells targeting CD33	NCT01864902	[73]
CART123	Chimeric Antigen Receptor-Transduced T Cells targeting CD123	NCT02159495	[74,75]
WT1 peptide vaccine	Vaccine targeting WT1	NCT00965224	[76,77]
WT1-specific CD8(+) T-cell infusion	Adoptive Cell Transfer	NCT01640301	[78–80]

Table 3. *Cont.*

Agent	Mechanism of Action	Ongoing Clinical Trial	Reference
Haploidentical NK cell infusion	Adoptive Cell Transfer	NCT01947322, NCT01385423, NCT01370213, NCT00303667, NCT01621477, NCT00526292, NCT00789776, NCT02259348, NCT01795378, NCT01898793, NCT01386619	[81]
AlloHSCT	Adoptive Cell Transfer	More than 40 active clinical trials identified	[82–85]
Donor lymphocyte infusion (post alloHCT)	Adoptive Cell Transfer	NCT01758367, NCT01390311, NCT00068718, NCT01523223, NCT01760655, NCT00534118, NCT00005799, NCT00448357	[86–89]

Source: www.clinicaltrials.gov.

Most commonly used induction regimens involve a combination of infusional cytarabine, an anthracycline, and perhaps an additional agent. Cytarabine, a deoxycytidine analog that is actively metabolized to arabinofuranosylcytidine triphosphate (ara-CTP), serves as the backbone for many commonly utilized salvage regimens, demonstrating efficacy in relapsed AML both as monotherapy when given in high doses (HIDAC), and in combination with other therapeutic agents [12,13]. In general, patients with a good performance status who have not yet received HIDAC can receive this treatment regimen in the salvage setting with or without an anthracycline, as per NCCN guidelines [90]. Patients who suffer a late relapse, especially one greater than 18 months from initial CR (CR1), can sometimes achieve a second CR (CR2) by retreatment with the same initial induction regimen [90]. With reported CR2 rates of only 32% to 47%, however, HIDAC monotherapy is far from an acceptable standard of care for relapsed disease [12,13].

FLA/FLAG—Fludarabine is a purine analog that acts by inhibiting ribonucleotide reductase (RNR), which augments the rate of synthesis of ara-CTP in circulating AML blasts when infused prior to cytarabine [91]. It has been studied in relapsed AML in combination with high-dose cytarabine (FLA), with or without granulocyte-colony stimulating factor (G-CSF), with reported CR rates ranging from 46% to 63% [14–16] (Table 1). Idarubicin, an anthracycline, is frequently added to FLAG and despite a lack of evidence of improved outcome is a reasonable option in select patients [16]. Notably, FLA did not produce superior CR rates in the salvage setting when compared to standard induction chemotherapy (cytarabine, daunorubicin, and etoposide) in the randomized MRC AML-HR trial (CR rates: 61% FLA *versus* 63% ADE, *p* = 0.8), and in fact survival at 4 years was significantly inferior using this approach (16% *versus* 27%, *p* = 0.05) [17]. Likewise, the addition of G-CSF to FLA in this trial failed to demonstrate improvement in outcomes over FLA alone (CR rates: 58% G-CSF *versus* 61% no G-CSF, *p* = 0.7). Nevertheless, FLAG ± idarubicin remains an accepted alternative to HIDAC monotherapy in relapsed AML.

CLAG/CLAG-M—Cladribine is another RNR-inhibiting purine analogue that was found to yield synergistic effects on inhibition of cell proliferation, induction of apoptosis, and disruption of mitochondrial membrane potential when combined with cytarabine [92]. It has been associated with CR rates ranging from 38% to 58% when combined with high-dose cytarabine and G-CSF (CLAG) in the relapsed setting [18–21] (Table 1), with the highest rates observed in those treated with mitoxantrone in addition to CLAG (CLAG-M) [21].

MEC/EMA-86/MAV—Combinations of mitoxantrone, etoposide and cytarabine have been extensively evaluated in relapsed AML with multiple variations in the dose and schedule (MEC, EMA-86, MAV), resulting in CR rates between 18% and 66% [20,22–25,27,28,93] (Table 1) with the highest rates seen when given as timed-sequential therapy [27,93]. A single-institution retrospective review by Price *et al.* evaluated 162 patients with RR-AML treated with CLAG *versus* MEC and found overall CR rates of 37.9% *versus* 23.8% ($p = 0.05$), with a median follow up of 20.3 months [20]. Although limited by the retrospective nature of the study, a possible superiority of CLAG is suggested. Notably, the addition of sirolimus to MEC was evaluated in an arm of the E1906 trial, a phase II study among patients with RR-AML, but closed to accrual early with 15% responses [30]. An ongoing phase II study (NCT01729845) is currently evaluating the effect of pre-treatment "priming" with decitabine, a hypomethylating agent, prior to MEC after a phase I study found a CR rate of 30% (9 of 30 patients; CR + CRp + CRi = 50%) with a treatment related mortality (TRM) of 20% [26].

GCLAC—Clofarabine is a second-generation deoxyadenosine analog that is characterized by high resistance to phosphorolytic cleavage by bacterial purine nucleoside phosphorylase, potent inhibition of DNA synthesis, prolonged retention of clofarabine triphosphate in leukemic blasts [34] and, similar to fludarabine and cladribine, can inhibit RNR reductase and increase the intracellular concentration of ara-CTP when administered prior to cytarabine [94]. Studies evaluating clofarabine with intermediate-dose cytarabine (1 gm/m^2) have found CR rates 35%–51% [33–35] (Table 1). GCLAC is a regimen containing clofarabine, high dose cytarabine (2 g/m^2), and G-CSF that has resulted in comparable CR rates (46% in a phase I/II study) [36] (Table 1). A retrospective study comparing 50 patients who received GCLAC to 101 patients who received FLAG or FLA demonstrated a superior CR rate for patients who received GCLAC, with an odds ratio of 9.57 ($p < 0.0001$) [37]. GCLAC also demonstrated impressive efficacy as initial induction therapy with an overall CR rate of 76% (CR + CRp = 82%) in a recently reported multicenter trial [95]. Further studies will be necessary to determine conclusively if GCLAC is superior to other approaches in RR-AML.

FLAD—Liposomal daunorubicin has been found to be at least as effective as free (non-liposomal) daunorubicin in leukemic cells and could have decreased toxicity [96,97]. This agent was evaluated in combination with cytarabine and fludarabine (FLAD), with an overall CR rate of 53% (CR in 73% of relapsed AML subjects *versus* 0% of refractory AML subjects) among 41 patients with RR-AML (including two patients with CML in myeloid blast crisis) [29]. Fifty-eight percent of patients who achieved CR were able to proceed to alloHSCT, which raises the possibility of this regimen being utilized as a bridge to transplant.

FLAM—Flavopiridol, a synthetic flavone derivative initially isolated from the stem bark of the Indian tree (*Dysoxylum binectariferum*), has properties as a cyclin-dependent kinase inhibitor and has been evaluated as timed sequential therapy in combination with cytarabine and mitoxantrone (FLAM) with a CR rate of 42.5% in a phase II study of 47 patients with RR-AML, including a CR rate of 75% in those with relapsed AML compared to only 9% in those with primary or multiply refractory disease [31] (Table 1). A phase I trial evaluating a "Hybrid FLAM" regimen, which administers Flavopiridol as a 30-min bolus followed by 4-h infusion, found a CR rate for relapsed AML patients of 92% (11 of 12 patients) at the maximum tolerated dose and 31% for primary refractory patients (5 of 16 patients) [32]. However, a randomized phase II study found an overall CR rate of 28% (six patients achieved CR, four patients CRi) among 36 patients, including patients with primary refractory AML and post-HSCT relapse [30]. This study randomized patients to either FLAM, carboplatin-topotecan (14% patients achieved CR or CRi), or sirolimus-MEC. Early FLAM-related mortality was 28% (with 4 of 10 deaths related to overwhelming tumor lysis and cytokine release syndrome from Flavopiridol), predominantly in patients older than 65 years. Thus this regimen holds promise for younger patients (<60–65 y/o) but may be excessively toxic for the older population.

HAA—Homoharringtonine is an alkaloid derived from *Cephalotaxus fortunei* that, when combined with cytarabine and the anthracycline aclarubicin, was shown to induce a CR rate of 76.1% after one cycle of treatment among 46 patients with RR-AML [38] (Table 1). Patients who did not respond or only had a partial response (PR) underwent an additional cycle of HAA, which increased the overall CR rate to 80.4%. In this study, no TRM was documented, but 89.1% of patients developed infections [38].

CPX351—CPX 351 is a bilamellar liposome that encapsulates cytarabine and daunorubicin in an optimally synergistic fixed molar ratio of 5:1 [39]. It was found to induce a CR in 10 of 43 patients (23%) in a phase I study [39] and yielded a CR rate of 49.3% (37% CR + 12.3% CRi) when compared with provider's-choice of intensive salvage therapy in adults with first relapse of AML (CR + CRi = 40.9%) in a phase II, multicenter, randomized trial [40] (Table 1). A possible clinical benefit for patients treated with CPX 351 was observed in subjects with poor-risk disease, as defined by European Prognostic Index [40].

Vosaroxin—Vosaroxin is a novel anticancer quinolone derivative that intercalates DNA and inhibits topoisomerase II [53]. It was evaluated in combination with cytarabine in a phase III randomized multinational study comprising 711 patients at 124 sites, where the combination was found to improve CR (30.1% *versus* 16.3%, $p = 0.00001$) and median OS (7.5 months *versus* 6.1 months, 2-sided stratified log-rank $p = 0.02$) when compared to the placebo/cytarabine group. Overall survival (OS) benefit was greatest in patients aged 60 years or older (7.1 months *versus* 5 months, $p = 0.003$) and those with early relapse (6.7 months *versus* 5.2 months, $p = 0.04$) [54]. A separate phase Ib/II study evaluating the same combination among patients with RR-AML found a combined CR + CRi rate of 28% [98]. Notably, the CR + CRi rate was 69% for patients whose initial CR lasted greater or equal to 12 months, while patients with initial CR >3 months and <12 months and patients with refractory disease had CR + CRi of 13% and 21%, respectively.

Elacytarabine is an elaidic acid ester of cytarabine that was compared against seven commonly used salvage regimens (investigator's choice) in a large phase III study but was not found to improve CR or OS rate [52]. Interestingly no significant difference with regards to OS was found among the different salvage treatment regimens.

3. Targeted Agents

Increased understanding of AML biology has led to the identification of deregulated pathways that drive blast proliferation. These discoveries have, in turn, given way to the development of agents targeting these molecular pathways.

Cancer Metabolism—Oncogenic mutations affecting two isoforms of the isocitrate dehydrogenase (IDH) enzyme, IDH1 and IDH2, have been reported in approximately 30% of de novo AML and appear to be an unfavorable prognostic factor [99]. AG-221 is an oral, potent, reversible, and selective inhibitor of the mutated IDH2 protein that is currently under evaluation, with early results of an ongoing phase I study revealing objective responses in 6 of 10 patients thus far including three CRs and two CRp (NCT01915498) [51]. An IDH1 inhibitor, AG-120, is also undergoing phase I testing in patients with RR-AML harboring an IDH1 mutation (NCT02074839).

CPI-613 is a lipoate derivative that disrupts mitochondrial metabolism by inhibiting pyruvate dehydrogenase and α-ketogluterate dehydrogenase [100]. When combined with HIDAC and mitoxantrone in a phase I study, 18 patients (50%) achieved a CR or CRi, while 14% of patients died in the first 30 days [59]. Notably, the CR + CRi rate was also 50% among patients 60 years of age or older [59].

Plerixafor—In an effort to disrupt the interaction between leukemic blasts and the bone marrow microenvironment, which is postulated to be an important mediator of chemotherapy resistance [101], plerixafor, a bicyclam that inhibits the CXCR4 chemokine receptor, was evaluated in combination with MEC for the treatment of RR-AML and was found to induce a CR + CRi rate of 46% in a phase I/II study [102]. A follow up study is currently underway evaluating the effect of G-CSF priming in addition to the abovementioned regimen (NCT00906945).

Kinase inhibition—Internal tandem duplication mutations resulting in constitutive activation of the FMS-like tyrosine kinase receptor 3 (FLT3-ITD) are present in approximately 20%–30% of cases of AML, represent a high-risk feature in normal karyotype AML, and are associated with a high risk of relapse following alloHSCT [103]. Pratz *et al.* examined the efficacy of six FLT3-ITD inhibitors for potency against mutant and wild-type FLT3 as well as for cytotoxic effect against a series of primary blast samples and found that the inhibitors could be ranked, from most to least selective against FLT3-ITD, as quizartinib, sorafenib, sunitinib, KW2449, and lestaurtinib [104].

Quizartinib (AC220) has been shown in a phase I trial to be safe and efficacious in patients with both FLT3-ITD negative and positive RR-AML, with most of the responses being PR or CRi and occurring in FLT3-ITD positive patients [105]. Multiple phase II trials for RR-AML have been conducted [106] but to date have only been reported in abstract form [107,108].

In the recently reported SAL-Soraml trial, sorafenib demonstrated safety and improved event free survival compared to placebo when used as an adjunct to standard induction chemotherapy in 267 younger (age <60) patients with newly diagnosed AML, only 17% of whom were FLT3-ITD mutated (3-year event-free survival 40% *versus* 22%, *p* = 0.013) [109]. It also demonstrated safety with early data suggesting a possible reduction in relapse rates when used as maintenance therapy in FLT3-ITD mutated AML patients after alloHSCT [110,111]. Additionally, sorafenib monotherapy exhibited antileukemic efficacy in patients with RR-AML, including patients who relapsed after alloHSCT, in a small retrospective study including 13 patients [112].

Unfortunately, mutations of the FLT3 kinase domain can arise and limit the efficacy of FLT3 inhibitors [113]. The most commonly observed FLT3 mutation occurs at the D835 residue, followed by the F691L [114]. Crenolanib (CP-868,596) is a novel tyrosine kinase inhibitor (TKI) that was originally developed as a selective and potent inhibitor of PDGFR α and β, but also has high affinity for other type III receptor tyrosine kinases such as FLT3. A preclinical study by Zimmerman *et al.* demonstrated that crenolanib has potent activity against FLT3-ITD as well as FLT3 D835 mutations in binding assays and in Ba/F3 cells from a mouse model. Several phase II trials evaluating crenolanib in patients with RR-AML and FLT3 mutations are ongoing (NCT01522469 and NCT01657682).

Another FLT3 inhibitor that has demonstrated inhibitory activity against FLT3-ITD/N676D, FLT3-ITD/F691L, and FLT3-D835Y mutants is G-749, which displayed potent antileukemic activity in bone marrow blasts from AML patients regardless of FLT3 mutation status [115]. AMG 925 is a FLT3/CDK4 dual kinase inhibitor that also demonstrated potent and selective activity *in vivo* in AML tumor models in preclinical studies [116].

JAK inhibition—The Janus kinase—signal transducer and activator of transcription (JAK-STAT) pathway has been found to be dysregulated in AML [117]. Ruxolitinib is a potent, selective JAK1 and JAK2 inhibitor that was found to be overall reasonably well tolerated in a phase I/II study, where 1 of 26 patients with RR-AML achieved a CRp [41]. A previous phase II study, on the other hand, found that 3 of 18 patients with post myeloproliferative disease-AML were able to achieve a CR or CRi [42].

mTOR inhibition—Mammalian target of rapamycin (mTOR) is a serine/threonine kinase involved in the regulation of cell growth and proliferation by translational control of key proteins [43]. Rapamycin is an mTOR inhibitor that has been evaluated as monotherapy, inducing a PR in four of nine patients [43], and in combination with decitabine, achieving a decline in blast percentage in 4 of 13 patients in a phase I trial [44]. Another mTOR inhibitor, RAD001 (everolimus), was evaluated in combination with 7 + 3 chemotherapy (daunorubicin 60 mg/m^2 d1 to d3, cytarabine 200 mg/m^2 d1 to d7) in a phase Ib study of 28 patients (age <65) with relapsed AML and produced a CR rate of 68% [45].

Vorinostat—Vorinostat is a histone deacetylase inhibitor that, despite promising data in phase I trials, was found in a phase II study to have a CR rate of only 4.5% in a group of 22 patients with RR-AML (16 patients) and untreated AML (6 patients) [48]. However, when given in combination with azacitidine and gemtuzumab ozogamicin, 42.3% of patients achieved a CR + CRi [49]. Another study evaluating vorinostat in combination with cytarabine and etoposide found a CR rate of 46% at the maximum tolerated dose of vorinostat 200 mg twice a day [50].

Statins—Interestingly, AML blasts frequently overexpress the genes for the low-density lipoprotein (LDL) receptor. Blockade of 3-hydroxy-3-methylglutaryl coenzyme reductase (HMG-CoAR) inhibits cholesterol uptake and synthesis and is believed to sensitize AML cells to cytotoxic therapy [55]. A phase II study evaluating pravastatin, intermediate-dose cytarabine, and idarubicin in patients with relapsed AML found a CR + CRi of 75%, which suggests that this approach may improve efficacy [56]. Notably, a study evaluating pravastatin in addition to idarubicin and cytarabine in patients with *de novo*, untreated AML did not find a significant improvement in CR rates when compared to historical results [118].

Proteasome Inhibition—Bortezomib, a proteasome inhibitor commonly utilized in multiple myeloma, was administered in combination with MEC chemotherapy in a phase I study, where 17 of 33 evaluable patients (52%) achieved either a CR or CRi and TRM was 9% [57]. Several clinical trials are currently evaluating bortezomib, either as monotherapy or in combination to other agents, in patients with RR-AML (Table 2).

Other Pathways—Tosedostat is a novel oral agent that inhibits aminopeptidase activity, resulting in the depletion of cellular amino acid pools selectively in tumor cells [46]. Several studies have evaluated the efficacy of tosedostat monotherapy in RR-AML with CR rates ranging from 10% to 17% [46,47]. It has been observed that, given the pharmacokinetic characteristics and mechanism of action of tosedostat, patients require treatment for at least 4 weeks (and possibly longer) for full therapeutic effect to be reached [47].

ABT-199 is a selective, orally bioavailable small molecule BCL-2 inhibitor that is currently under evaluation in a phase II study with preliminary data revealing a CR + CRi rate of 15.5% among 32 patients [60].

Hedgehog pathway—Aberrant activation of the hedgehog (Hh) pathway was found to be a feature of some CD34-positive myeloid leukemic cells in a preclinical study, where inhibition of Hh signaling was found to induce apoptosis in Hh-responsive CD34 cells [119]. Several studies utilizing Hh inhibitors in RR-AML are currently ongoing.

4. Immunotherapy

Unlike conventional chemotherapy, which primarily targets dividing cells, or small molecules that target specific pathways within blasts, immunotherapeutic interventions aim at directing an immune response against tumor cells. Several immunotherapeutic modalities are currently under evaluation and are detailed below and in Table 3.

Antibodies—Two targets in AML have served as the main focus for monoclonal antibody studies: CD123 and CD33. The latter is expressed on blasts in 80%–90% of patients with AML [61]. Gemtuzumab ozogamicin (GO), a CD33-directed antibody linked to the antibiotic cytotoxin calicheamicin, received accelerated approval by the FDA in 2000 but was withdrawn from the U.S. market in 2010 after an interim analysis of SWOG S0106 failed to demonstrate a benefit of adding GO to standard induction chemotherapy, while finding an increased rate of fatal adverse events (5.8% *versus* 0.8%, $p = 0.002$) [62]. Although subsequent studies evaluating GO alone or in combination have produced mixed results in RR-AML, one recent study using fractionated doses of GO combined with standard dose cytarabine found a CR + CRp rate of 75% and 2-year survival of 51% with a low TRM (8.3%) [63]. Further studies will be necessary to determine the safety of GO when administered in fractionated doses.

Other anti-CD33 antibodies include lintuzumab, an unconjugated humanized murine monoclonal antibody that failed to improve CR rates when combined with MEC in a phase III randomized multicenter study [66], and SGN-CD33A, a monoclonal antibody conjugated to a novel synthetic pyrrolobenzodiazepine dimer, which is a potent DNA cross-linking cytotoxin. Following favorable results in a preclinical study [64], an ongoing phase I trial of SGN-CD33A in relapsed AML or patients who decline conventional induction/consolidation therapy has found evidence of antileukemic activity, with 47% of patients achieving blast clearance (CR + CRi + morphologic leukemia-free state), with no maximum tolerated dose identified at this interim analysis (NCT01902329) [65].

CSL362 is a humanized second-generation anti-CD123 antibody with favorable preclinical data [67] that was found to be safe and well tolerated as maintenance therapy in a phase I study of AML patients with CR + CRp and high risk of relapse (NCT01632852) [68]. A phase 2 study of CSL362 is planned.

Bispecific T-cell-engaging (BiTE) antibodies are single-chain antibodies designed to direct cytotoxic T lymphocytes at a predefined surface antigen on tumor cells. AMG 330 is a human BiTE antibody against CD33 and CD3 that has demonstrated potent cytolysis *in vitro* against human AML cells proportional to the level of cell-surface CD33 expression [69], which varied by cytogenetic and molecular subtype [120]. It has also been shown to improve the survival of NOD/SCID mice with leukemia caused by human MOLM-13 AML cells [70]. Meanwhile, a phase I trial is currently underway to further evaluate MGD 006, a humanized Dual Affinity Re-Targeting (DART) bispecific antibody-based molecule directed against CD123 and CD3 (NCT02152956) [71].

Natural Killer (NK) cells are effector lymphocytes of the innate immune system capable of exerting anti-AML activity, as exemplified by its role in the graft-versus-leukemia (GVL) effect after alloHSCT [72]. A humanized bispecific killer cell engager (BiKE) antibody containing binding sites for CD16 and CD33 (CD16x33 BiKE) has been shown to trigger NK cell activation in preclinical studies and could potentially enhance and direct the GVL effect in patients with CD33+ AML after transplant, especially after CMV reactivation [72]. Another study seeking to exploit the anti-AML activity of NK cells has focused on the adoptive transfer of haploidentical NK cells into patients with poor-prognosis AML, where these cells have successfully expanded *in vivo* and induced CR in 5 of 19 patients [81].

Adoptive Cell Therapy—Following favorable ongoing studies in lymphoid malignancies, chimeric antigen receptor-transduced T cells (CART), which are synthetic transmembrane constructs that combine the specificity of antibody target recognition with the potent effector mechanisms of T-cell immunity, have been designed to target CD33 (CART33) and CD123 (CART123) in AML. A study by Wang *et al.*, in which CART33 cells were administered to a patient with relapsed AML, found a temporal decrease in blast ratio from >50% to <6% two weeks after infusion. Unfortunately, the patient then developed cytokine release syndrome requiring a TNF-α inhibitor and subsequently died from disease progression 13 weeks after CART33 infusion [73]. On the other hand, CART123 cells have demonstrated antileukemic activity in animal studies [74,121] and could potentially be superior to CART33 based on their lower toxicity profile against normal hematopoietic cells and identical killing profile against malignant myeloid cells [75]. A phase I study evaluating CART123 in patients with RR-AML is reportedly scheduled to begin soon (NCT02159495).

The Wilms tumor 1 (WT1) gene, a zinc finger transcription factor implicated in leukemogenesis, is overexpressed in 70% of AML patients [78,79] and has been targeted through the adoptive transfer of WT1-specific CD8(+) cytotoxic T-cell clones. In post-transplant patients, these T-cells were found to be safe and able to persist, with evidence of antileukemic activity in some patients [80].

Donor lymphocyte infusion (DLI) can be considered for patients who relapse after undergoing an alloHSCT in an attempt to induce a GVL effect. Generally patients who achieve a CR prior to DLI have a better chance of achieving a durable remission [86,87]. Interestingly, animal studies suggest a possible immunomodulatory effect of azacitidine that might attenuate graft-*versus*-host disease (GVHD) after DLI [88]. A recent phase I study evaluated azacitidine after DLI in eight patients with relapsed AML after alloHSCT and found six CRs and only grade 1 or 2 acute GVHD, which suggests that azacitidine after salvage chemotherapy and DLI is well tolerated and does not appear to hinder neutrophil recovery [89].

Vaccines—A number of studies have looked at vaccination with different leukemia-associated antigens including WT1, PR1, proteinase 3, and RHAMM, with the goal of establishing an immunological response capable of eradicating malignant cells [122]. These studies have generally demonstrated safety and immune correlates but no clinical efficacy. However, a recent phase I/II study of 30 AML patients (3 in PR, 27 in CR with high-risk of relapse) administered a dendritic cell WT1 vaccine in the adjuvant setting and found that 8 of 23 patients with elevated WT1 transcript had a molecular response following vaccination, with five of these eight patients subsequently maintaining remission at a median follow-up of 63 months [76]. This included one patient who was in PR at time of vaccination and is reportedly still in CR more than 5 years after initial diagnosis. A separate phase II study evaluating a multivalent WT1 peptide vaccine in patients with AML in CR is currently underway (NCT01266083).

Allogeneic Hematopoietic Stem Cell Transplant—AlloHSCT is an aggressive intervention that provides patients with RR-AML who have a good performance status and an adequate donor with the best chance of achieving a durable remission [82,123]. Relapsed AML patients entering an alloHSCT in CR have significantly superior OS compared to those with residual detectable disease [82,124]. However, patients with RR-AML who are not in CR prior to undergoing an alloHSCT can still experience improved long-term survival as evidenced by Duval *et al.*, who found an OS of 19% at 3 years among 1673 patients [125]. Patients lacking a suitable matched-related donor have other options for stem cell sources available, including matched unrelated donor, double cord blood units, and haploidentical (haplo) family donor. Notably, haplo-identical donors are often readily available from family members, providing a rapid alternative route to transplantation with acceptable toxicity in relapsed AML patients without a matched related donor option [29,126,127]. Unfortunately a large number of patients with RR-AML are elderly or have less than ideal performance status, which restricts their ability to undergo an alloHSCT with myeloablative conditioning (MAC). Reduced-intensity conditioning (RIC) regimens have been designed to address this problem and, in general, are thought to be associated with decreased TRM at the expense of increased risk of relapse when compared to MAC [83]. A recent retrospective study comparing RIC *versus* MAC alloHSCT among 132 patients aged 35 years or older with AML (including patients in CR1, CR2 or greater, or with refractory disease) found a lower 4-year non-relapse mortality with RIC (13% *versus* 28%, $p = 0.009$), a similar 4-year relapse rate (44% *versus* 33%, $p = 0.22$) and similar overall survival (50% *versus* 43%, $p = 0.38$) [84]. Survival of AML patients relapsing after transplantation is dismal. Response rates for patients who receive intensive salvage therapy after relapse, which offers the best chance for response, is approximately 30% [85]. When post-alloHSCT patients do achieve CR, outcomes have been found to be better with the use of donor cells for consolidation: 2 year OS 55% ± 11% in patients who received either DLI or second HSCT, as compared to 20% ± 10% in patients who only received initial salvage chemotherapy [85]. Azacitidine monotherapy can also be utilized and was found to induce a CR in 15% of patients (CR + PR = 22%) from a total of 204 patients with AML/MDS who relapsed after undergoing an alloHSCT [128].

5. Low-Intensity Therapy

Not all patients with RR-AML will be good candidates for the aggressive salvage therapy as described above due to reasons such as poor performance status, comorbidities, or cumulative toxicity from prior therapies. Treatment options in this setting are often palliative in nature and include best supportive care or less aggressive therapies such as hypomethylating agents or low-dose cytarabine (LDAC), which can induce CR rates of around 17% [129].

Hypomethylating agents—The hypomethylating agents 5-azacitidine and decitabine are cytidine analogs that act in part by inhibiting DNA methyltransferases [130] and are increasingly used during induction or salvage therapy in patients who are not good candidates for "aggressive" treatment [90]. A retrospective review encompassing three institutions in France found a CR rate of 21% with 11% PR and an overall survival of 9 months (median OS not reached for responders, 4.5 months OS for non-responders) among 47 patients with RR-AML receiving azacitidine 75 mg/m^2 days 1–7, while patients were able to proceed with an alloHSCT with reduced intensity conditioning [131]. Decitabine, on the other hand, was found to have a CR rate of 15.7% and a median OS of 177 days among 102 patients with RR-AML in a retrospective study by Ritchie *et al.* [132]. Interestingly, TET2 mutations have recently been proposed as a predictive biomarker of responsiveness to hypomethylating agents in myelodysplastic syndrome (MDS) and low blast count AML [133,134]. It remains to be seen if the identification of TET2 mutations will be useful in patients with AML regardless of blast count.

6. Discussion

Most patients who are diagnosed with AML will die of AML. Even within the favorable-risk subgroup of patients, as currently defined by cytogenetic and molecular criteria, many do not enjoy long-term survival. Although standard induction and consolidation chemotherapy regimens are undoubtedly intensive, a fundamental problem in the treatment of AML is not that available therapies are toxic but rather they are not effective enough [135]. Moreover, this therapeutic failure has been masked by the lack of progress in high sensitivity treatment response criteria [136]; a recent review of almost 5000 patients treated on clinical trials and/or in leukemia centers of excellence showed that most patients (mean 79%) treated with curative intent induction chemotherapy had achieved a "complete remission" endpoint as we currently define it, despite a median overall survival of only 20 months for the group [2]. Compounding the difficulty in curing AML is the fact that it is predominantly a disease of older adults who are less likely to be treated intensively [137,138]. While the outcomes for untreated and refractory AML are dire, those for relapsed AML are only slightly better with less than 30% of patients surviving 12 months after relapse [5,7,85].

In RR-AML patients with poor performance status, prohibitive comorbidities, or those who do not wish to undergo aggressive therapy, options are currently limited to best supportive care or low-intensity therapy with palliative intent. Although patients who are good candidates for aggressive treatment have a significant number of salvage therapy options available to them, none has categorically proven to offer superior outcomes and participation in clinical trials should be encouraged (Figure 1). In general, aggressive salvage therapies are given with the intent of maximally "debulking" the disease burden prior to proceeding with an alloHSCT. Indeed, the depth of remission when entering alloHSCT (as measured by minimal residual disease, or MRD), rather than its chronological setting (CR1 *versus* CR2), may be most predictive of overall survival [124]. Unfortunately, with a median age at diagnosis of 67, many AML patients are poor candidates for traditional alloHSCT due to comorbidity or poor performance status. However, despite a significant non-relapse mortality risk, alloHSCT provides the best chance of achieving a durable response at this time [85,125]. Patients who relapse after alloHSCT have a grim prognosis [85].

AML has historically been approached as a homogeneous diagnostic entity with a resulting "one size fits all" treatment strategy, often resulting in disappointing outcomes. In reality, the acute myeloid leukemias are a heterogeneous group of diseases with distinct molecular and phenotypic characteristics. While factors such as patient age, secondary AML, WBC count at presentation, and cytogenetic and molecular markers all are *associated* with treatment resistance, they offer suboptimal predictive power for the individual patient [2]. Heterogeneity in disease biology explains, in part, the unpredictable sensitivity to a particular treatment among AML patients. It is plausible that advances in genome sequencing technology will allow for timely and economically feasible personalized therapy based on molecular profiling and *ex vivo* drug sensitivity and resistance testing [139–141]. It is tempting to speculate that such an ability to accurately tailor therapy might eventually abrogate the need for future "salvage therapy".

In addition to AML clone biology characteristics that are postulated to contribute to therapy resistance and disease relapse, the bone marrow microenvironment has also been shown to affect therapeutic efficacy in patients with AML. A recent study found that AML cells can educate bone marrow-derived stromal cells to secrete Gas6, which fosters AML cell growth and chemoresistance via the receptor tyrosine kinase Axl [101]. Overexpression of CXCR4, a chemokine receptor, has been correlated with poor survival and its inhibition is the focus of several studies [142]. Combination therapy strategies that also target the microenvironment may be necessary in order to improve outcomes.

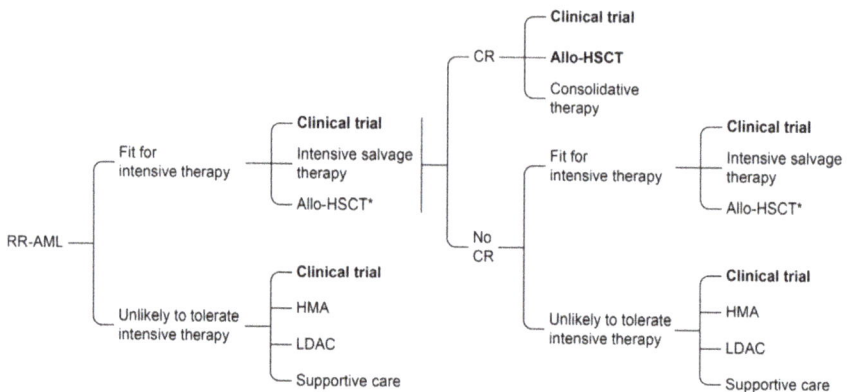

Figure 1. Treatment algorithm for patients with RR-AML in 2015. There is no standard of care for the treatment of relapsed or refractory AML. A clinical trial is always the preferred option. The above algorithm is based on current clinical practice and will hopefully change in coming years due to improvements. In particular the targeted and immunotherapeutic agents detailed in this review may ultimately have utility in (1) initial therapy; (2) as a bridge to, or as a temporizing measure before, allo-HSCT; and/or (3) as part of consolidative therapy. * Achievement of a complete remission (CR) prior to undergoing alloHSCT is associated with best survival and is generally preferred. The survival of patients with residual disease undergoing alloHSCT varies considerably however and this therapy may be a reasonable option in selected patients not in CR [125]. HMA: Hypomethylating agent. LDAC: Low-dose cytosine arabinoside. Allo-HSCT: Allogeneic Hematopoietic Stem Cell Transplant.

7. Conclusions

"Relapse" of AML is predicated on the concept of remission. The development of increasingly sensitive minimal or measurable residual disease (MRD) assays has demonstrated that current remission criteria, originally proposed in 1956, do not provide sensitive assessment of AML disease burden [136], as evidenced by the disconnect between the apparent success of current induction therapy in achieving complete remission in most patients and the stark reality of median overall survival times of less than two years [2]. Furthermore, studies evaluating remission status and subsequent relapse risk have shown traditional morphologic assessment is inferior when compared with newer methods such as flow cytometry [143–145] or PCR based detection of AML associated mutations [146] or gene over-expression [79,147,148]. Nevertheless, while it is clear that clinically evident relapsed AML represents an end-stage, advanced process that could potentially be detected at an earlier time utilizing a sensitive MRD assay, it is unclear how much more effective treatment at this earlier timepoint will be compared to treatment in the conventional salvage setting described herein [110,149,150]. It is likely that many patients experiencing AML "relapse" are in fact manifesting the clinical outgrowth of a refractory clone that has persisted despite apparently successful initial therapy [9]. We would argue, at least conceptually, that the main problem of AML relapse is not that we cannot adequately prevent or treat relapse, but rather that our apparently successful initial treatment was not as effective as we had hoped. Relapse is therefore not a sign that an initial successful treatment has now failed, but rather simply that it was not a successful treatment. It is in this context that the modest success of the aforementioned second-line therapies for relapsed AML should be judged and, in the absence of any obvious standard of care, we suggest that all patients with refractory or relapsed AML be offered a referral to an appropriate clinical trial whenever possible.

Acknowledgments: This work was supported by the Intramural Research Program of the National Heart, Lung, Blood Institute of the National Institutes of Health.

J. Clin. Med. **2015**, *4*, 665–695

Author Contributions: Nestor R. Ramos performed the literature search and wrote the first and final drafts. Clifton C. Mo, Judith E. Karp and Christopher S. Hourigan provided expert comments and editing.

Conflicts of Interest: Judith E. Karp is an advisor to Tolero. All other authors report no relevant conflict of interest.

References

1. American Cancer Society. *Cancer Facts & Figures 2015*; American Cancer Society: Atlanta, GA, USA, 2015; p. 4.
2. Walter, R.B.; Othus, M.; Burnett, A.K.; Lowenberg, B.; Kantarjian, H.M.; Ossenkoppele, G.J.; Hills, R.K.; Ravandi, F.; Pabst, T.; Evans, A.; *et al.* Resistance prediction in aml: Analysis of 4601 patients from MRC/NCRI, HOVON/SAKK, SWOC and MD Anderson Cancer Center. *Leukemia* **2014**, *29*, 312–320. [CrossRef] [PubMed]
3. Lowenberg, B.; Downing, J.R.; Burnett, A. Acute myeloid leukemia. *N. Engl. J. Med.* **1999**, *341*, 1051–1062. [CrossRef] [PubMed]
4. Bergua, J.M.; Montesinos, P.; Martinez-Cuadrón, D.; Fernández-Abellán, P.; Serrano, J.; Sayas, M.J.; Prieto-Fernandez, J.; Garcia, R.; Garcia-Huerta, A.J.; Barrios, M.; *et al.* A prognostic index for patients with refractory or in first relapsed acute myeloid leukemia treated with FLAG-ida or FLAGO-ida. *Blood* **2014**, *124*, 1049.
5. Breems, D.A.; Van Putten, W.L.; Huijgens, P.C.; Ossenkoppele, G.J.; Verhoef, G.E.; Verdonck, L.F.; Vellenga, E.; De Greef, G.E.; Jacky, E.; Van der Lelie, J.; *et al.* Prognostic index for adult patients with acute myeloid leukemia in first relapse. *J. Clin. Oncol.* **2005**, *23*, 1969–1978. [CrossRef] [PubMed]
6. Kurosawa, S.; Yamaguchi, T.; Miyawaki, S.; Uchida, N.; Sakura, T.; Kanamori, H.; Usuki, K.; Yamashita, T.; Okoshi, Y.; Shibayama, H.; *et al.* Prognostic factors and outcomes of adult patients with acute myeloid leukemia after first relapse. *Haematologica* **2010**, *95*, 1857–1864. [CrossRef] [PubMed]
7. Pemmaraju, N.; Kantarjian, H.; Garcia-Manero, G.; Pierce, S.; Cardenas-Turanzas, M.; Cortes, J.; Ravandi, F. Improving outcomes for patients with acute myeloid leukemia in first relapse: A single center experience. *Am. J. Hematol.* **2015**, *90*, 27–30. [CrossRef] [PubMed]
8. Genomic and epigenomic landscapes of adult *de novo* acute myeloid leukemia. *N. Engl. J. Med.* **2013**, *368*, 2059–2074.
9. Ding, L.; Ley, T.J.; Larson, D.E.; Miller, C.A.; Koboldt, D.C.; Welch, J.S.; Ritchey, J.K.; Young, M.A.; Lamprecht, T.; McLellan, M.D.; *et al.* Clonal evolution in relapsed acute myeloid leukaemia revealed by whole-genome sequencing. *Nature* **2012**, *481*, 506–510. [CrossRef] [PubMed]
10. Meggendorfer, M.; Alpermann, T.; Porglerová, K.; Kern, W.; Schnittger, S.; Haferlach, C.; Haferlach, T. Genetic patterns of relapsed aml differ significantly from first manifestation and are dependent on cytogenetic risk groups at diagnosis: Results in 175 patients with paired samples. *Blood* **2014**, *124*, 1029. [CrossRef] [PubMed]
11. Hourigan, C.S.; Karp, J.E. New considerations in the design of clinical trials for the treatment of acute leukemia. *Clin. Investig.* **2011**, *1*, 509–517. [CrossRef]
12. Karanes, C.; Kopecky, K.J.; Head, D.R.; Grever, M.R.; Hynes, H.E.; Kraut, E.H.; Vial, R.H.; Lichtin, A.; Nand, S.; Samlowski, W.E.; *et al.* A phase III comparison of high dose ARA-C (HIDAC) *versus* HIDAC plus mitoxantrone in the treatment of first relapsed or refractory acute myeloid leukemia Southwest Oncology Group Study. *Leuk. Res.* **1999**, *23*, 787–794. [CrossRef] [PubMed]
13. Herzig, R.H.; Lazarus, H.M.; Wolff, S.N.; Phillips, G.L.; Herzig, G.P. High-dose cytosine arabinoside therapy with and without anthracycline antibiotics for remission reinduction of acute nonlymphoblastic leukemia. *J. Clin. Oncol.* **1985**, *3*, 992–997. [PubMed]
14. Lee, S.R.; Yang, D.H.; Ahn, J.S.; Kim, Y.K.; Lee, J.J.; Choi, Y.J.; Shin, H.J.; Chung, J.S.; Cho, Y.Y.; Chae, Y.S.; *et al.* The clinical outcome of flag chemotherapy without idarubicin in patients with relapsed or refractory acute myeloid leukemia. *J. Korean Med. Sci.* **2009**, *24*, 498–503. [CrossRef] [PubMed]
15. Montillo, M.; Mirto, S.; Petti, M.C.; Latagliata, R.; Magrin, S.; Pinto, A.; Zagonel, V.; Mele, G.; Tedeschi, A.; Ferrara, F. Fludarabine, cytarabine, and G-CSF (FLAG) for the treatment of poor risk acute myeloid leukemia. *Am. J. Hematol.* **1998**, *58*, 105–109. [CrossRef] [PubMed]
16. Virchis, A.; Koh, M.; Rankin, P.; Mehta, A.; Potter, M.; Hoffbrand, A.V.; Prentice, H.G. Fludarabine, cytosine arabinoside, granulocyte-colony stimulating factor with or without idarubicin in the treatment of high risk acute leukaemia or myelodysplastic syndromes. *Br. J. Haematol.* **2004**, *124*, 26–32. [CrossRef] [PubMed]

17. Milligan, D.W.; Wheatley, K.; Littlewood, T.; Craig, J.I.; Burnett, A.K. Fludarabine and cytosine are less effective than standard ade chemotherapy in high-risk acute myeloid leukemia, and addition of G-CSF and ATRA are not beneficial: Results of the MRC AML-HR randomized trial. *Blood* **2006**, *107*, 4614–4622. [CrossRef] [PubMed]

18. Martin, M.G.; Welch, J.S.; Augustin, K.; Hladnik, L.; DiPersio, J.F.; Abboud, C.N. Cladribine in the treatment of acute myeloid leukemia: A single-institution experience. *Clin. Lymphoma Myeloma* **2009**, *9*, 298–301. [CrossRef] [PubMed]

19. Wrzesien-Kus, A.; Robak, T.; Lech-Maranda, E.; Wierzbowska, A.; Dmoszynska, A.; Kowal, M.; Holowiecki, J.; Kyrcz-Krzemien, S.; Grosicki, S.; Maj, S.; *et al.* A multicenter, open, non-comparative, phase II study of the combination of cladribine (2-chlorodeoxyadenosine), cytarabine, and G-CSF as induction therapy in refractory acute myeloid leukemia—A report of the polish adult leukemia group (PALG). *Eur. J. Haematol.* **2003**, *71*, 155–162. [CrossRef] [PubMed]

20. Price, S.L.; Lancet, J.E.; George, T.J.; Wetzstein, G.A.; List, A.F.; Ho, V.Q.; Fernandez, H.F.; Pinilla-Ibarz, J.; Kharfan-Dabaja, M.A.; Komrokji, R.S. Salvage chemotherapy regimens for acute myeloid leukemia: Is one better? Efficacy comparison between CLAG and MEC regimens. *Leuk. Res.* **2011**, *35*, 301–304. [CrossRef] [PubMed]

21. Wierzbowska, A.; Robak, T.; Pluta, A.; Wawrzyniak, E.; Cebula, B.; Holowiecki, J.; Kyrcz-Krzemien, S.; Grosicki, S.; Giebel, S.; Skotnicki, A.B.; *et al.* Cladribine combined with high doses of arabinoside cytosine, mitoxantrone, and G-CSF (CLAG-M) is a highly effective salvage regimen in patients with refractory and relapsed acute myeloid leukemia of the poor risk: A final report of the polish adult leukemia group. *Eur. J. Haematol.* **2008**, *80*, 115–126. [CrossRef] [PubMed]

22. Amadori, S.; Arcese, W.; Isacchi, G.; Meloni, G.; Petti, M.C.; Monarca, B.; Testi, A.M.; Mandelli, F. Mitoxantrone, etoposide, and intermediate-dose cytarabine: An effective and tolerable regimen for the treatment of refractory acute myeloid leukemia. *J. Clin. Oncol.* **1991**, *9*, 1210–1214. [PubMed]

23. Trifilio, S.M.; Rademaker, A.W.; Newman, D.; Coyle, K.; Carlson-Leuer, K.; Mehta, J.; Altman, J.; Frankfurt, O.; Tallman, M.S. Mitoxantrone and etoposide with or without intermediate dose cytarabine for the treatment of primary induction failure or relapsed acute myeloid leukemia. *Leuk. Res.* **2012**, *36*, 394–396. [CrossRef] [PubMed]

24. Greenberg, P.L.; Lee, S.J.; Advani, R.; Tallman, M.S.; Sikic, B.I.; Letendre, L.; Dugan, K.; Lum, B.; Chin, D.L.; Dewald, G.; *et al.* Mitoxantrone, etoposide, and cytarabine with or without valspodar in patients with relapsed or refractory acute myeloid leukemia and high-risk myelodysplastic syndrome: A phase III trial (E2995). *J. Clin. Oncol.* **2004**, *22*, 1078–1086. [CrossRef] [PubMed]

25. Kohrt, H.E.; Patel, S.; Ho, M.; Owen, T.; Pollyea, D.A.; Majeti, R.; Gotlib, J.; Coutre, S.; Liedtke, M.; Berube, C.; *et al.* Second-line mitoxantrone, etoposide, and cytarabine for acute myeloid leukemia: A single-center experience. *Am. J. Hematol.* **2010**, *85*, 877–881. [CrossRef] [PubMed]

26. Halpern, A.B.; Estey, E.H.; Othus, M.; Orlowski, K.F.; Powell, M.A.; Chen, T.L.; Becker, P.S.; Scott, B.L.; Hendrie, P.C.; Ostronoff, F.; *et al.* Mitoxantrone, etoposide, and cytarabine (MEC) following epigenetic priming with decitabine in adults with relapsed/refractory acute myeloid leukemia (AML) or high-risk myelodysplastic syndrome (MDS): A phase 1 study. *Blood* **2014**, *124*, 3730. [CrossRef] [PubMed]

27. Archimbaud, E.; Thomas, X.; Leblond, V.; Michallet, M.; Fenaux, P.; Cordonnier, C.; Dreyfus, F.; Troussard, X.; Jaubert, J.; Travade, P.; *et al.* Timed sequential chemotherapy for previously treated patients with acute myeloid leukemia: Long-term follow-up of the etoposide, mitoxantrone, and cytarabine-86 trial. *J. Clin. Oncol.* **1995**, *13*, 11–18. [PubMed]

28. Link, H.; Freund, M.; Diedrich, H.; Wilke, H.; Austein, J.; Henke, M.; Wandt, H.; Fackler-Schwalbe, E.; Schlimok, G.; Hoffmann, R.; *et al.* Mitoxantrone, cytosine arabinoside, and vp-16 in 36 patients with relapsed and refractory acute myeloid leukemia. *Haematol. Blood Transfus.* **1990**, *33*, 322–325. [PubMed]

29. De Astis, E.; Clavio, M.; Raiola, A.M.; Ghiso, A.; Guolo, F.; Minetto, P.; Galaverna, F.; Miglino, M.; Di Grazia, C.; Ballerini, F.; *et al.* Liposomal daunorubicin, fludarabine, and cytarabine (FLAD) as bridge therapy to stem cell transplant in relapsed and refractory acute leukemia. *Ann. Hematol.* **2014**, *93*, 2011–2018. [CrossRef] [PubMed]

30. Litzow, M.R.; Wang, X.V.; Carroll, M.P.; Karp, J.E.; Ketterling, R.; Kaufmann, S.H.; Lazarus, H.M.; Luger, S.M.; Paietta, E.M.; Rowe, J.M.; *et al.* A randomized phase II trial of three novel regimens for relapsed/ refractory acute myeloid leukemia (AML) demonstrates encouraging results with a flavopiridol-based regimen: Results of eastern cooperative oncology group (ECOG) trial E1906. *Blood* **2014**, *124*, 3742.

31. Karp, J.E.; Smith, B.D.; Levis, M.J.; Gore, S.D.; Greer, J.; Hattenburg, C.; Briel, J.; Jones, R.J.; Wright, J.J.; Colevas, A.D. Sequential flavopiridol, cytosine arabinoside, and mitoxantrone: A phase II trial in adults with poor-risk acute myelogenous leukemia. *Clin. Cancer Res.* **2007**, *13*, 4467–4473. [CrossRef] [PubMed]

32. Karp, J.E.; Smith, B.D.; Resar, L.S.; Greer, J.M.; Blackford, A.; Zhao, M.; Moton-Nelson, D.; Alino, K.; Levis, M.J.; Gore, S.D.; *et al.* Phase 1 and pharmacokinetic study of bolus-infusion flavopiridol followed by cytosine arabinoside and mitoxantrone for acute leukemias. *Blood* **2011**, *117*, 3302–3310. [CrossRef] [PubMed]

33. Faderl, S.; Gandhi, V.; O'Brien, S.; Bonate, P.; Cortes, J.; Estey, E.; Beran, M.; Wierda, W.; Garcia-Manero, G.; Ferrajoli, A.; *et al.* Results of a phase 1-2 study of clofarabine in combination with cytarabine (ARA-C) in relapsed and refractory acute leukemias. *Blood* **2005**, *105*, 940–947. [CrossRef] [PubMed]

34. Scappini, B.; Gianfaldoni, G.; Caracciolo, F.; Mannelli, F.; Biagiotti, C.; Romani, C.; Pogliani, E.M.; Simonetti, F.; Borin, L.; Fanci, R.; *et al.* Cytarabine and clofarabine after high-dose cytarabine in relapsed or refractory AML patients. *Am. J. Hematol.* **2012**, *87*, 1047–1051. [CrossRef] [PubMed]

35. Faderl, S.; Wetzler, M.; Rizzieri, D.; Schiller, G.; Jagasia, M.; Stuart, R.; Ganguly, S.; Avigan, D.; Craig, M.; Collins, R.; *et al.* Clofarabine plus cytarabine compared with cytarabine alone in older patients with relapsed or refractory acute myelogenous leukemia: Results from the classic I trial. *J. Clin. Oncol.* **2012**, *30*, 2492–2499. [CrossRef] [PubMed]

36. Becker, P.S.; Kantarjian, H.M.; Appelbaum, F.R.; Petersdorf, S.H.; Storer, B.; Pierce, S.; Shan, J.; Hendrie, P.C.; Pagel, J.M.; Shustov, A.R.; *et al.* Clofarabine with high dose cytarabine and granulocyte colony-stimulating factor (G-CSF) priming for relapsed and refractory acute myeloid leukaemia. *Br. J. Haematol.* **2011**, *155*, 182–189. [CrossRef] [PubMed]

37. Becker, P.S.; Kantarjian, H.M.; Appelbaum, F.R.; Storer, B.; Pierce, S.; Shan, J.; Faderl, S.; Estey, E.H. Retrospective comparison of clofarabine *versus* fludarabine in combination with high-dose cytarabine with or without granulocyte colony-stimulating factor as salvage therapies for acute myeloid leukemia. *Haematologica* **2013**, *98*, 114–118. [CrossRef] [PubMed]

38. Yu, W.; Mao, L.; Qian, J.; Qian, W.; Meng, H.; Mai, W.; Tong, H.; Tong, Y.; Jin, J. Homoharringtonine in combination with cytarabine and aclarubicin in the treatment of refractory/relapsed acute myeloid leukemia: A single-center experience. *Ann. Hematol.* **2013**, *92*, 1091–1100. [CrossRef] [PubMed]

39. Feldman, E.J.; Lancet, J.E.; Kolitz, J.E.; Ritchie, E.K.; Roboz, G.J.; List, A.F.; Allen, S.L.; Asatiani, E.; Mayer, L.D.; Swenson, C.; *et al.* First-in-man study of CPX-351: A liposomal carrier containing cytarabine and daunorubicin in a fixed 5:1 molar ratio for the treatment of relapsed and refractory acute myeloid leukemia. *J. Clin. Oncol.* **2011**, *29*, 979–985. [CrossRef] [PubMed]

40. Cortes, J.E.; Goldberg, S.L.; Feldman, E.J.; Rizzeri, D.A.; Hogge, D.E.; Larson, M.; Pigneux, A.; Recher, C.; Schiller, G.; Warzocha, K.; *et al.* Phase II, multicenter, randomized trial of CPX-351 (cytarabine:Daunorubicin) liposome injection *versus* intensive salvage therapy in adults with first relapse AML. *Cancer* **2015**, *121*, 234–242. [CrossRef] [PubMed]

41. Pemmaraju, N.; Kantarjian, H.; Kadia, T.; Cortes, J.; Borthakur, G.; Newberry, K.; Garcia-Manero, G.; Ravandi, F.; Jabbour, E.; Dellasala, S.; *et al.* A phase I/II study of the janus kinase (JAK) 1 and 2 inhibitor ruxolitinib in patients with relapsed or refractory acute myeloid leukemia. *Clin. Lymphoma Myeloma Leuk.* **2015**, *15*, 171–176. [CrossRef] [PubMed]

42. Eghtedar, A.; Verstovsek, S.; Estrov, Z.; Burger, J.; Cortes, J.; Bivins, C.; Faderl, S.; Ferrajoli, A.; Borthakur, G.; George, S.; *et al.* Phase 2 study of the JAK kinase inhibitor ruxolitinib in patients with refractory leukemias, including postmyeloproliferative neoplasm acute myeloid leukemia. *Blood* **2012**, *119*, 4614–4618. [CrossRef] [PubMed]

43. Recher, C.; Beyne-Rauzy, O.; Demur, C.; Chicanne, G.; Dos Santos, C.; Mas, V.M.; Benzaquen, D.; Laurent, G.; Huguet, F.; Payrastre, B. Antileukemic activity of rapamycin in acute myeloid leukemia. *Blood* **2005**, *105*, 2527–2534. [CrossRef] [PubMed]

44. Liesveld, J.L.; O'Dwyer, K.; Walker, A.; Becker, M.W.; Ifthikharuddin, J.J.; Mulford, D.; Chen, R.; Bechelli, J.; Rosell, K.; Minhajuddin, M.; *et al.* A phase I study of decitabine and rapamycin in relapsed/refractory AML. *Leuk. Res.* **2013**, *37*, 1622–1627. [CrossRef] [PubMed]

45. Park, S.; Chapuis, N.; Saint Marcoux, F.; Recher, C.; Prebet, T.; Chevallier, P.; Cahn, J.Y.; Leguay, T.; Bories, P.; Witz, F.; *et al.* A phase Ib GOELAMS study of the mTOR inhibitor RAD001 in association with chemotherapy for aml patients in first relapse. *Leukemia* **2013**, *27*, 1479–1486. [CrossRef] [PubMed]
46. Lowenberg, B.; Morgan, G.; Ossenkoppele, G.J.; Burnett, A.K.; Zachee, P.; Duhrsen, U.; Dierickx, D.; Muller-Tidow, C.; Sonneveld, P.; Krug, U.; *et al.* Phase I/II clinical study of tosedostat, an inhibitor of aminopeptidases, in patients with acute myeloid leukemia and myelodysplasia. *J. Clin. Oncol.* **2010**, *28*, 4333–4338. [CrossRef] [PubMed]
47. Cortes, J.; Feldman, E.; Yee, K.; Rizzieri, D.; Advani, A.S.; Charman, A.; Spruyt, R.; Toal, M.; Kantarjian, H. Two dosing regimens of tosedostat in elderly patients with relapsed or refractory acute myeloid leukaemia (OPAL): A randomised open-label phase 2 study. *Lancet Oncol.* **2013**, *14*, 354–362. [CrossRef] [PubMed]
48. Schaefer, E.W.; Loaiza-Bonilla, A.; Juckett, M.; DiPers, J.F.; Roy, V.; Slack, J.; Wu, W.T.; Laumann, K.; Espinoza-Delgado, I.; Gore, S.D.; *et al.* A phase 2 study of vorinostat in acute myeloid leukemia. *Haematol. Hematol. J.* **2009**, *94*, 1375–1382. [CrossRef]
49. Walter, R.B.; Medeiros, B.C.; Gardner, K.M.; Orlowski, K.F.; Gallegos, L.; Scott, B.L.; Hendrie, P.C.; Estey, E.H. Gemtuzumab ozogamicin in combination with vorinostat and azacitidine in older patients with relapsed or refractory acute myeloid leukemia: A phase I/II study. *Haematologica* **2014**, *99*, 54–59. [CrossRef] [PubMed]
50. Gojo, I.; Tan, M.; Fang, H.B.; Sadowska, M.; Lapidus, R.; Baer, M.R.; Carrier, F.; Beumer, J.H.; Anyang, B.N.; Srivastava, R.K.; *et al.* Translational phase I trial of vorinostat (suberoylanilide hydroxamic acid) combined with cytarabine and etoposide in patients with relapsed, refractory, or high-risk acute myeloid leukemia. *Clin. Cancer Res.* **2013**, *19*, 1838–1851. [CrossRef] [PubMed]
51. Stein, E.; Tallman, M.; Pollyea, D.A.; Flinn, I.W.; Fathi, A.T.; Stone, R.M.; Levine, R.L.; Agresta, S.; Schenkein, D.; Yang, H.; *et al.* Clinical safety and activity in a phase I trial of AG-221, a first in class, potent inhibitor of the IDH2-mutant protein, in patients with IDH2 mutant positive advanced hematologic malignancies. In Proceedings of the 105th Annual Meeting of the American Association for Cancer Research, San Diego, CA, USA, 6–8 April 2014.
52. Roboz, G.J.; Rosenblat, T.; Arellano, M.; Gobbi, M.; Altman, J.K.; Montesinos, P.; O'Connell, C.; Solomon, S.R.; Pigneux, A.; Vey, N.; *et al.* International randomized phase III study of elacytarabine *versus* investigator choice in patients with relapsed/refractory acute myeloid leukemia. *J. Clin. Oncol.* **2014**, *32*, 1919–1926. [CrossRef] [PubMed]
53. Lancet, J.E.; Ravandi, F.; Ricklis, R.M.; Cripe, L.D.; Kantarjian, H.M.; Giles, F.J.; List, A.F.; Chen, T.; Allen, R.S.; Fox, J.A.; *et al.* A phase Ib study of vosaroxin, an anticancer quinolone derivative, in patients with relapsed or refractory acute leukemia. *Leukemia* **2011**, *25*, 1808–1814. [CrossRef] [PubMed]
54. Ravandi, F.; Ritchie, E.; Sayar, H.; Lancet, J.; Craig, M.D.; Vey, N.; Strickland, S.A.; Schiller, G.; Jabbour, E.; Erba, H.P.; *et al.* Improved survival in patients with first relapsed or refractory acute myeloid leukemia (AML) treated with vosaroxin plus cytarabine *versus* placebo plus cytarabine: Results of a phase 3 double-blind randomized controlled multinational study (VALOR). *Blood* **2014**, *124*, LBA 6.
55. Kornblau, S.M.; Banker, D.E.; Stirewalt, D.; Shen, D.; Lemker, E.; Verstovsek, S.; Estrov, Z.; Faderl, S.; Cortes, J.; Beran, M.; *et al.* Blockade of adaptive defensive changes in cholesterol uptake and synthesis in AML by the addition of pravastatin to idarubicin + high-dose ARA-C: A phase 1 study. *Blood* **2007**, *109*, 2999–3006. [PubMed]
56. Advani, A.S.; McDonough, S.; Copelan, E.; Willman, C.; Mulford, D.A.; List, A.F.; Sekeres, M.A.; Othus, M.; Appelbaum, F.R. SWOG0919: A phase 2 study of idarubicin and cytarabine in combination with pravastatin for relapsed acute myeloid leukaemia. *Br. J. Haematol.* **2014**, *167*, 233–237. [CrossRef] [PubMed]
57. Advani, A.S.; Elson, P.; Kalaycio, M.E.; Mukherjee, S.; Gerds, A.T.; Hamilton, B.K.; Hobson, S.; Smith, A.; Rush, M.L.; Bogati, S.; *et al.* Bortezomib + MEC (mitoxantrone, etoposide, cytarabine) for relapsed/refractory acute myeloid leukemia: Final results of an expanded phase 1 trial. *Blood* **2014**, *124*, 978.
58. Chen, Y.; Kantarjian, H.; Estrov, Z.; Faderl, S.; Ravandi, F.; Rey, K.; Cortes, J.; Borthakur, G. A phase II study of lenalidomide alone in relapsed/refractory acute myeloid leukemia or high-risk myelodysplastic syndromes with chromosome 5 abnormalities. *Clin. Lymphoma Myeloma Leuk.* **2012**, *12*, 341–344. [CrossRef] [PubMed]
59. Pardee, T.S.; Stadelman, K.; Isom, S.; Ellis, L.R.; Berenzon, D.; Hurd, D.D.; Harrelson, R.; Manuel, M.; Dralle, S.; Lyerly, S.; *et al.* The mitochondrial metabolism inhibitor CPI-613 is highly active in combination with high dose ARA-C (HIDAC) and mitoxantrone in a phase I study for relapsed or refractory acute myeloid leukemia (AML). *Blood* **2014**, *124*, 3744.

60. Konopleva, M.; Pollyea, D.A.; Potluri, J.; Chyla, B.J.; Busman, T.; McKeegan, E.; Salem, A.; Zhu, M.; Ricker, J.L.; Blum, W.; *et al.* A phase 2 study of ABT-199 (GDC-0199) in patients with acute myelogenous leukemia (AML). *Blood* **2014**, *124*, 118.

61. Thol, F.; Schlenk, R.F. Gemtuzumab ozogamicin in acute myeloid leukemia revisited. *Expert. Opin. Biol. Ther.* **2014**, *14*, 1185–1195. [CrossRef] [PubMed]

62. Petersdorf, S.; Kopecky, K.; Stuart, R.K.; Larson, R.A.; Nevill, T.J.; Stenke, L.; Slovak, M.L.; Tallman, M.S.; Willman, C.L.; Erba, H.; *et al.* Preliminary results of Southwest Oncology Group Sstudy S0106: An international intergroup phase 3 randomized trial comparing the addition of gemtuzumab ozogamicin to standard induction therapy *versus* standard induction therapy followed by a second randomization to post-consolidation gemtuzumab ozogamicin *versus* no additional therapy for previously untreated acute myeloid leukemia. *Blood* **2009**, *114*, 326–327.

63. Pilorge, S.; Rigaudeau, S.; Rabian, F.; Sarkozy, C.; Taksin, A.L.; Farhat, H.; Merabet, F.; Ghez, S.; Raggueneau, V.; Terre, C.; *et al.* Fractionated gemtuzumab ozogamicin and standard dose cytarabine produced prolonged second remissions in patients over the age of 55 years with acute myeloid leukemia in late first relapse. *Am. J. Hematol.* **2014**, *89*, 399–403. [CrossRef] [PubMed]

64. Sutherland, M.S.K.; Walter, R.B.; Jeffrey, S.C.; Burke, P.J.; Yu, C.P.; Kostner, H.; Stone, I.; Ryan, M.C.; Sussman, D.; Lyon, R.P.; *et al.* SGN-CD33A: A novel CD33-targeting antibody-drug conjugate using a pyrrolobenzodiazepine dimer is active in models of drug-resistant AML. *Blood* **2013**, *122*, 1455–1463. [CrossRef] [PubMed]

65. Stein, E.M.; Stein, A.; Walter, R.B.; Fathi, A.T.; Lancet, J.E.; Kovacsovics, T.J.; Advani, A.S.; DeAngelo, D.J.; O'Meara, M.M.; Zhao, B.; *et al.* Interim analysis of a phase 1 trial of SGN-CD33A in patients with CD33-positive acute myeloid leukemia (AML). *Blood* **2014**, *124*, 623. [CrossRef] [PubMed]

66. Feldman, E.J.; Brandwein, J.; Stone, R.; Kalaycio, M.; Moore, J.; O'Connor, J.; Wedel, N.; Roboz, G.J.; Miller, C.; Chopra, R.; *et al.* Phase III randomized multicenter study of a humanized anti-CD33 monoclonal antibody, lintuzumab, in combination with chemotherapy, *versus* chemotherapy alone in patients with refractory or first-relapsed acute myeloid leukemia. *J. Clin. Oncol.* **2005**, *23*, 4110–4116. [CrossRef] [PubMed]

67. Busfield, S.J.; Biondo, M.; Wong, M.; Ramshaw, H.S.; Lee, E.M.; Ghosh, S.; Braley, H.; Panousis, C.; Roberts, A.W.; He, S.Z.; *et al.* Targeting of acute myeloid leukemia *in vitro* and *in vivo* with an anti-CD123 mAB engineered for optimal ADCC. *Leukemia* **2014**, *28*, 2213–2221. [CrossRef] [PubMed]

68. Smith, B.D.; Roboz, G.J.; Walter, R.B.; Altman, J.K.; Ferguson, A.; Curcio, T.J.; Orlowski, K.F.; Garrett, L.; Busfield, S.J.; Barnden, M.; *et al.* First-in man, phase 1 study of CSL362 (anti-IL3Rα/anti-CD123 monoclonal antibody) in patients with CD123+ acute myeloid leukemia (AML) in CR at high risk for early relapse. *Blood* **2014**, *124*, 120.

69. Laszlo, G.S.; Gudgeon, C.J.; Harrington, K.H.; Dell'Aringa, J.; Newhall, K.J.; Means, G.D.; Sinclair, A.M.; Kischel, R.; Frankel, S.R.; Walter, R.B. Cellular determinants for preclinical activity of a novel CD33/CD3 bispecific T-cell engager (BiTE) antibody, AMG 330, against human AML. *Blood* **2014**, *123*, 554–561. [CrossRef] [PubMed]

70. Friedrich, M.; Henn, A.; Raum, T.; Bajtus, M.; Matthes, K.; Hendrich, L.; Wahl, J.; Hoffmann, P.; Kischel, R.; Kvesic, M.; *et al.* Preclinical characterization of AMG 330, a CD3/CD33-bispecific T-cell-engaging antibody with potential for treatment of acute myelogenous leukemia. *Mol. Cancer Ther.* **2014**, *13*, 1549–1557. [CrossRef] [PubMed]

71. Uy, G.; Stewart, S.; Baughman, J.; Rettig, M.; Chichili, G.; Bonvini, E.; Wigginton, J.; Lechleider, R.; DiPersio, J. A phase I trial of MGD006 in patients with relapsed acute myeloid leukemia (AML). *J. Immun. Ther. Cancer* **2014**, *2*, 87. [CrossRef]

72. Wiernik, A.; Foley, B.; Zhang, B.; Verneris, M.R.; Warlick, E.; Gleason, M.K.; Ross, J.A.; Luo, X.; Weisdorf, D.J.; Walcheck, B.; *et al.* Targeting natural killer cells to acute myeloid leukemia *in vitro* with a CD16 × 33 bispecific killer cell engager and ADAM17 inhibition. *Clin. Cancer Res.* **2013**, *19*, 3844–3855. [CrossRef] [PubMed]

73. Wang, Q.S.; Wang, Y.; Lv, H.Y.; Han, Q.W.; Fan, H.; Guo, B.; Wang, L.L.; Han, W.D. Treatment of CD33-directed chimeric antigen receptor-modified T cells in one patient with relapsed and refractory acute myeloid leukemia. *Mol. Ther.* **2015**, *23*, 184–191. [CrossRef] [PubMed]

74. Gill, S.; Tasian, S.K.; Ruella, M.; Shestova, O.; Li, Y.; Porter, D.L.; Carroll, M.; Danet-Desnoyers, G.; Scholler, J.; Grupp, S.A.; *et al.* Preclinical targeting of human acute myeloid leukemia and myeloablation using chimeric antigen receptor-modified T cells. *Blood* **2014**, *123*, 2343–2354. [CrossRef] [PubMed]

75. Pizzitola, I.; Anjos-Afonso, F.; Rouault-Pierre, K.; Lassailly, F.; Tettamanti, S.; Spinelli, O.; Biondi, A.; Biagi, E.; Bonnet, D. Chimeric antigen receptors against CD33/CD123 antigens efficiently target primary acute myeloid leukemia cells *in vivo*. *Leukemia* **2014**, *28*, 1596–1605. [CrossRef] [PubMed]

76. Berneman, Z.N.; Van de Velde, A.L.; Willemen, Y.; Anguille, S.; Saevels, K.; Germonpré, P.; Huizing, M.T.; Peeters, M.; Snoeckx, A.; Parizel, P.; *et al.* Vaccination with WT1 mRNA-electroporated dendritic cells: Report of clinical outcome in 66 cancer patients. *Blood* **2014**, *124*, 310. [CrossRef] [PubMed]

77. Rosenblat, T.L.; Frattini, M.G.; Chanel, S.M.; Dao, T.; Bernal, Y.; Jurcic, J.G.; Zhang, R.; Simancek, P.; Tallman, M.S.; Scheinberg, D.A.; *et al.* Phase II trial of WT1 analog peptide vaccine in patients with acute myeloid leukemia (AML) in complete remission (CR). *Blood* **2012**, *120*, 3624.

78. Goswami, M.; Hensel, N.; Smith, B.D.; Prince, G.T.; Qin, L.; Levitsky, H.I.; Strickland, S.A.; Jagasia, M.; Savani, B.N.; Fraser, J.W.; *et al.* Expression of putative targets of immunotherapy in acute myeloid leukemia and healthy tissues. *Leukemia* **2014**, *28*, 1167–1170. [CrossRef] [PubMed]

79. Cilloni, D.; Renneville, A.; Hermitte, F.; Hills, R.K.; Daly, S.; Jovanovic, J.V.; Gottardi, E.; Fava, M.; Schnittger, S.; Weiss, T.; *et al.* Real-time quantitative polymerase chain reaction detection of minimal residual disease by standardized WT1 assay to enhance risk stratification in acute myeloid leukemia: A European LeukemiaNet study. *J. Clin. Oncol.* **2009**, *27*, 5195–5201. [CrossRef] [PubMed]

80. Chapuis, A.G.; Ragnarsson, G.B.; Nguyen, H.N.; Chaney, C.N.; Pufnock, J.S.; Schmitt, T.M.; Duerkopp, N.; Roberts, I.M.; Pogosov, G.L.; Ho, W.Y.; *et al.* Transferred WT1-reactive CD8+ T cells can mediate antileukemic activity and persist in post-transplant patients. *Sci. Transl. Med.* **2013**, *5*. [CrossRef]

81. Miller, J.S.; Soignier, Y.; Panoskaltsis-Mortari, A.; McNearney, S.A.; Yun, G.H.; Fautsch, S.K.; McKenna, D.; Le, C.; Defor, T.E.; Burns, L.J.; *et al.* Successful adoptive transfer and *in vivo* expansion of human haploidentical NK cells in patients with cancer. *Blood* **2005**, *105*, 3051–3057. [CrossRef] [PubMed]

82. Armistead, P.M.; de Lima, M.; Pierce, S.; Qiao, W.; Wang, X.; Thall, P.F.; Giralt, S.; Ravandi, F.; Kantarjian, H.; Champlin, R.; *et al.* Quantifying the survival benefit for allogeneic hematopoietic stem cell transplantation in relapsed acute myelogenous leukemia. *Biol. Blood Marrow Transplant.* **2009**, *15*, 1431–1438. [CrossRef] [PubMed]

83. Shimoni, A.; Hardan, I.; Shem-Tov, N.; Yerushalmi, R.; Nagler, A. Allogeneic hematopoietic stem-cell transplantation in AML and MDS using myeloablative *versus* reduced-intensity conditioning: Long-term follow-up. *Leukemia* **2010**, *24*, 1050–1052. [CrossRef] [PubMed]

84. Sebert, M.; Porcher, R.; Robin, M.; Ades, L.; Boissel, N.; Raffoux, E.; Xhaard, A.; Dhedin, N.; Larghero, J.; Himberlin, C.; *et al.* Equivalent outcomes using reduced intensity or conventional myeloablative conditioning transplantation for patients aged 35 years and over with AML. *Bone Marrow Transplant.* **2015**, *50*, 74–81. [CrossRef] [PubMed]

85. Bejanyan, N.; Oran, B.; Shanley, R.; Warlick, E.; Ustun, C.; Vercellotti, G.; Verneris, M.; Wagner, J.E.; Weisdorf, D.; Brunstein, C. Clinical outcomes of aml patients relapsing after matched-related donor and umbilical cord blood transplantation. *Bone Marrow Transplant.* **2014**, *49*, 1029–1035. [CrossRef] [PubMed]

86. Itonaga, H.; Tsushima, H.; Taguchi, J.; Fukushima, T.; Taniguchi, H.; Sato, S.; Ando, K.; Sawayama, Y.; Matsuo, E.; Yamasaki, R.; *et al.* Treatment of relapsed adult T-cell leukemia/lymphoma after allogeneic hematopoietic stem cell transplantation: The Nagasaki Transplant Group experience. *Blood* **2013**, *121*, 219–225. [CrossRef] [PubMed]

87. Takami, A.; Yano, S.; Yokoyama, H.; Kuwatsuka, Y.; Yamaguchi, T.; Kanda, Y.; Morishima, Y.; Fukuda, T.; Miyazaki, Y.; Nakamae, H.; *et al.* Donor lymphocyte infusion for the treatment of relapsed acute myeloid leukemia after allogeneic hematopoietic stem cell transplantation: A retrospective analysis by the adult acute myeloid leukemia working group of the Japan Society for Hematopoietic Cell Transplantation. *Biol. Blood Marrow Transplant.* **2014**, *20*, 1785–1790. [CrossRef] [PubMed]

88. Schroeder, T.; Czibere, A.; Platzbecker, U.; Bug, G.; Uharek, L.; Luft, T.; Giagounidis, A.; Zohren, F.; Bruns, I.; Wolschke, C.; *et al.* Azacitidine and donor lymphocyte infusions as first salvage therapy for relapse of AML or MDS after allogeneic stem cell transplantation. *Leukemia* **2013**, *27*, 1229–1235. [CrossRef] [PubMed]

89. Ghobadi, A.; Fiala, M.A.; Abboud, C.N.; Cashen, A.F.; Eissenberg, L.; Graubert, T.; Jacoby, M.A.; Pusic, I.; Schroeder, M.A.; Stockerl-Goldstein, K.E.; *et al.* A phase I study of azacitidine after donor lymphocyte infusion for relapsed acute myeloid leukemia post allogeneic stem cell transplantation. *Blood* **2013**, *122*, 3320.

90. O'Donnell, M.R.; Tallman, M.S.; Abboud, C.N.; Altman, J.K.; Appelbaum, F.R.; Arber, D.A.; Attar, E.; Borate, U.; Coutre, S.E.; Damon, L.E.; *et al.* Acute myeloid leukemia, version 2.2013. *J. Nat. Compr. Cancer Netw.* **2013**, *11*, 1047–1055.

91. Gandhi, V.; Estey, E.; Keating, M.J.; Plunkett, W. Fludarabine potentiates metabolism of cytarabine in patients with acute myelogenous leukemia during therapy. *J. Clin. Oncol.* **1993**, *11*, 116–124. [PubMed]

92. Chow, K.U.; Boehrer, S.; Napieralski, S.; Nowak, D.; Knau, A.; Hoelzer, D.; Mitrou, P.S.; Weidmann, E. In AML cell lines ARA-C combined with purine analogues is able to exert synergistic as well as antagonistic effects on proliferation, apoptosis and disruption of mitochondrial membrane potential. *Leuk. Lymphoma* **2003**, *44*, 165–173. [CrossRef] [PubMed]

93. Thomas, X.; Fenaux, P.; Dombret, H.; Delair, S.; Dreyfus, F.; Tilly, H.; Vekhoff, A.; Cony-Makhoul, P.; Leblond, V.; Troussard, X.; *et al.* Granulocyte-macrophage colony-stimulating factor (GM-CSF) to increase efficacy of intensive sequential chemotherapy with etoposide, mitoxantrone and cytarabine (EMA) in previously treated acute myeloid leukemia: A multicenter randomized placebo-controlled trial (EMA91 trial). *Leukemia* **1999**, *13*, 1214–1220. [CrossRef] [PubMed]

94. Cooper, T.; Ayres, M.; Nowak, B.; Gandhi, V. Biochemical modulation of cytarabine triphosphate by clofarabine. *Cancer Chemother. Pharmacol.* **2005**, *55*, 361–368. [CrossRef] [PubMed]

95. Becker, P.S.; Medeiros, B.C.; Stein, A.S.; Othus, M.; Appelbaum, F.R.; Forman, S.J.; Scott, B.L.; Hendrie, P.C.; Gardner, K.M.; Pagel, J.M.; *et al.* G-CSF priming, clofarabine, and high dose cytarabine (GCLAC) for upfront treatment of acute myeloid leukemia, advanced myelodysplastic syndrome or advanced myeloproliferative neoplasm. *Am. J. Hematol.* 2014. [CrossRef]

96. Verdonck, L.F.; Lokhorst, H.M.; Roovers, D.J.; van Heugten, H.G. Multidrug-resistant acute leukemia cells are responsive to prolonged exposure of daunorubicin: Implications for liposome-encapsulated daunorubicin. *Leuk. Res.* **1998**, *22*, 249–256. [CrossRef] [PubMed]

97. Ermacora, A.; Michieli, M.; Pea, F.; Visani, G.; Bucalossi, A.; Russo, D. Liposome encapsulated daunorubicin (daunoxome) for acute leukemia. *Haematologica* **2000**, *85*, 324–325.

98. Lancet, J.E.; Roboz, G.J.; Cripe, L.D.; Michelson, G.C.; Fox, J.A.; Leavitt, R.D.; Chen, T.; Hawtin, R.; Craig, A.R.; Ravandi, F.; *et al.* A phase 1b/2 study of combination vosaroxin and cytarabine in patients with relapsed or refractory acute myeloid leukemia. *Haematologica* **2014**, *100*, 231–237. [CrossRef] [PubMed]

99. Marcucci, G.; Maharry, K.; Wu, Y.Z.; Radmacher, M.D.; Mrozek, K.; Margeson, D.; Holland, K.B.; Whitman, S.P.; Becker, H.; Schwind, S.; *et al.* IDH1 and IDH2 gene mutations identify novel molecular subsets within *de novo* cytogenetically normal acute myeloid leukemia: A Cancer and Leukemia Group B study. *J. Clin. Oncol.* **2010**, *28*, 2348–2355. [CrossRef] [PubMed]

100. Stuart, S.D.; Schauble, A.; Gupta, S.; Kennedy, A.D.; Keppler, B.R.; Bingham, P.M.; Zachar, Z. A strategically designed small molecule attacks alpha-ketoglutarate dehydrogenase in tumor cells through a redox process. *Cancer Metab.* **2014**, *2*. [CrossRef]

101. Ben-Batalla, I.; Schultze, A.; Wroblewski, M.; Erdmann, R.; Heuser, M.; Waizenegger, J.S.; Riecken, K.; Binder, M.; Schewe, D.; Sawall, S.; *et al.* Axl, a prognostic and therapeutic target in acute myeloid leukemia mediates paracrine crosstalk of leukemia cells with bone marrow stroma. *Blood* **2013**, *122*, 2443–2452. [CrossRef] [PubMed]

102. Uy, G.L.; Rettig, M.P.; Motabi, I.H.; McFarland, K.; Trinkaus, K.M.; Hladnik, L.M.; Kulkarni, S.; Abboud, C.N.; Cashen, A.F.; Stockerl-Goldstein, K.E.; *et al.* A phase 1/2 study of chemosensitization with the CXCR4 antagonist plerixafor in relapsed or refractory acute myeloid leukemia. *Blood* **2012**, *119*, 3917–3924. [CrossRef] [PubMed]

103. Konig, H.; Levis, M. Targeting FLT3 to treat leukemia. *Expert Opin. Ther. Targets* **2015**, *19*, 37–54. [CrossRef] [PubMed]

104. Pratz, K.W.; Sato, T.; Murphy, K.M.; Stine, A.; Rajkhowa, T.; Levis, M. FLT3-mutant allelic burden and clinical status are predictive of response to FLT3 inhibitors in AML. *Blood* **2010**, *115*, 1425–1432. [CrossRef] [PubMed]

105. Cortes, J.E.; Kantarjian, H.; Foran, J.M.; Ghirdaladze, D.; Zodelava, M.; Borthakur, G.; Gammon, G.; Trone, D.; Armstrong, R.C.; James, J.; *et al.* Phase I study of quizartinib administered daily to patients with relapsed or refractory acute myeloid leukemia irrespective of FMS-like tyrosine kinase 3-internal tandem duplication status. *J. Clin. Oncol.* **2013**, *31*, 3681–3687. [CrossRef] [PubMed]

106. Wander, S.A.; Levis, M.J.; Fathi, A.T. The evolving role of FLT3 inhibitors in acute myeloid leukemia: Quizartinib and beyond. *Ther. Adv. Hematol.* **2014**, *5*, 65–77. [CrossRef] [PubMed]

107. Cortes, J.E.; Tallman, M.S.; Schiller, G.; Trone, D.; Gammon, G.; Goldberg, S.; Perl, A.E.; Marie, J.P.; Martinelli, G.; Levis, M. Results of a phase 2 randomized, open-label, study of lower doses of quizartinib (AC220; ASP2689) in subjects with FLT3-ITD positive relapsed or refractory acute myeloid leukemia (AML). *Blood* **2013**, *122*, 494.

108. Levis, M.J.; Perl, A.E.; Dombret, H.; Dohner, H.; Steffen, B.; Rousselot, P.; Martinelli, G.; Estey, E.H.; Burnett, A.K.; Gammon, G.; *et al.* Final results of a phase 2 open-label, monotherapy efficacy and safety study of quizartinib (AC220) in patients with FLT3-ITD positive or negative relapsed/refractory acute myeloid leukemia after second-line chemotherapy or hematopoietic stem cell transplantation. *Blood* **2012**, *120*, 673.

109. Röllig, C.; Müller-Tidow, C.; Hüttmann, A.; Noppeney, R.; Kunzmann, V.; Baldus, C.D.; Brandts, C.H.; Krämer, A.; Schäfer-Eckart, K.; Neubauer, A.; *et al.* Sorafenib *versus* placebo in addition to standard therapy in younger patients with newly diagnosed acute myeloid leukemia: Results from 267 patients treated in the randomized placebo-controlled SAL-Soraml trial. **2014**, *124*, 6.

110. Hourigan, C.S.; McCarthy, P.; de Lima, M. Back to the future! The evolving role of maintenance therapy after hematopoietic stem cell transplantation. *Biol. Blood Marrow Transplant.* **2014**, *20*, 154–163. [CrossRef] [PubMed]

111. Chen, Y.B.; Li, S.; Lane, A.A.; Connolly, C.; Del Rio, C.; Valles, B.; Curtis, M.; Ballen, K.; Cutler, C.; Dey, B.R.; *et al.* Phase I trial of maintenance sorafenib after allogeneic hematopoietic stem cell transplantation for FMS-like tyrosine kinase 3 internal tandem duplication acute myeloid leukemia. *Biol. Blood Marrow Transplant.* **2014**, *20*, 2042–2048. [CrossRef] [PubMed]

112. Sammons, S.L.; Pratz, K.W.; Smith, B.D.; Karp, J.E.; Emadi, A. Sorafenib is tolerable and improves clinical outcomes in patients with FLT3-ITD acute myeloid leukemia prior to stem cell transplant and after relapse post-transplant. *Am. J. Hematol.* **2014**, *89*, 936–938. [CrossRef] [PubMed]

113. Grunwald, M.R.; Levis, M.J. FLT3 inhibitors for acute myeloid leukemia: A review of their efficacy and mechanisms of resistance. *Int. J. Hematol.* **2013**, *97*, 683–694. [CrossRef] [PubMed]

114. Zimmerman, E.I.; Turner, D.C.; Buaboonnam, J.; Hu, S.; Orwick, S.; Roberts, M.S.; Janke, L.J.; Ramachandran, A.; Stewart, C.F.; Inaba, H.; *et al.* Crenolanib is active against models of drug-resistant FLT3-ITD-positive acute myeloid leukemia. *Blood* **2013**, *122*, 3607–3615. [CrossRef] [PubMed]

115. Lee, H.K.; Kim, H.W.; Lee, I.Y.; Lee, J.; Lee, J.; Jung, D.S.; Lee, S.Y.; Park, S.H.; Hwang, H.; Choi, J.S.; *et al.* G-749, a novel FLT3 kinase inhibitor, can overcome drug resistance for the treatment of acute myeloid leukemia. *Blood* **2014**, *123*, 2209–2219. [CrossRef] [PubMed]

116. Keegan, K.; Li, C.; Li, Z.H.; Ma, J.; Ragains, M.; Coberly, S.; Hollenback, D.; Eksterowicz, J.; Liang, L.M.; Weidner, M.; *et al.* Preclinical evaluation of AMG 925, a FLT3/CDK4 dual kinase inhibitor for treating acute myeloid leukemia. *Mol. Cancer Ther.* **2014**, *13*, 880–889. [CrossRef] [PubMed]

117. Xiang, Z.; Zhao, Y.; Mitaksov, V.; Fremont, D.H.; Kasai, Y.; Molitoris, A.; Ries, R.E.; Miner, T.L.; McLellan, M.D.; DiPersio, J.F.; *et al.* Identification of somatic JAK1 mutations in patients with acute myeloid leukemia. *Blood* **2008**, *111*, 4809–4812. [CrossRef] [PubMed]

118. Shadman, M.; Mawad, R.; Dean, C.; Shannon-Dorcy, K.; Sandhu, V.; Hendrie, P.C.; Scott, B.L.; Walter, R.B.; Becker, P.S.; Pagel, J.; *et al.* Idarubicin, cytarabine and pravastatin as induction therapy for untreated acute myeloid leukemia and high-risk myelodysplastic syndrome. *Blood* **2014**, *124*, 3732.

119. Kobune, M.; Takimoto, R.; Murase, K.; Iyama, S.; Sato, T.; Kikuchi, S.; Kawano, Y.; Miyanishi, K.; Sato, Y.; Niitsu, Y.; *et al.* Drug resistance is dramatically restored by hedgehog inhibitors in CD34+ leukemic cells. *Cancer Sci.* **2009**, *100*, 948–955. [CrossRef] [PubMed]

120. Krupka, C.; Kufer, P.; Kischel, R.; Zugmaier, G.; Bögeholz, J.; Köhnke, T.; Lichtenegger, F.S.; Schneider, S.; Metzeler, K.H.; Fiegl, M.; *et al.* CD33 target validation and sustained depletion of AML blasts in long-term cultures by the bispecific T-cell-engaging antibody AMG 330. *Blood* **2014**, *123*, 356.

121. Mardiros, A.; Dos Santos, C.; McDonald, T.; Brown, C.E.; Wang, X.; Budde, L.E.; Hoffman, L.; Aguilar, B.; Chang, W.-C.; Bretzlaff, W.; *et al.* T cells expressing CD123-specific chimeric antigen receptors exhibit specific cytolytic effector functions and antitumor effects against human acute myeloid leukemia. *Blood* **2013**, *122*, 3138–3148. [CrossRef] [PubMed]

122. Hourigan, C.S.; Levitsky, H.I. Evaluation of current cancer immunotherapy: Hemato-oncology. *Cancer J. (Sudbury, Mass.)* **2011**, *17*, 309–324. [CrossRef]

123. Jabbour, E.; Daver, N.; Champlin, R.; Mathisen, M.; Oran, B.; Ciurea, S.; Khouri, I.; Cornelison, A.M.; Ghanem, H.; Cardenas-Turanzas, M.; *et al.* Allogeneic stem cell transplantation as initial salvage for patients with acute myeloid leukemia refractory to high-dose cytarabine-based induction chemotherapy. *Am. J. Hematol.* **2014**, *89*, 395–398. [CrossRef] [PubMed]

124. Walter, R.B.; Buckley, S.A.; Pagel, J.M.; Wood, B.L.; Storer, B.E.; Sandmaier, B.M.; Fang, M.; Gyurkocza, B.; Delaney, C.; Radich, J.P.; *et al.* Significance of minimal residual disease before myeloablative allogeneic hematopoietic cell transplantation for AML in first and second complete remission. *Blood* **2013**, *122*, 1813–1821. [CrossRef] [PubMed]

125. Duval, M.; Klein, J.P.; He, W.; Cahn, J.Y.; Cairo, M.; Camitta, B.M.; Kamble, R.; Copelan, E.; de Lima, M.; Gupta, V.; *et al.* Hematopoietic stem-cell transplantation for acute leukemia in relapse or primary induction failure. *J. Clin. Oncol.* **2010**, *28*, 3730–3738. [CrossRef] [PubMed]

126. Luznik, L.; O'Donnell, P.V.; Symons, H.J.; Chen, A.R.; Leffell, M.S.; Zahurak, M.; Gooley, T.A.; Piantadosi, S.; Kaup, M.; Ambinder, R.F.; *et al.* HLA-haploidentical bone marrow transplantation for hematologic malignancies using nonmyeloablative conditioning and high-dose, posttransplantation cyclophosphamide. *Biol. Blood Marrow Transplant.* **2008**, *14*, 641–650. [CrossRef] [PubMed]

127. Raiola, A.M.; Dominietto, A.; di Grazia, C.; Lamparelli, T.; Gualandi, F.; Ibatici, A.; Bregante, S.; Van Lint, M.T.; Varaldo, R.; Ghiso, A.; *et al.* Unmanipulated haploidentical transplants compared with other alternative donors and matched sibling grafts. *Biol. Blood Marrow Transplant.* **2014**, *20*, 1573–1579. [CrossRef] [PubMed]

128. Craddock, C.; Labopin, M.; Houhou, M.; Robin, M.; Finke, J.; Chevallier, P.; Yakoub-Agha, I.; Bourhis, J.-H.; Sengelov, H.; Blaise, D.; *et al.* Activity and tolerability of azacitidine in patients who relapse after allogeneic stem cell transplantation (allo-SCT) for acute myeloid leukemia (AML) and myelodysplasia (MDS): A survey from the european society for blood and marrow transplantation (EBMT). *Blood* **2014**, *124*, 2506–2506.

129. Sarkozy, C.; Gardin, C.; Gachard, N.; Merabet, F.; Turlure, P.; Malfuson, J.V.; Pautas, C.; Micol, J.B.; Thomas, X.; Quesnel, B.; *et al.* Outcome of older patients with acute myeloid leukemia in first relapse. *Am. J. Hematol.* **2013**, *88*, 758–764. [CrossRef] [PubMed]

130. Tawfik, B.; Sliesoraitis, S.; Lyerly, S.; Klepin, H.D.; Lawrence, J.; Isom, S.; Ellis, L.R.; Manuel, M.; Dralle, S.; Berenzon, D.; *et al.* Efficacy of the hypomethylating agents as frontline, salvage, or consolidation therapy in adults with acute myeloid leukemia (AML). *Ann. Hematol.* **2014**, *93*, 47–55. [CrossRef] [PubMed]

131. Ivanoff, S.; Gruson, B.; Chantepie, S.P.; Lemasle, E.; Merlusca, L.; Harrivel, V.; Charbonnier, A.; Votte, P.; Royer, B.; Marolleau, J.P. 5-azacytidine treatment for relapsed or refractory acute myeloid leukemia after intensive chemotherapy. *Am. J. Hematol.* **2013**, *88*, 601–605. [CrossRef] [PubMed]

132. Ritchie, E.K.; Feldman, E.J.; Christos, P.J.; Rohan, S.D.; Lagassa, C.B.; Ippoliti, C.; Scandura, J.M.; Carlson, K.; Roboz, G.J. Decitabine in patients with newly diagnosed and relapsed acute myeloid leukemia. *Leuk. Lymphoma* **2013**, *54*, 2003–2007. [CrossRef] [PubMed]

133. Bejar, R.; Lord, A.; Stevenson, K.; Bar-Natan, M.; Perez-Ladaga, A.; Zaneveld, J.; Wang, H.; Caughey, B.; Stojanov, P.; Getz, G.; *et al.* TET2 mutations predict response to hypomethylating agents in myelodysplastic syndrome patients. *Blood* **2014**, *124*, 2705–2712. [CrossRef] [PubMed]

134. Itzykson, R.; Kosmider, O.; Cluzeau, T.; Mansat-De Mas, V.; Dreyfus, F.; Beyne-Rauzy, O.; Quesnel, B.; Vey, N.; Gelsi-Boyer, V.; Raynaud, S.; *et al.* Impact of TET2 mutations on response rate to azacitidine in myelodysplastic syndromes and low blast count acute myeloid leukemias. *Leukemia* **2011**, *25*, 1147–1152. [CrossRef] [PubMed]

135. Estey, E.H. Primacy of resistance rather than toxicity in determining outcome of therapy for AML. *Clin. Lymphoma Myeloma Leuk.* **2014**, *14*, S56–S58. [CrossRef] [PubMed]

136. Hourigan, C.S.; Karp, J.E. Minimal residual disease in acute myeloid leukaemia. *Nat. Rev. Clin. Oncol.* **2013**, *10*, 460–471. [CrossRef] [PubMed]

137. Meyers, J.; Yu, Y.; Kaye, J.A.; Davis, K.L. Medicare fee-for-service enrollees with primary acute myeloid leukemia: An analysis of treatment patterns, survival, and healthcare resource utilization and costs. *Appl. Health Econ. Health Policy* **2013**, *11*, 275–286. [CrossRef] [PubMed]

138. Hourigan, C.S.; Karp, J.E. Development of therapeutic agents for older patients with acute myelogenous leukemia. *Curr. Opin. Investig. Drugs* **2010**, *11*, 669–677. [PubMed]

139. Pemovska, T.; Kontro, M.; Yadav, B.; Edgren, H.; Eldfors, S.; Szwajda, A.; Almusa, H.; Bespalov, M.M.; Ellonen, P.; Elonen, E.; *et al.* Individualized systems medicine strategy to tailor treatments for patients with chemorefractory acute myeloid leukemia. *Cancer Discov.* **2013**, *3*, 1416–1429. [CrossRef] [PubMed]

140. Becker, P.S.; Oehler, V.; Estey, E.H.; Martins, T.; Perdue, A.; David, J.; Chien, S.; Hendrie, P.C.; Ostronoff, F.; Blau, C.A. Feasibility trial of individualized therapy for relapsed or refractory acute myeloid leukemia based on a high throughput *in vitro* drug sensitivity assay. *Blood* **2014**, *124*, 3748. [CrossRef] [PubMed]

141. Hourigan, C.S.; Karp, J.E. Personalized therapy for acute myeloid leukemia. *Cancer Discov.* **2013**, *3*, 1336–1338. [CrossRef] [PubMed]

142. Konoplev, S.; Rassidakis, G.Z.; Estey, E.; Kantarjian, H.; Liakou, C.I.; Huang, X.; Xiao, L.; Andreeff, M.; Konopleva, M.; Medeiros, L.J. Overexpression of CXCR4 predicts adverse overall and event-free survival in patients with unmutated FLT3 acute myeloid leukemia with normal karyotype. *Cancer* **2007**, *109*, 1152–1156. [CrossRef] [PubMed]

143. Freeman, S.D.; Virgo, P.; Couzens, S.; Grimwade, D.; Russell, N.; Hills, R.K.; Burnett, A.K. Prognostic relevance of treatment response measured by flow cytometric residual disease detection in older patients with acute myeloid leukemia. *J. Clin. Oncol.* **2013**, *31*, 4123–4131. [CrossRef] [PubMed]

144. Inaba, H.; Coustan-Smith, E.; Cao, X.; Pounds, S.B.; Shurtleff, S.A.; Wang, K.Y.; Raimondi, S.C.; Onciu, M.; Jacobsen, J.; Ribeiro, R.C.; *et al.* Comparative analysis of different approaches to measure treatment response in acute myeloid leukemia. *J. Clin. Oncol.* **2012**, *30*, 3625–3632. [CrossRef] [PubMed]

145. Grimwade, D.; Freeman, S.D. Defining minimal residual disease in acute myeloid leukemia: Which platforms are ready for "prime time"? *Blood* **2014**, *124*, 3345–3355. [CrossRef] [PubMed]

146. Ivey, A.; Hills, R.K.; Simpson, M.A.; Jovanovic, J.V.; Gilkes, A.F.; Patel, Y.; Bhudia, N.; Farah, H.; Mason, J.; Wall, K.; *et al.* Molecular detection of minimal residual disease provides the most powerful independent prognostic factor irrespective of clonal architecture in nucleophosmin (NPML) mutant acute myeloid leukemia. **2014**, *124*, 70.

147. Steinbach, D.; Bader, P.; Willasch, A.; Bartholomae, S.; Debatin, K.M.; Zimmermann, M.; Creutzig, U.; Reinhardt, D.; Gruhn, B. Prospective validation of a new method of monitoring minimal residual disease in childhood acute myeloid leukemia. *Clin. Cancer Res.* **2015**, *15*, 1353–1359. [CrossRef]

148. Goswami, M.; McGowan, K.S.; Lu, K.; Jain, N.; Candia, J.; Hensel, N.F.; Tang, J.; Calvo, K.R.; Battiwalla, M.; Barrett, A.J.; *et al.* A multigene array for measurable residual disease detection in AML patients undergoing SCT. *Bone Marrow Transplant.* 2015. [CrossRef]

149. Platzbecker, U.; Wermke, M.; Radke, J.; Oelschlaegel, U.; Seltmann, F.; Kiani, A.; Klut, I.M.; Knoth, H.; Rollig, C.; Schetelig, J.; *et al.* Azacitidine for treatment of imminent relapse in MDS or AML patients after allogeneic HSCT: Results of the relaza trial. *Leukemia* **2012**, *26*, 381–389. [CrossRef] [PubMed]

150. De Lima, M.; Giralt, S.; Thall, P.F.; de Padua Silva, L.; Jones, R.B.; Komanduri, K.; Braun, T.M.; Nguyen, H.Q.; Champlin, R.; Garcia-Manero, G. Maintenance therapy with low-dose azacitidine after allogeneic hematopoietic stem cell transplantation for recurrent acute myelogenous leukemia or myelodysplastic syndrome: A dose and schedule finding study. *Cancer* **2010**, *116*, 5420–5431. [CrossRef] [PubMed]

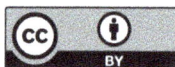

MDPI

St. Alban-Anlage 66

4052 Basel

Switzerland

Tel. +41 61 683 77 34

Fax +41 61 302 89 18

www.mdpi.com

Journal of Clinical Medicine Editorial Office

E-mail: jcm@mdpi.com

www.mdpi.com/journal/jcm

www.ingramcontent.com/pod-product-compliance
Lightning Source LLC
Chambersburg PA
CBHW051848210326
41597CB00033B/5818